Fracture Management:

A Practical Approach

Fracture Management:
A Practical Approach

J. TED HARTMAN, M.D.

Professor and Chairman
Department of Orthopaedic Surgery
Texas Tech University
Lubbock, Texas

Lea & Febiger • *1978* • *Philadelphia*

Library of Congress Cataloging in Publication Data

Hartman, James Ted, 1925–
  Fracture management.

  Bibliography.
  Includes index.
  1. Fractures.   2. Dislocations.   I. Title.
[DNLM: 1. Dislocations—Therapy.   2. Fractures—
Therapy. WE175 H333f]
RD101.H37   1977   617′.15   77-24292
ISBN 0-8121-0601-6

Published in Great Britain by Henry Kimpton Publishers, London

Printed in the United States of America

Print number   3   2   1

To my family—
    my wife, Jean
    and our children, Jim, Tom, and Martha

PREFACE

This book has been planned and written especially as a handbook to aid in the diagnosis and management of fractures and dislocations. It covers the subjects in a complete and useful fashion but is not meant to be an exhaustive compendium for the management of trauma to the musculoskeletal system. Rather it is more for the casualty officer in the emergency room and for the medical student learning a method of assessing and managing trauma to the musculoskeletal system.

General principles to be used in the management of any fracture or dislocation are outlined. All of the injuries are grouped into regional sections. The pertinent anatomic features of the region are pointed out in the first part of each chapter. This section is followed by detailed individual discussion of injuries that occur in the region under consideration. Factors to be noted in the history and examination of the individual injuries are then noted. The points necessary or helpful in accurate assessment of roentgenograms are next discussed. Methods of management of the specific injury are then outlined.

Fractures in children are sufficiently different to warrant a special consideration in each chapter. This discussion is at the end of the chapter and covers injuries specific to the geographic region covered by that chapter.

Many of the factors to consider in treatment of fractures and dislocations were known to the early surgeon because of knowledge gained from experience and from postmortem dissections. However, truly accurate understanding and treatment of these injuries had to await discovery of the roentgenogram and its subsequent improvements. In addition, the decision to manage certain injuries by operation could not be justified until the principles of asepsis and antisepsis were developed. Prior to the use of chloroform general anesthesia, all procedures were performed with analgesic agents, an only partially satisfactory method. Contemporary anesthesia has added much to our capability for managing the fracture or dislocation.

Lastly, in today's world of high speed, the multiply injured patient has become more commonplace. The management of this patient's injuries often requires crossing the boundary lines of many specialties. The coordination of the various disciplines involved in the effective care of the multiply injured patient is an art unto itself and requires a person of broad general background.

The general surgeon most often assumes this role; the sophisticated trauma unit has arisen to provide the vehicle to meet this special need. The well-organized effective trauma unit has saved many lives and decreased the disabilities in scores of others.

Lubbock, Texas   J. Ted Hartman

ACKNOWLEDGMENTS

Many persons have contributed selflessly to this undertaking. First, appreciation must be expressed to my own family for its fullest support. To Theresa Moorhouse, who has tirelessly typed and retyped the manuscript goes my deepest thanks. Thanks also go to our office staff—Beverly Nix, Barbara Gray, Jim Rockenbach, and Terri Ullrich—for ready willingness to perform any task, no matter how onerous.

The acquisition of appropriate illustrations is never without trial. This task has been made much easier, thanks to the beautiful illustrative talent of Gary Bishop. As well, the author is deeply indebted to Raymond Bagg, M.D., of El Paso, Texas, Leon Love, M.D., Professor and Chairman of the Department of Radiology at Loyola University in Maywood, Illinois, and Donald Bricker, M.D., Clinical Professor of Cardiothoracic Surgery at Texas Tech University in Lubbock, for many of the roentgenographic illustrations. Thanks are also due Mark Nickel for the detailed photographic work necessary for quality illustrations.

Charles Sargent has helped in planning illustrations and material, and Ann Gilmer has provided extensive and accurate reference support. Alvin Buhr, M.D., counseled and forwarded to the author a reference book unavailable in this country. To each of them, many thanks.

It has been said that no publication should go to press without critical review. This book is no exception, having received such attention from George S. Phalen, M.D., of Dallas, Henry V. Crock, M.D., of Melbourne, Victoria, Australia, and Michael F. Schafer, M.D., of Chicago. To each of them the author is beholden for undertaking this somewhat tedious and often onerous task.

Many of the ideas and much of the material expressed in this book are the product of experiences while the author was Chief of the Orthopaedic Surgery Service at Cook County Hospital in Chicago. Special appreciation is expressed to those members of the staff who helped mold many of the ideas herein expressed. Although no point of direct identification can be made, much of the warp and woof of this material reflects the influence of the late Carl E. Badgley, M.D., who was Chief of Orthopaedic Surgery at the University of Michigan while the author was in residency training there. The same must be said for Professor Joseph Trueta, Nuffield Professor Emeritus of Orthopaedic Surgery at

Oxford University, and J. I. Kendrick, M.D., Chairman Emeritus, and George S. Phalen, M.D., of the Department of Orthopaedic Surgery at the Cleveland Clinic. This book is mute expression of appreciation to these men of influence in the author's career as an orthopaedic surgeon.

And, last, thanks to Edward H. Wickland, Jr., Executive Editor of Lea & Febiger whose vision of this task was accurate and whose support toward its completion was unending.

J.T.H.

CONTENTS

1

GENERAL ASSESSMENT OF THE INJURED PATIENT

Before an injury can be treated, it must be established that the patient is in condition to tolerate and respond to treatment. His general condition should first be evaluated; that is, (1) the mechanism of injury should be ascertained, (2) emergent conditions (airway obstruction, bleeding, coma) should be given immediate attention, and (3) the injured part should be examined carefully by all methods necessary to establish an accurate diagnosis.

HISTORY OF PRESENT INJURY

To be able to understand a subject as vast as injuries to the bones and joints, there must be methods by which various bits of information are gleaned, assessed and organized. The journalists have long used a short poem to help them determine the accuracy and completeness of their stories. It runs:

> I keep six honest serving-men
> (They taught me all I knew);
> Their names are What and Why and When
> And How and Where and Who.
> Kipling: *The Elephant's Child*

If the same questions are accurately answered in a medical history, then much of the information for assessment of the patient and his injury is at hand.

Has the patient observed any unusual feelings of warmth, cold, or no feeling at all since the present injury occurred? Did the patient observe the preparations to extricate and remove him from the scene of the accident to the site for emergency care?

Other historical information to be asked the patient should include whether or not the involved part was normal prior to this injury. Is the patient receiving treatment for any other condition(s)? Has there been known neoplasm? Does some type of endocrine imbalance exist?

The history from the patient is helpful when ascertaining the mechanism of injury, but the patient may not always be sufficiently conscious to provide accurate and useful information. Any observers of the injury-producing episode may be helpful in giving information leading to a more complete assessment of the mechanism of injury.

To know how the injury occurred often enables the physician to anticipate the full extent of injury, including associated injuries of importance. Appropriate treatment almost always depends upon knowledge of the mechanism of

1

injury. For example, in a patient with a complete tear of the posterior ligamentous complex from an accident induced flexion injury to the cervical spine, the intact anterior ligamentous complex should provide a stabilizing effect. Hence, the cervical spine is extended to achieve the needed stability.

PHYSICAL EXAMINATION

A broad quick evaluation or triage of the patient should be first performed by the ABC (airway, bleeding, comatose) system. The airway is the first area to receive attention. Is an accessory airway needed? Is the patient breathing with adequate respiratory control and exchange? Following control of this area, one observes and controls any external hemorrhage (bleeding). Only after securing this area of potential trouble is attention directed to the patient's cardiovascular status (comatose). Is the patient in shock? What is the blood pressure? The pulse rate?

An intravenous catheter should be inserted if there is reason for giving any type of intravenous fluid. In addition, one may need to monitor the central venous pressure. Any question about the need for measurement of central venous pressure should be resolved by inserting the catheter for such monitoring (Fig. 1–1). The insertion of a venous catheter provides for easy withdrawal of a specimen of blood to send to the blood bank for typing (and crossmatching if indicated). Following insertion, the catheter is kept open with 5% dextrose in Ringer's lactate until further assessment of fluid needs can be made.

The examination of the injured part should start with observation. Is the skin intact? Is there obvious deformity of the involved part? Is the color of the skin

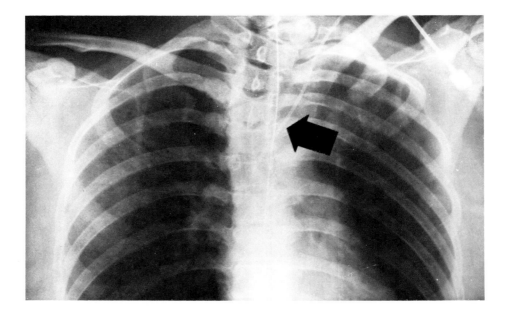

Fig. 1–1. Anteroposterior chest roentgenogram with catheter (arrow) in vena cava for monitoring the central venous pressure.

overlying and distal to the injured area normal? Of course, in injuries to a limb usually the opposite member is available for comparison.

What is the status of the peripheral pulse(s) distal to the injury? Is sensation and motor strength intact distal to the site of injury? In case of spinal injury, are reflexes normal distal to the injury? Is the injured part adequately splinted for temporary care while the assessment is being completed?

The general physical examination is an essential part of any evaluation of a patient following injury. Other injuries that are not as obvious may be found during examination. Traumatic inguinal hernias have been found to exist without specific complaint from the patient. Evidence of abrasions and contusions to the thoracic or abdominal walls may alert the examiner to underlying pathologic conditions.

ASSESSMENT OF FRACTURES

A fracture may be defined as a break in the continuity of bone or cartilage. On a roentgenogram the break may vary from an almost imperceptible line to many fracture lines with obvious loss of the normal shape of the bone. In an effort to describe the fracture more accurately, a number of descriptive and modifying adjectives have been devised. Some of these terms are obvious as to meaning while others need explanation.

1. Incomplete fracture—the fracture line cannot be seen to cross all cortices of bone on roentgenograms (Fig. 1–2).
2. Complete fracture—the evident fracture line crosses all cortices of bone as seen on roentgenograms (Fig. 1–3).

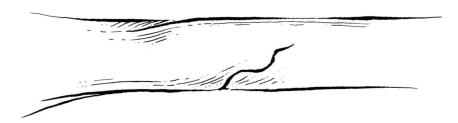

Fig. 1–2. Incomplete fracture.

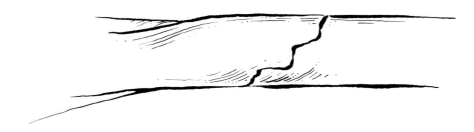

Fig. 1–3. Complete fracture.

3. Undisplaced fracture—although a complete fracture exists, the distal fragment(s) does not shift from its normal relationship with the proximal fragment as seen on roentgenograms (Fig. 1–4).
4. Displaced fracture—on roentgenograms, the distal fragment(s) is shifted away from its usual relationship to the proximal fragment (Fig. 1–5).
5. Angulated fracture—the longitudinal axis of the bone distal to the fracture site is angled away from that of the proximal bone on observation and/or roentgenograms (Fig. 1–6).
6. Rotation—description of rotation of the distal fragment along its longitudinal axis in relation to the proximal fragment; a situation judged by observation and on roentgenograms (Fig. 1–7).
7. Simple fracture—a single line of break exists in one bone.

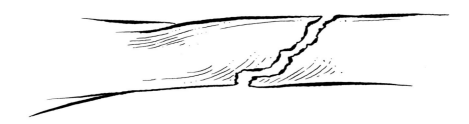

Fig. 1–4. Undisplaced fracture.

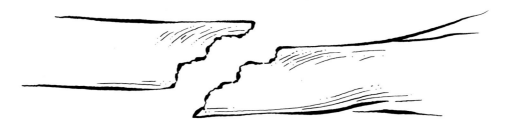

Fig. 1–5. Displaced fracture.

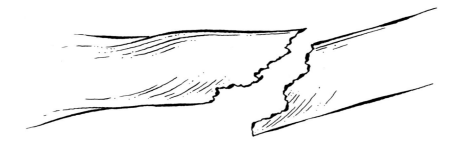

Fig. 1–6. Angulated fracture.

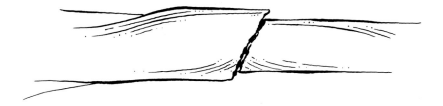

Fig. 1–7. Rotational deformity.

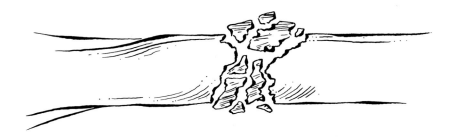

Fig. 1–8. Comminuted fracture.

8. Comminuted fracture—more than one fracture line exists in one bone (Fig. 1–8).
9. Closed fracture—the fracture fragment(s) has not penetrated the skin.
10. Open fracture (formerly called compound fracture)—the fracture communicates externally to air through a break in the skin. The bone may penetrate through the skin (within-out) or an external object may penetrate the skin down to bone (without-in).
11. Type of fracture—descriptive terminology as judged on roentgenograms.
    a. Transverse—the line of the break is transverse in relation to the longitudinal axis of the shaft (Fig. 1–9).
    b. Oblique—the line of the break is oblique in relation to the longitudinal axis of the shaft (Fig. 1–10).
    c. Spiral—this fracture is spiral in relation to the longitudinal axis of the bone (Fig. 1–11).
    d. Impacted—the distal fracture fragment is compressed into the proximal fragment. Impaction often produces a certain amount of stability at the fracture site (Figs. 1–12).
    e. Greenstick fracture—the fracture occurs in a person who has not yet achieved full growth and can create an angulation deformity (Fig. 1–13).
    f. Torus fracture—the fracture is caused by longitudinal compression in a person who has not achieved full growth. A compression fracture in which the cortex buckles (Fig. 1–14).

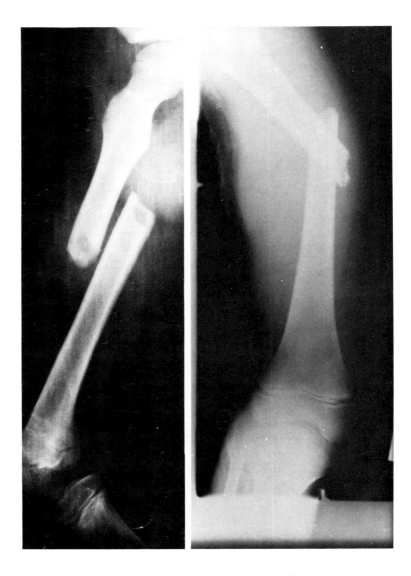

Fig. 1–9. Fairly transverse fracture of child's femur, which was treated in Russell's traction. Bayonet apposition will be best position in which the two fragments could unite. After early union was palpated at three weeks, a spica cast was applied until full union was present at ten weeks.

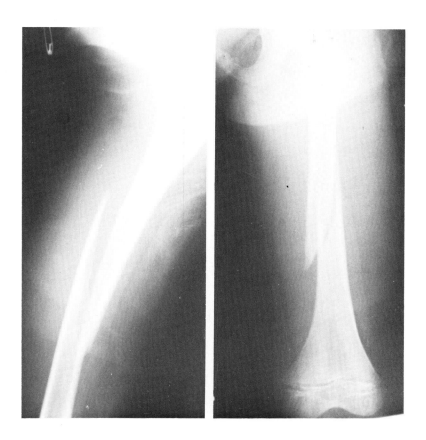

Fig. 1–10.   Long oblique fracture in child's femur, which was treated in Russell's traction with modest overriding allowed. After fracture began early union at three weeks, a spica cast was applied for eight weeks.

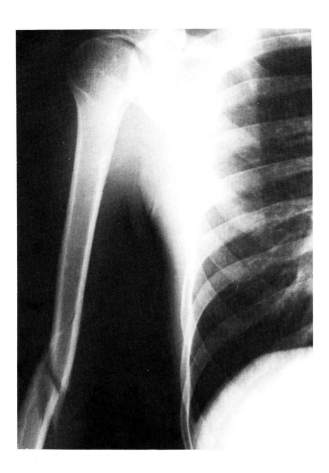

Fig. 1–11.   Spiral fracture at junction of middle and distal one thirds of the humerus. A light hanging arm cast was used to treat this fracture.

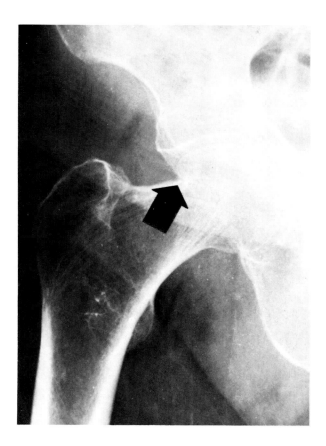

Fig. 1–12. Impacted fracture of femoral neck. Note that superior femoral neck and head meet at an acute angle (arrow). Three pins were used to retain position of fracture fragments while union of fracture ensued.

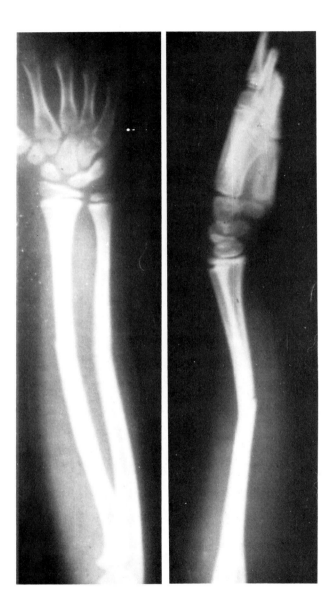

Fig. 1–13. Greenstick fractures of radius and ulna in child.

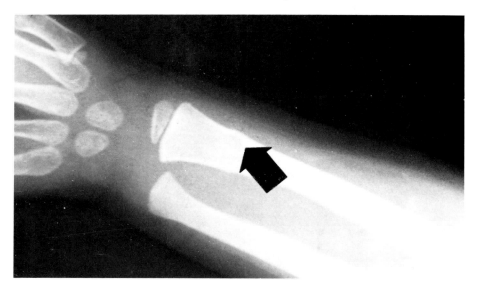

Fig. 1–14. Torus fracture of radius. Cortex bulges where fractured bone is impacted. Simple immobilization for four to six weeks should suffice for treatment of this fracture.

12. Anatomic location within a specific bone.
    a. Shaft (diaphysis)—central portion of a long bone.
    b. Metaphysis—toward the growth plate of a long bone.
    c. Epiphyseal—within the growth segment of a long bone.
    d. Fracture of a process of a bone—described in anatomic terms (Fig. 1–15).
    e. Articular—fracture into a joint.
    f. Subcapital—inferior to the head of a specific bone (Fig. 1–16a).
    g. Cervical (neck)—along the neck of a specific bone, e.g., scapula, femur, humerus (Fig. 1–16b).
    h. Intertrochanteric—between the greater and lesser trochanters of the femur (Fig. 1–16c).
    i. Subtrochanteric—inferior to the trochanters of the femur (Fig. 1–16d).
    j. Supracondylar—above the condyles, e.g., humerus or femur (Fig. 1–17a).
    k. Intercondylar—between the condyles (humerus and femur) (Fig. 1–17b).
    l. Plateau—usually refers to the proximal tibia (Fig. 1–18).
    m. Malleolar—process of distal tibia medially or fibula laterally at the ankle (Fig. 1–19).
13. Pathologic—implying preexisting pathology within a bone, e.g., neoplasm replacing the portion of bone in which a fracture has occurred (Fig. 1–20).

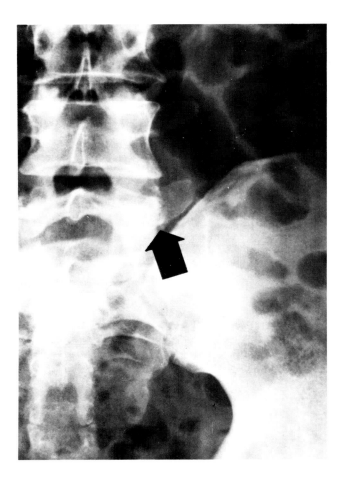

Fig. 1–15. Fracture of transverse process of fifth lumbar vertebra (arrow).

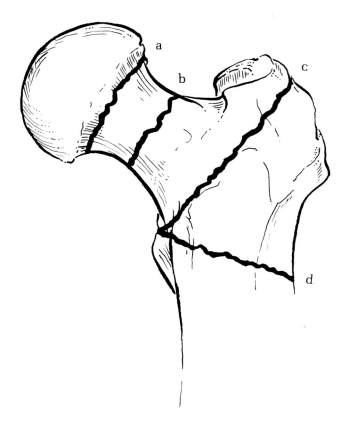

Fig. 1–16. Fractures of femur: subcapital fracture of femoral neck (a); transcervical fracture of femur (b); intertrochanteric fracture of femur (c); subtrochanteric fracture of the femur (d).

1-17

1-18

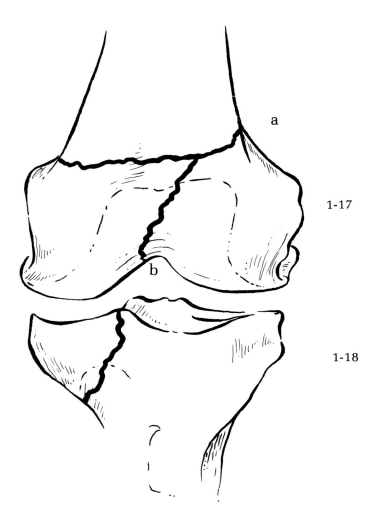

Fig. 1–17. Fractures of distal femur: supracondylar fracture (a); intercondylar fracture (b).

Fig. 1–18. Tibial plateau fracture.

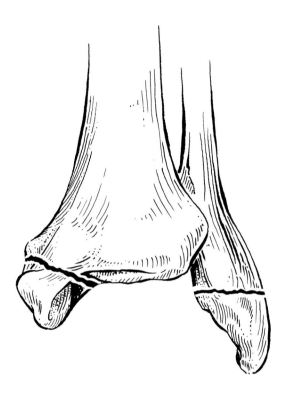

Fig. 1-19. Malleolar fractures.

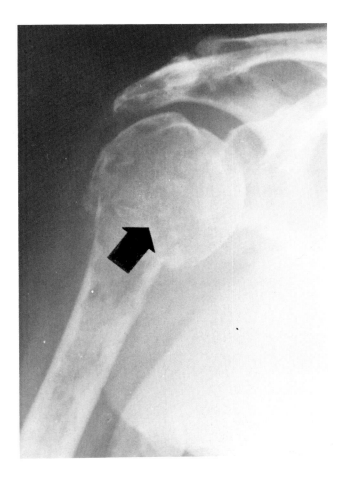

Fig. 1–20. Pathologic fracture of proximal humerus. Fracture (arrow) has occurred through area of bone invaded by neoplasm.

Full evaluation of the individual fracture utilizes a number of features. In any part of a limb in which two bones provide the stability, a fracture of one bone with displacement can only occur if the other bone of the two-bone system is fractured or if a ligamentous separation between the two bones occurs at the joint proximal to or distal to the site of fracture (Fig. 1–21). This same both bone principle is in effect within the pelvis. Any fracture of the "perfect circle" of the pelvis in which displacement occurs must be accompanied by a fracture elsewhere within that circle (Fig. 1–22). This is also seen within the bony structures encasing the smaller circles of the obturator foramina.

In fractures of the long bones, as pointed out by Charnley (Fig. 1–23A), the periosteum on the concave side of the bony deformity often is intact. In treating these injuries, the reduction is accomplished by increasing the deformity and

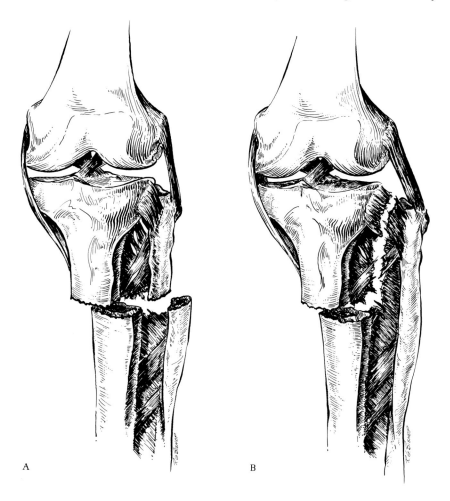

A   B

Fig. 1–21.   Result of displacement of one bone when two parallel and rigid rods are attached to each other firmly at both ends. A, obligatory displacement of the other bone. B, their attachment at one end must "give way." This is the both bone principle so important in managing forearm and lower leg fractures.

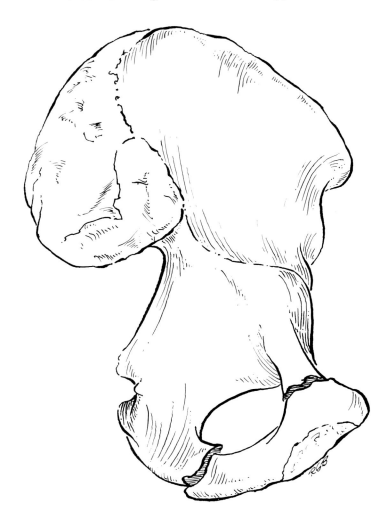

Fig. 1–22. Rigid circle concept of pelvis. Fracture *with* displacement anywhere in circle must be accompanied by fracture or separation elsewhere in circle. This applies to major foramen of pelvis as well as to both of its obturator foramina.

Fig. 1–23. Steps in reducing fracture of long bone. A, Periosteum is often intact on concave side of deformity and separated on convex side. B, Cortex of distal fragment on concave side of deformity is brought to meet like cortex of proximal fragment. C, Cortices are held together, and ⟶ distal fragment is brought from its exaggerated position down to neutral. D and E, Reduction is then maintained by applying cast which utilizes three-point fixation shown here.

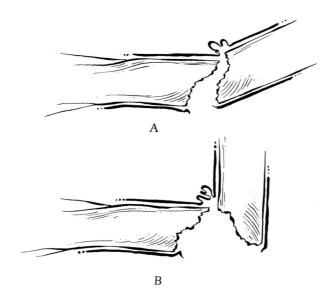

A

B

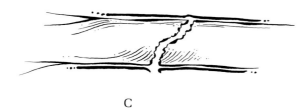

C

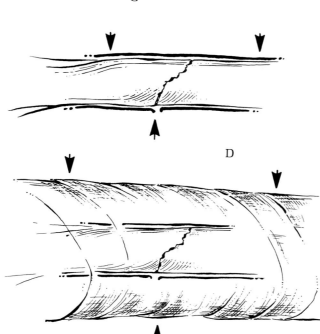

D

E

manipulating the two fractured tips of the cortices on the concave side to meet each other (Fig. 1–23B). The distal fragment is then brought to neutral position to tauten the intact periosteum (Fig. 1–23C). The principle of three-point fixation is achieved by application of a plaster of Paris cast to maintain reduction (Fig. 1–23D). This causes a pressure toward the intact periosteum at the fracture site and a force opposite this at the two ends of the immobilizing device (Fig. 1–23E).

When it is not possible to depend upon intact periosteum because of the massiveness of the injury, one may rely upon fixation methods utilizing Steinmann pins or Kirschner wires through the fractured bone above and below the fracture site. These wires are then incorporated into the plaster cast to achieve more effective fixation. This method is called external skeletal fixation. In any instance, the best alternative may be to operate, openly reduce the fractures, and internally fix it by some device, such as a plate or an intramedullary rod.

Blood Supply

The blood supply into the area of fracture must be considered in any thoughtful evaluation of a fracture. The arterial supply into a long bone is known to occur from the periosteum and the endosteum. There is an adequate anastomosis between these two sources in long bones as shown by Crock (Fig. 1–24), so that any obstruction from one source may be compensated by the

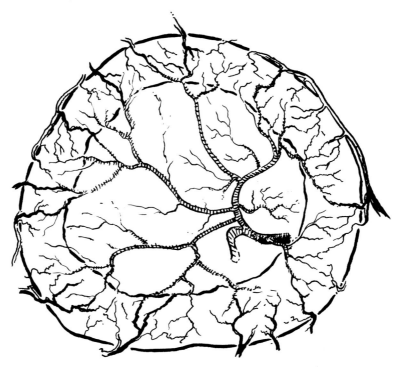

Fig. 1–24. Illustration (after Crock) of periosteal and endosteal circulation on cross section of tubular bone.

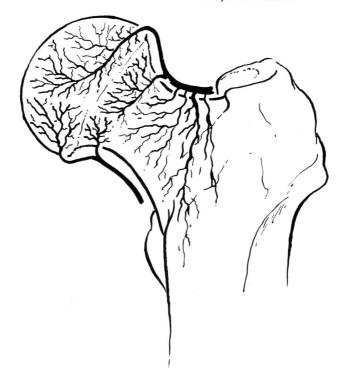

Fig. 1–25. Blood supply of femoral neck and head (after Trueta and Crock). Note that circulation into femoral head travels from distal to proximal up femoral neck.

other. However, the blood supply into the distal tibia is generally considered poor. In addition, the magnitude of the initial trauma may play a significant role in determining the sufficiency of the blood supply to the fracture site. In some areas, such as the femoral head, a segment of bone is purely intra-articular and for nutrition must rely upon vessels coming in from outside (Fig. 1–25). The early and accurate reduction of these fractures and dislocations plays a role in the long-term good results of this group of patients.

The importance of the blood supply is recognized when one realizes that the first stage of fracture repair is the hematoma formed at the time of fracture. This hematoma must organize and then undergo transformation directly into fibrous bone or else into cartilage and then into fibrous bone. The fibrous bone then gradually remodels into the type of bone consistent with the demands placed upon it. These are the stages of fracture repair (Fig. 1–26). They are mute evidence of the living nature of bone.

Roentgenograms

The classification of any fracture can be accomplished with accuracy only after roentgenograms are studied. These roentgenograms, to be adequate, must include the joint above and the joint below the fracture site. In addition, there must be at least two views of the fracture site taken at 90 degree angles from

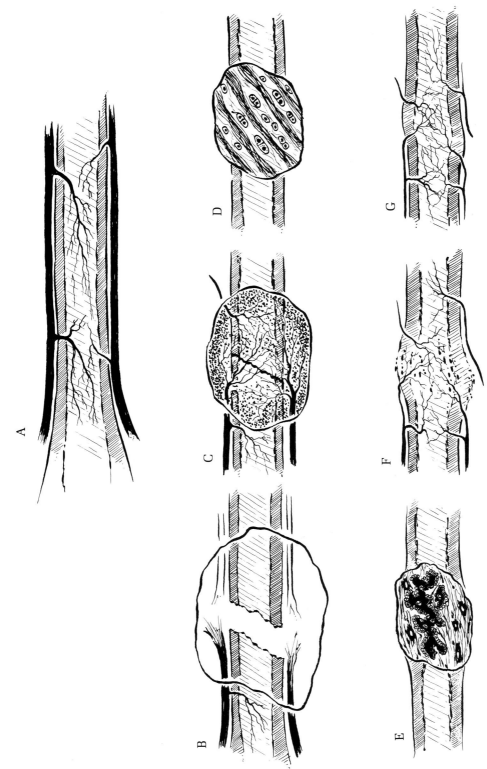

Fig. 1–26. Illustration of stages of fracture healing. A, Normal bone and its blood supply. B and C, Bleeding into fracture site clots. D, E, and F, Hematoma then is gradually replaced by ossification process. G, Remodelling.

22

each other. These allow a review of the fracture site, the joint above, and the joint below in two separate planes at 90 degrees to each other. An initial assessment may require special supplementary views such as oblique views (as tibial plateau) or tomograms (occasionally necessary to fully evaluate tibial plateau and certain spinal fractures).

APPROACH TO TREATMENT

The appropriate treatment plan varies according to the individual fracture and cannot be developed until the full circumstances of the fracture are known. Having taken a history, including the mechanism of injury and having examined the area of injury, the treating physician has valuable information to be used in the development of a plan of treatment. Knowing the mechanism of injury will often provide knowledge as to position of instability (that position recreated by this mechanism). Conversely, an opposite position will probably enhance stability.

Visualization of the patient and the injured part will help determine treatment. Does an open wound overlie the fracture? The open wound requires special consideration. Is a deformity present? Is this deformity caused by angulation of the bone fragments? How much angulation can be accepted? Is this deformity a rotational one that cannot be accepted? What vascular or neurologic complications are present?

Prior to development of the treatment plan, study of the roentgenogram is essential. The roentgenogram must be taken at 90 degree planes from each other and include the joint above and the joint below the fracture site. Quality of the roentgenogram must be sufficiently good to fully assess the bony injury. Nothing less can be accepted.

Operative Indications. There are relative and absolute indications for operating upon fractures. If the surgeon is not able to reduce and/or maintain adequate reduction of a fracture by nonoperative means, then operation is absolutely indicated. The open fracture is an absolute indication for wound excision and as accurate a fracture reduction as possible. If experience indicates that the best results are obtained by open reduction and/or internal fixation of certain types of fractures, then that would be a relative indication for operation. These relative and absolute indications may vary from one surgeon to another and from one area to another.

Anesthesia. The choice of an anesthetic is an individual one determined by the fracture and by the managing surgeon and the anesthesiologist. This decision is reached after assessment of the general condition of the patient, determination of the type of manipulation necessary to reduce the fracture or dislocation, estimation of the time involved in this reduction, and choice of the type of fixation to be used. For reducing the Colles' fracture I prefer a local anesthetic injected into the hematoma after a surgical "prep." Other surgeons believe that a general anesthetic is essential for management of this problem.

Immobilization. Immobilization is also a matter of preference for the surgeon. In the Colles' fracture, some surgeons use a "sugar tong" (Fig. 1–27); others prefer a long arm cast (Fig. 1–28). The result of immobilization is the same, but the method for accomplishing this varies. The objective is to secure union across the fracture site, however achieved.

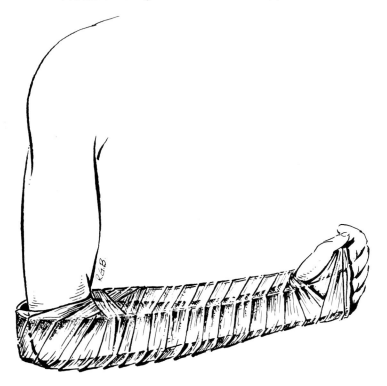

Fig. 1–27. Sugar tong splint to maintain reduction of wrist fractures. It circles around distal upper arm to prevent pronation and supination. Its distal extension maintains three-point fixation. Gauze surrounding sugar tong splint can be easily cut if excessive swelling ensues.

Following reduction, the fracture must be immobilized until one can see evidence on roentgenograms of ensuing union. In long bone fractures, the usual time for union runs from about ten weeks to about four months. The evidence of union roentgenographically includes a generalized loss of clear-cut fracture lines and presence of callus as well as its maturity. Before union can be considered complete one must see bony trabeculae coursing across the site of the former fracture. In an immaculately reduced and immobilized long bone one seldom sees much in the way of callous formation and must rely on the fading of the original distinct fracture-line. In the early weight-bearing treatment of the femoral shaft or of the tibia with the cast brace, Dehne and Scully rely on the time in cast and palpable stability more than they do on roentgenographic evidence of union of the fracture. This, however, is a matter of experience.

The dislocated joint, once reduced, must be kept immobile in a stable position for the time necessary to achieve capsular healing. This may be as short as ten days for some small joints in the hand and foot and up to eight weeks for major joints.

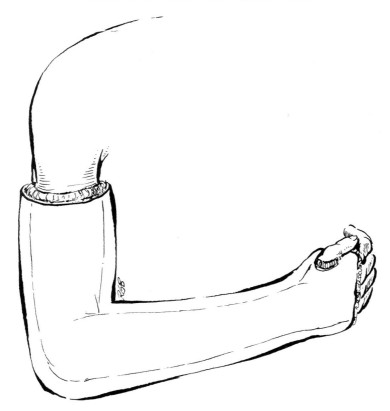

Fig. 1–28. Long arm cast, a completely encircling cylinder of plaster which prevents pronation and supination by virtue of its above elbow extension. The fracture is held reduced by three-point fixation. This cast often needs to be univalved along one side to allow for undue soft tissue swelling.

Instructing the Patient. After the extent of injury is known, the treatment plan has been evolved, and the anesthetic has been chosen, the physician must discuss these proposed plans with the patient. This discussion should include whether the patient need be hospitalized and, if so, for how long. The patient should be given an estimate of the time during which he will be immobilized in a cast or other device. Potential problems of the particular fracture or dislocation should be related to the patient so that he can consider himself informed before giving consent for the proposed treatment.

Follow-up. As soon as immobilization of the fracture or the dislocation can be discontinued, an intensive thoughtful exercise program must be developed to regain full motion and strength of the affected part. The treating physician has the responsibility to continue follow-up care in a patient until the preinjury status is reached or until optimum recovery has taken place.

COMPLICATIONS

The complications for any fracture may be considered under immediate and late categories. The late group can be broken down into intermediate and truly late.

Immediate Complications

The immediate group of complications encompasses those problems occurring concomitant to the fracture, i.e., open fracture, vascular impairment, neurologic deficit, tendon or muscular injury, visceral injuries, and prior loss of bone substance.

Open Fracture. When the fractured bone ends communicate to the air, the contamination of such a wound is inescapable, the extent varying according to circumstances. Obviously, the open fracture containing gravel and debris from the roadside has a greater tendency to become infected than does the wound caused by the fractured tibia penetrating the skin. Complacency has *no* role in the management of the open fracture, however small the wound. Uncontrollable gas gangrene and tetanus infections following open fracture have caused the amputation of more than one limb.

As mentioned previously, the open fracture is an absolute indication for operation—wound excision, excision of all evident necrotic tissue, and copious irrigation followed by reduction. Judicious use of a minimal amount of metal for fixation when combined with external fixation is not contraindicated in selected open fractures.

The preoperative use of tetanus toxoid booster is strongly urged. Tetanus antitoxin and gas gangrene antitoxin have not proved as effective as once hoped, and the allergic reactions to them have not been inconsequential. In addition, since the use of a broad spectrum antibiotic intraoperatively and postoperatively has proved effective in controlling many gas gangrene and tetanus infections, routine use of well selected antibiotic coverage is urged in the treatment of the open fracture. Antibiotic therapy should continue for a period of about two weeks from the initial pickup of debris. Because specific potentially infecting organisms are usually unknown, a broader spectrum antibiotic such as ampicillin (Polycillin) is my preference.

Vascular Impairment. The loss of or a diminished circulation to the extremity distal to a fracture is a most serious complication and one that must be fully evaluated as to extent. Interruption of circulation can be caused by (1) swelling of soft tissues at the area of the fracture or by (2) traumatic severance of a major vessel at the point of injury. Partial severance of an artery can cause massive hemorrhage into the soft tissues, whereas total severance of the artery more often allows retraction and muscular occlusion of the artery. Repair of the injured major vessel is indicated, if not essential, for a functional extremity distal to the injury. When combined with vascular injury, the fracture is often best managed by internal fixation to remove as much stress as possible from the vascular repair.

Neurologic Deficit. The presence of any neurologic deficit peripheral to the injury must be determined *prior* to treatment. The possibility of nerve injury from the fracture fragments exists but is not common. On the other hand, certain injuries, by virtue of anatomic relationships, are prone to cause neurologic deficits, and these must be documented *prior* to treatment.

Tendon and/or Muscular Injury. Injuries to tendons and/or muscles may occur with any fracture in the extremity but are particularly prone to occur in the open fracture. These, too, should be documented prior to initiation of any treatment.

Visceral Injuries. In any patient with multiple injuries visceral injuries must be suspected, particularly when there is evidence of abrasion and contusion of the thoracoabdominal walls. In the pelvic fractures, particularly those involving the pubic ramus and/or the ischium, one must consider urethral injury. Catheterization of the bladder with an indwelling catheter is appropriate in this situation. Should there be difficulty in passing the catheter, or should the urine returned be bloody, suspicion of a urethral injury must exist, and appropriate attention must be given to exclude this diagnosis or to provide proper treatment.

Pathologic Fracture. A fracture may occur through an area where bone substance has been lost because of endocrine or neoplastic disorders. When a fracture occurs in such an area, fixation of the fracture by operative means is often the treatment of choice. This then allows early mobilization of the patient and treatment of the underlying condition as indicated.

Late Complications, Intermediate in Time

In the delayed group of complications, there is a category of intermediate occurrences that requires attention. They are listed not necessarily in order of occurrence or magnitude of problem but by approximate time of occurrence.

Fatty Emboli. Within 48 hours to 96 hours, fatty emboli tend to appear if they are going to occur. The earlier the appearance, generally, the more profound is the potential seriousness of this complication. The best treatment so far has been supportive and includes maintaining an airway and sufficient oxygen exchange associated with fast-acting steroid therapy.

Silent Venous Thrombosis. Although it can occur any time, silent venous thrombosis most commonly occurs after 96 hours. If inadequately controlled, pulmonary embolism can occur. Other problems from this are residual poor venous return and extremity swelling. Silent venous thrombosis is a particularly well-recognized complication in supracondylar femur and tibial plateau fractures at the knee, as well as in hip fractures (Fig. 1–29). The use of anticoagulants has helped prevent this complication, as has elevation of the foot of the bed to 20 or 25 degrees.

Volkmann's Ischemic Contracture. This poorly understood syndrome is heralded by unrelenting pain in the involved extremity. The arterial supply to that segment of the limb is interrupted by spasm of the arteries, large and small, as well as of the arterioles. If unrelieved, the end result can be necrosis of muscles and nerves with consequent loss of sensation and motor control in the involved part (Fig. 1–30). This is notably seen in the forearm and is associated with supracondylar fractures of the humerus; it has been reported in the calf following use of Bryant's traction for femoral fracture.

Appropriate treatment must be actively pursued once this condition is identified. Surgical release of the fascia of the involved compartment is

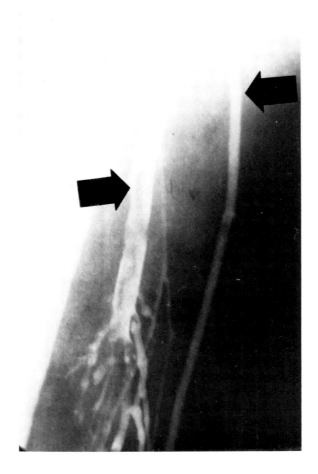

Fig. 1–29. Venogram performed in patient after fracture of femoral neck. Left arrow points to thrombus trailing proximally up deep femoral vein(s). Right arrow is pointing to clearly seen saphenous vein—an occurrence fairly common when deep venous return is decreased.

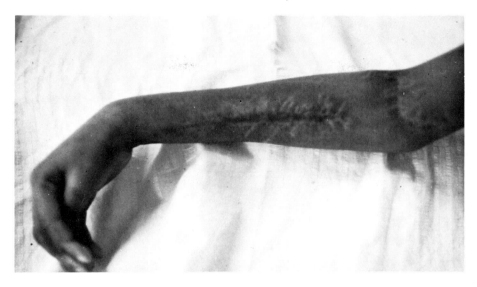

Fig. 1–30. Forearm in which complication of Volkmann's ischemic contracture has occurred. Operative scars from open reduction and forearm fasciotomy are clearly visible. Necrosis of some of volar forearm musculature has forced palmar flexed wrist.

essential. Elevation of the involved artery(ies) from its bed and injection of 1% local anesthetic around the periphery of the vessel as well as in the lumen has been beneficial. If operative treatment has been necessary, then reduction of the fracture under direct vision followed by internal fixation is indicated to improve stability and more effectively splint the soft tissues.

Late Complications, Delayed

Late delayed complications include delayed union, reflex sympathetic dystrophy, malunion, and nonunion.

Delayed Union. The fracture has not united in the time usually expected for that particular fracture. Immobilization may be continued as previously if a reasonable chance exists that union can occur. The alternative to this method of treatment would be an operative approach to add stimulus by a bone graft and/or to immobilize by some form of internal fixation.

Reflex Sympathetic Dystrophy (Sudeck's Atrophy). The dominant features of reflex sympathetic dystrophy are unrelenting pain in the limb following fracture treatment, multiple joint pericapsulitis, and thin appearing, cold, clammy skin. Roentgenograms show a patchy osteoporosis of the involved extremity. Its true cause is unknown, no evident common denominator existing between the type of fracture or severity of injury. Treatment, once the diagnosis is established, is to give a series of sympathetic nerve blocks and pursue an intensive physical therapy program of active and active assistive exercises following an application of heat (most effective appears to be paraffin baths). When not contraindicated, an orally administered monamine oxidase inhibitor, an unlikely drug, has nevertheless been helpful in many instances. This

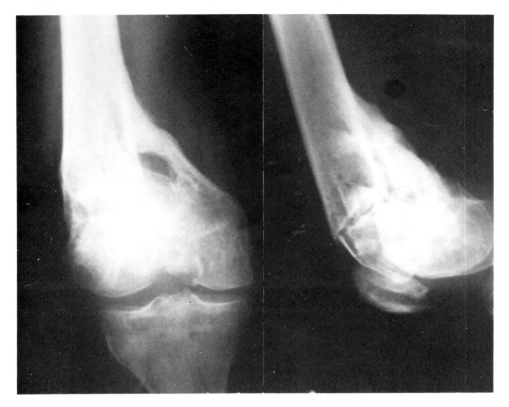

Fig. 1–31. Malunion following severely comminuted femoral supracondylar fracture. This allows adequate, though not normal, range of motion.

syndrome tends to occur more commonly following union of a Colles' fracture but can occur after any extremity injury.

Malunion. The fracture has healed, but the distal fragment is not in normal anatomic relationship to the proximal fragment (Fig. 1–31). The deformity is usually an angular one but can be a deformity caused by rotation of the distal fragment on the longitudinal axis. Malunion may be sufficiently disabling to warrant operative sectioning of the bone followed by realignment in a more anatomic position.

Nonunion. The fragments fail to achieve bony union (Fig. 1–32). Although the causes for failure of union of a fracture are not positively known, several factors probably contribute to its development. The magnitude of the initial injury almost surely plays some role in this condition; the greater the initial damage, the more likely that nonunion will ensue. Inadequate immobilization appears to enhance nonunion. The adequacy of the blood supply into a bone at the fracture site must be a factor in nonunion, as we know that fracture healing requires an adequate hematoma in its first stage. Another finding common to some ununited fractures is presence of a low grade infection. A sine qua non for achievement of union in this instance is control of the infection. A last but not

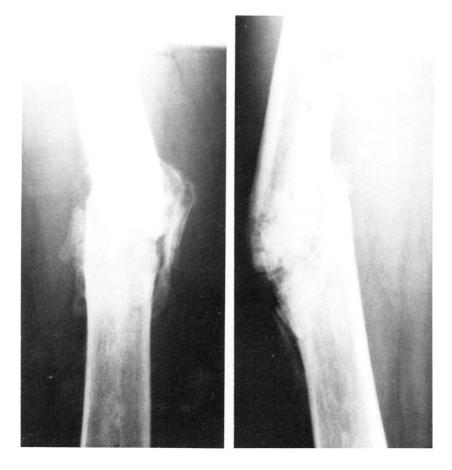

Fig. 1–32. Laminogram through area of nonunion of femoral shaft fracture. Note bony overgrowth about periphery, as well as increased density in nonunion site. The nonunion is seen as meandering oblique dark line.

to be ignored fact is that failure to achieve bone-to-bone contact often contributes to nonunion.

There have been a number of definitions setting forth specific time intervals before declaring nonunion to exist. Gregory pointed out that nonunion in effect exists at that point in time when union of the fracture cannot be anticipated to occur without its being provided an extra stimulus. This extra stimulus most commonly is a bone graft across the site of nonunion. I prefer a modified Phemister type of bone graft, each end of the united bone being trimmed and fish-scaled back to bleeding bone prior to laying on strips of cancellous bone from the iliac crest. In this method it is important to retain about one third of the fibrous nonunion for stability (Badgley). Trueta maintains that another essential maneuver in any operation for nonunion is to medullarize both fragments—that is, to curet all fibrous tissue from the medullary canal adjacent to the site of nonunion in order to provide blood supply to the bone graft fragments. Continued immobilization is also necessary. Some surgeons succeed in treatment of the nonunion by applying rigid compression plate(s) across the site of nonunion; others may use intramedullary fixation at this point.

PLASTER OF PARIS CASTS

Once reduction has been effected, plaster of Paris is often used to immobilize the injured part. For this purpose, the Egyptians, over a thousand years ago, used a linen material stiffened with starch, albumin, and clay. The relatively recent incorporation of the plaster into gauze, along with standardization of available sizes and lengths, has simplified the application of a cast.

In most instances, prior to application of the plaster, a padding material is used. This padding material is a nonwoven material made usually of cotton or cellulose and has the property of stretching to fit over prominences and varying shapes. Its use is to prevent undue pressure against any point in the cast and at the same time allow adequate immobilization by the cast.

Unpadded casts are used by some surgeons in treating fractures. However, this technique, requiring experience and precision, is best avoided by those not well versed in its use.

For an extremity, the cast should extend distally beyond the joint below the fracture and proximally above the joint proximal to the fracture. Any arm cast that includes the hand should extend to the metacarpal bases and usually include a thenar strip from the palm to the dorsum of the hand between the thumb and index finger. This supports the hand properly, prevents supination and pronation, and usually allows a maximum of comfort.

In general, any cast that includes the foot should include the metatarsal heads. I always bring a plantar extension of the cast to support all toes to their tips. The dorsal side of the cast is cut back to the metatarsal necks to provide a ''bumper'' to protect the toes and at the same time prevent flexion contractures of any toes.

Plaster of Paris is commonly provided in rolls with widths of 2, 3, 4, 5, and 6 inches. Splints for reinforcement come in the following sizes: 3" × 15", 4" × 15", 5" × 30", and 5" × 45".

The technique of wetting a roll of plaster of Paris is to place the roll into lukewarm water (37 to 40°C) with the end up. Once the roll has been saturated with water, the bubbles that have been coming from the roll will cease. One finger should then be placed in the center hole at the end of each roll while the end of the roll is grasped by the other fingers; the roll is then compressed lightly between the two hands. The roll is next unwound onto the previously prepared (usually padded) extremity. The encircling turns are laid on the surface, not pulled tightly. To change the direction of the roll, place a finger under the end of the plaster strip in the direction toward which it is desired to turn and take a backward tuck. This creates a wedge-shaped fold in the plaster and changes direction of the roll. After several layers of a roll of plaster are used, plaster splints may be placed to increase the thickness and strength of the cast. More plaster is unrolled over the splints to secure them and help incorporate them into the cast. The hand that is not rolling is always smoothing the newly applied plaster. To create a stronger homogeneous mass all of the cast must have been completed before the plaster dries. A laminated cast is a structurally weak cast.

Once the plaster has been completely rolled on, the cast is rubbed and molded to assume the required contour. Care must be taken not to indent the cast while it is setting, as an indentation can create an unrelenting pressure. Pressure sores have been caused by just such an indentation.

The plaster of Paris cast starts to set within 10 to 15 minutes and gives off considerable heat from the exothermic reaction of the plaster with water. Although the cast feels hard at 20 to 30 minutes, the full strength of plaster of Paris is not reached until most of the water has evaporated. Evaporation requires 36 to 48 hours and is the basis for requesting patients in walking casts not to walk on the cast until 48 hours after application.

Postreduction Care

After a cast has been applied to a recently reduced fracture, that part should be elevated to minimize swelling. If significant swelling is anticipated, or occurs, the cast should be split on one side from the proximal to the distal point. The side to be split will be that side toward which the extremity distal to the injury could move without endangering the reduction. For example, the cast of the newly reduced Colles' fracture is split on the ulnar side, that being the side toward which stability of reduction is maintained. Occasionally even the split cast gives insufficient relief for swelling. In this instance the cast must be spread sufficiently to decompress the pressure of swelling. A well-reduced fracture is of no benefit when circulation to its surrounding soft tissues has been compromised by such unrelieved swelling.

Instructions to the patient should include keeping the cast dry. A plastic bag placed temporarily over the casted extremity will allow the patient to bathe or shower. It will also keep the distal lower extremity dry in inclement weather. Patients with the foot encased in a cast usually have to be told not to walk on the cast unless a walking heel has been incorporated in the cast. For early and relatively brief weight bearing, one may use the cast boot or an inexpensive oversized tennis shoe (easily found in a discount store) on the casted foot. Weight bearing in this instance can be begun as soon as the plaster is well hardened (4 hours).

REFERENCES

1. Adams, J. C.: Outline of Fractures, Including Joint Injuries, 6th ed. Baltimore, Williams & Wilkins, 1972.
2. Badgley, C. E., Personal Communication.
3. Charnley, J.: Closed Treatment of Common Fractures, 3rd ed. Edinburgh, Livingstone, 1961.
4. Crock, H. V.: The Blood Supply to the Lower Limb Bones in Man. Edinburgh, Livingstone, 1967.
5. Dehne, E. and Torp, R. P.: Treatment of joint injuries by immediate mobilization. Clin. Orthop. 77:219, 1971.
6. Gregory, C.: Resident Conferences, Parkland Hospital, Dallas, 1974.
7. Ralston, E. L.: Handbook of Fractures. St. Louis, C. V. Mosby Co., 1967.
8. Rockwood, C. A., and Green, D. P.: Fractures. Philadelphia, J. B. Lippincott Co., 1975.
9. Scully, T. J.: Ambulant, nonoperative management of femoral shaft fractures, Part I. Clin. Orthop. 100:195, 1974.
10. Scully, T. J.: Ambulant, nonoperative management of femoral shaft fractures, Part II. Clin. Orthop. 100:204, 1974.

11. Trueta, J.: Studies of the Development and Decay of the Human Frame. Philadelphia, W. B. Saunders Co., 1968.
12. Watson-Jones, R.: Fractures and Joint Injuries, 4th ed. Baltimore, Williams & Wilkins Co., 1952-1955.

2

FRACTURES IN CHILDREN

Fractures in children are different. Not only must the treating physician reduce the fracture to an acceptable position, but he must do so with full knowledge of the potential damage to vital anatomic structures adjacent to the fracture, with full knowledge of potential alteration to growth caused by injury to the germinal cells of the epiphyseal plate nearby, and also with full knowledge of the propensity for growth and remodeling in poorly reduced fractures. The fracture in a child must be given a totally different consideration than would a similar fracture in an adult.

In order to adequately evaluate the fracture of a limb in a child, the roentgenograms must be taken at planes varying from each other by 90 degrees and must include the joint above and the joint below the fracture. In addition, views of the opposite extremity must be obtained which are as accurate a mirror of the views of the injured limb as possible. Only in this way can one assess with accuracy the fracture and the ossific centers of the epiphyses. The necessity of obtaining roentgenograms that are accurate mirror images cannot be overemphasized.

In general, because of increased plasticity, the child's skeleton can sustain, without injury, a force that would fracture the mature bone of an adult.

ANGULAR AND ROTATIONAL DEFORMITIES

Growth and remodeling can correct many of the deformities occurring following fractures in the child. However, one cannot fail to recognize the lack of potential for spontaneous correction in fractures at certain locations. Several factors contribute to correction of an angular deformity:

1. The age of the child at the time of an injury has a significant bearing on the outcome of a fracture. Obviously the older a child is at the time of injury, the less epiphyseal growth can occur and hence the less is the potential for spontaneous correction.
2. The distance of the fracture from the epiphyseal plate plays a role in the ultimate result. Blount has shown conclusively that the closer a fracture is to the epiphyseal plate, the greater are the chances of correction of any angulation deformity. Thus, a midshaft angulation will have less chance for spontaneous correction than would a fracture nearer the epiphyseal plate.

3. The amount of angulation after reduction will affect the end result. The greater an angulation, the less will be its potential for spontaneous correction.

The greatest potential for spontaneous correction of an angular deformity is present when the deformity occurs in the plane of motion of a nearby ginglymus (hinge) joint (Fig. 2–1). Gradual correction of the deformity usually occurs, but with little note of deformity by the patient in the meantime because it is in the axis of motion of the joint.

Rotational deformities about the longitudinal axis of a long bone, however, cannot be accepted, and an accurate reduction of a rotational deformity is advisable because the child has no growth mechanism to correct it. One method of identifying a rotational deformity is by comparing the roentgenographic details of the joint above and the joint below the fracture with

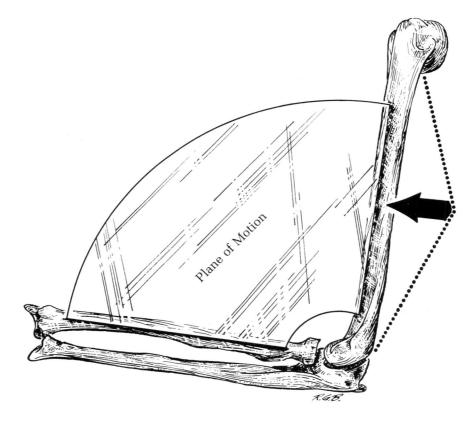

Lateral View

Fig. 2–1. Illustration of plane of motion of forearm on upper arm. Following fracture of forearm or humerus in the child, residual angulation is more acceptable in this plane. There will be a tendency toward self-correction with time.

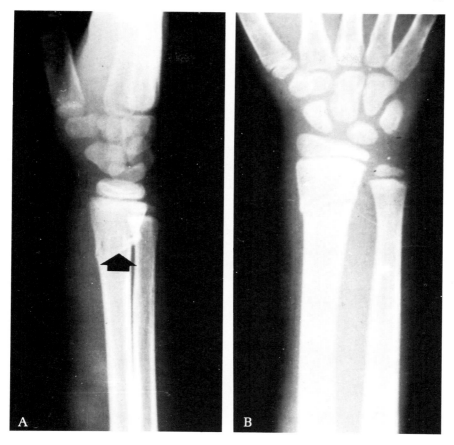

Fig. 2–2. Rotational fracture. A, In lateral view distal radius appears wider than shaft just proximal to fracture (arrow). Because radius is somewhat oval-shaped at this point, lack of apparent equal width on roentgenogram is excellent indication of rotary deformity. B, Anteroposterior roentgenogram of wrist is not so revealing as is lateral view. Since the growth potential for a child's bone cannot accommodate for a rotational deformity, an accurate reduction is advisable.

roentgenographic details of the uninjured side. Another means is to measure on the roentgenogram the width of the proximal and distal fragments near the fracture site. These fragments, of course, should be equal. However, if any rotational deformity exists, one fragment may be wider than the other, and the cross section of the bone near the fracture line will be oval, not round (Fig. 2–2).

INJURIES OF EPIPHYSIS, EPIPHYSEAL PLATE, AND METAPHYSIS

Injuries involving the epiphysis, the epiphyseal plate (physis), and the metaphysis were for many years poorly understood. But with the work of Aitken, and then more recently that of Salter and Harris, and Siffert, the sequence of events of individual injuries may be predicted with relative accuracy. The scheme of Salter and Harris is most commonly used today and will be used in this book. It describes five different types of epiphyseal injuries and gives justification for the necessary method of treatment (Fig. 2–3). It also provides some element of prognosis as to growth alteration.

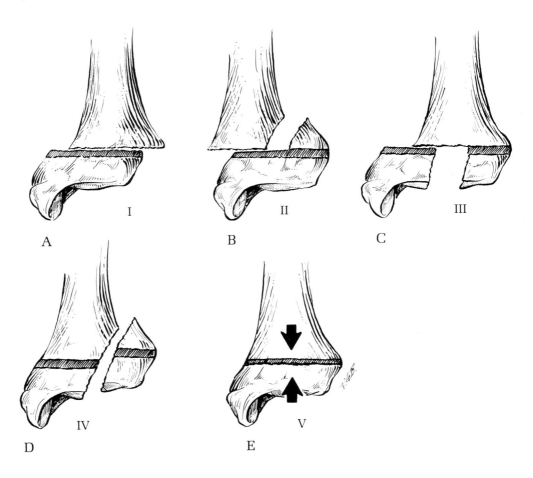

Fig. 2–3. Salter-Harris classification of epiphyseal injuries. A, Type I injury is pure slip through hypertrophic layer of cells. Gentle reduction is necessary, and a slightly imperfect reduction can be accepted. B, In type II injury partial separation has occurred through layer of hypertrophic cells of epiphyseal plate. The injuring force then appears to turn into the metaphysis, leaving epiphyseal plate intact between that segment of metaphysis and epiphysis. Gentle reduction as accurate as is feasible is required. Residual growth is seldom altered. C, In type III injury, epiphysis fractures, and one segment separates across plate. Accurate reduction is required for sake of joint congruity, even if open reduction is necessary. D, In type IV epiphyseal injury shearing force fractures across epiphysis, across plate, and continues through metaphysis to its cortex. Because of potential for growth alteration, perfect reduction must be accomplished and maintained, even though this may require open reduction and internal fixation with small Kirschner wires. E, Type V injury is caused by compression force that crushes germinal potential of epiphysis, causing cessation of growth. This may be suspected from history of injury but more often is a retrospective diagnosis.

The Salter-Harris Classification is as follows:

Type I (Fig. 2–3A). A slip occurs across the epiphyseal plate so that the metaphysis and the epiphysis change their positional relationship. This slip occurs through the zone of hypertrophic cells, and no change in the growth pattern would be expected.

Type II (Fig. 2–3B). A line of force causes a separation through a portion of the epiphyseal plate and then turns into the metaphysis, leaving a portion of the metaphysis with the epiphysis. Because the separation of the epiphyseal plate occurs through the zone of hypertrophic cells, any change in the growth pattern would be unlikely.

Type III (Fig. 2–3C). A fracture splits the epiphysis and then turns to complete its force across the epiphyseal plate. Displacement of one portion of the epiphysis occurs from the other part of the epiphysis, as well as from its adjacent metaphyseal relationship. The epiphyseal separation is at the level of the hypertrophic cells. This injury rarely causes any growth alteration once reasonable reduction is obtained.

Type IV (Fig. 2–3D). A shearing force fractures longitudinally through the epiphysis, across the epiphyseal plate, and up the metaphysis to the cortex. Reduction of this fragment must be perfect to prevent an alteration of growth. Imperfect reduction allows bony union of a part of the metaphysis to the epiphysis adjacent to it, stopping growth at that point but unable to change growth elsewhere in the epiphyseal plate. If this fracture cannot be perfectly reduced by closed means, or if perfect reduction cannot be maintained, it is essential to openly reduce the fragments and transfix them with small threaded Kirschner wires. The wires across the interior of the plate will not significantly alter growth, but they should be removed at six weeks.

Type V (Fig. 2–3E). This injury to the epiphysis is caused by a compressive force which in effect crushes the germinal cells. Roentgenograms do not show any change. This injury may be suspected from the history given by the patient. Examination reveals swelling and pain over the epiphyseal plate region. Time and failure of growth alone confirm the diagnosis.

Review of the histologic detail of the epiphyseal plate (Fig. 2–4) indicates the existence of germinal layers of cartilage cells in the epiphysis proper. As we study the section of the epiphyseal plate from the epiphyseal side toward the metaphyseal side, we note dividing cells followed by enlarging cells and then areas of amorphous calcium between the cartilage cells (zone of provisional calcification). On the metaphyseal side of this are seen death of the cartilage cells and farther along, toward the diaphysis, an ingrowth of blood vessels, osteoid tissue, and osteoblasts. Finally, on the metaphyseal side, calcium salts are laid down in the osteoid seams to form bone. Logically, we could assume that any injury in the germinal cell level would destroy growth potential and that injury toward the metaphyseal side of the germinal layer of cartilage cells would likely allow continuation of the growth pattern of the involved bone.

Fortunately, most injuries to the epiphysis occur at the zone of hypertrophic cells and if treated with proper diligence should provide a minimal chance for growth irregularity. A crushing injury to the epiphyseal plate can, however, injure the cells of the germinal layer and retard growth. The slipping in the slipped capital femoral epiphysis of nontraumatic origin occurs in the germinal layer, as well as in the dividing and hypertrophic areas and appears to be due to some defect in the basic protein organization. This changing position is stopped by pin fixation which allows union to ensue across the epiphyseal plate.

The injury occurring at the epiphysis of the child from infancy up to about six months of age is typically a type I slip. This is often difficult to diagnose, but continuing irritability, localized pain, and often splinting of an extremity in a child of this age group should cause suspicion of this injury. Comparison roentgenograms of the opposite limb are mandatory for accurate assessment.

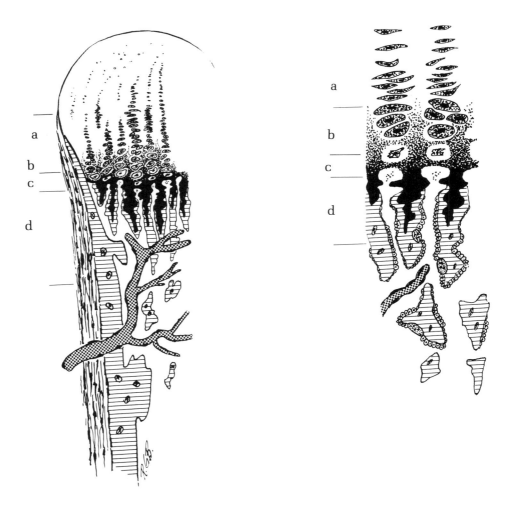

Fig. 2–4. Illustration of typical epiphyseal plate. Inset at right shows plate in greater detail. Resting cells (a), hypertrophic zone (b), zone of provisional calcification (c), and zone of osteoid ingrowth and the zone of ossification (d).

Immobilization for six to eight weeks is usually sufficient for the epiphyseal injury once it has been properly reduced.

Concern for growth potential is of no greater import than is the regard for the vascularity of the involved bone. The epiphysis receives its blood supply by multiple vessels about the periphery from the periosteum. Few if any vessels penetrate the epiphyseal plate, so that its nutrition will depend upon adequate circulation from the metaphysis or from the periosteal vessels about the periphery of the epiphyseal plate coursing into the epiphysis and ultimately reaching the plate.

The purely intra-articular position of some of the epiphyses serves to cause greater concern in certain injuries because of potentially precarious blood

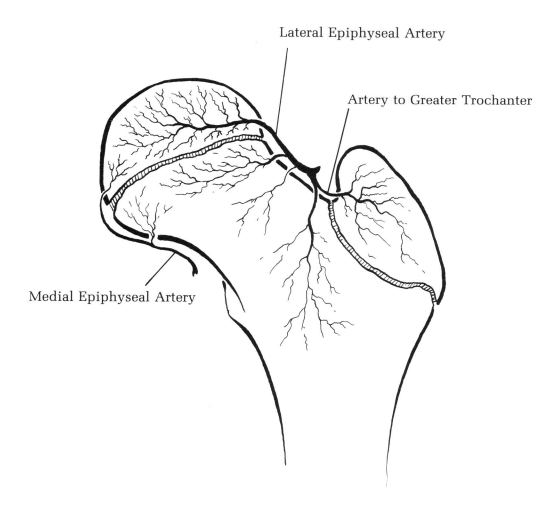

Fig. 2–5. Illustration of blood supply into femoral head and neck (after Crock) of child. Note arterial blood flow from distal to proximal in neck and potential for loss of that circulation from dislocation of hip, traumatic slip of the capital femoral epiphysis, or from certain hip fractures.

supply. For example, the capital femoral epiphysis is totally intra-articular (Fig. 2–5) and must rely upon retinacular vessel(s) for its nutrition. The retinacular vessel(s) arise from a terminal branch of the medial femoral circumflex artery and course along the periphery of the neck of the femur. Any significant displacement of the capital femoral epiphysis or of the femoral head could lead to loss of circulation. In like manner, a posterior dislocation may interrupt the circulation to the femoral head. Because of this fact alone, the acute slipped capital femoral epiphysis, traumatic or otherwise, and the dislocated hip in the child constitute two of the few real emergencies in orthopaedic surgery. Restoration of the proper anatomic relationship as soon as it can be accomplished must be the goal.

Other bones and processes lying intra-articular are the humeral head, the odontoid process of the axis, and the carpal navicular. Appropriate consideration must be given to fractures and dislocations occurring at these areas.

GREENSTICK FRACTURES

The construction of the child's bone is such as to permit more deformity before reaching its point of maximum elasticity. When this point is surpassed, an angular deformity can occur which is almost as though the bone were "bent." Thus is created the greenstick fracture (Fig. 2–6). This fracture does not remodel quickly, and if the angulation is of any consequence at all, completion of the fracture followed by reduction and then applying a cast until the fracture is united is the treatment of choice. Particularly is this necessary in the midforearm (site of most greenstick fractures) where the radius must be able to rotate freely about the ulna in supination and pronation.

Another type of fracture in the greenstick group is the torus fracture (Fig. 2–7). This is seen as a buckling of the cortex and occurs from a longitudinal compressive force. This is a stable fracture and need be supported by a cast or splint for only four to six weeks.

INJURIES TO LIGAMENTS

In the child and adolescent, injuries to the ligaments about a joint are not common, but do occur. Particularly does the ligament tear in the weight bearing joints of the knee and the ankle, especially during competitive sports. In fact, an avulsion bony injury may occur in preference to ligament tearing in a child or an adolescent. Once a diagnosis of ligamentous injury is made, that part should be put to rest by an appropriate immobilizing device. Orthopaedic surgeons who manage a multitude of these injuries in varying age groups stress the infrequent necessity to consider an operative approach for effective treatment in the young age group.

OPERATIONS

The need for nonoperative management of most children's fractures or dislocations cannot be overstressed. However, there are circumstances in which operative management is absolutely indicated. These include:

1. Acute slipped capital femoral epiphysis.
2. Displaced femoral neck fracture.
3. Irreducible dislocations of the hip.

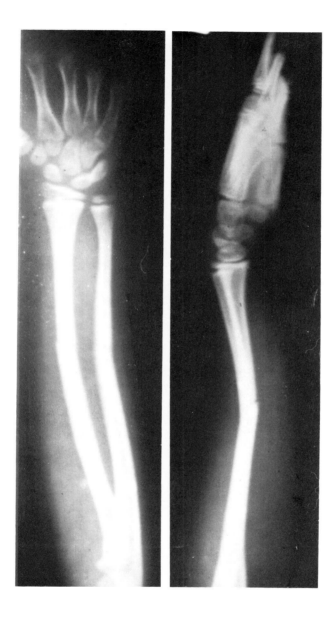

Fig. 2–6. Anteroposterior and lateral roentgenograms of typical greenstick fractures of both bones of forearm. This angulation might be acceptable in the younger child with considerable growth potential, but if much greater, the break would need to be completed and the fracture reduced and immobilized in a cast.

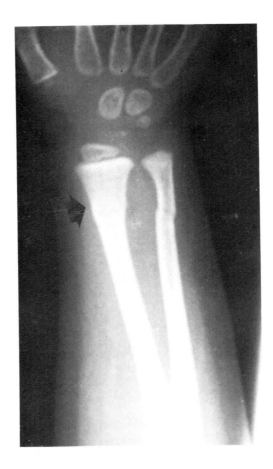

Fig. 2–7. Anteroposterior roentgenogram of torus fracture of radius. Note that cortices bulge at fracture site.

4. Open fracture of any bone.
5. Avulsion fracture of the tibial tubercle.
6. Irreducible totally displaced radial head fragment.
7. Volkmann's ischemic contracture—developing.

Other types of injury provide a relative indication for operation depending on individual circumstances. These would include:

1. Supracondylar fracture of humerus with a deepening nerve deficit or weakening pulse.
2. Salter type IV epiphyseal injury (Fig. 2–8). This must be openly reduced and internally fixed if reduction is unobtainable or cannot be maintained closed.

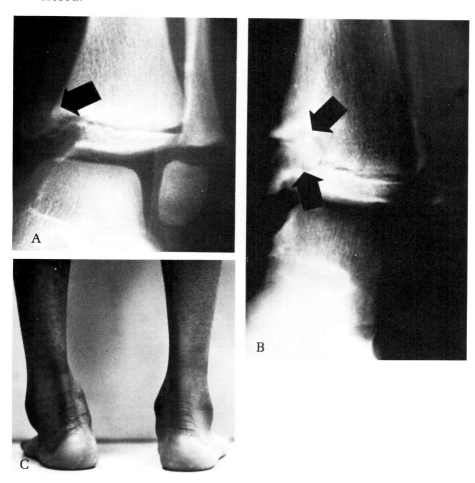

Fig. 2–8. Consequences of inadequately recognized and thus poorly reduced Type IV fracture. A, In original anteroposterior roentgenogram, note malleolar fracture crossing epiphyseal plate into metaphysis of distal tibia (arrow). B, Anteroposterior view two years after treatment. Two different levels of epiphyseal plate are seen at medial side of distal tibia (arrows). Joint line is oblique from superomedial to inferolateral side. C, Mute evidence of growth decrease at medial distal tibial epiphysis of left ankle.

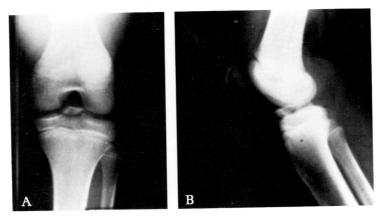

Fig. 2–9. Fracture of tibial spine in a child. A, Anteroposterior view. B, Lateral view. Full extension usually reduces and maintains reduction of this fracture.

3. Avulsion of tibial spines (Fig. 2–9)—if irreducible closed.
4. Fractures of the capitulum that are not well reduced.
5. Avulsion separation of 5mm or greater of the medial humeral epicondyle which cannot be reduced, or in which reduction cannot be maintained.

Specific details of consideration and treatment for individual fractures and dislocations will be discussed under the heading of that injury in the chapter on the geographical area involved.

REFERENCES

1. Aitken, A. P.: The end results of the fractured distal radial epiphysis. J. Bone Joint Surg. *17*:302, 1935.
2. Aitken, A.P.: The end results of fractures of the proximal humeral epiphysis. J. Bone Joint Surg. *18*:1036, 1936.
3. Aitken, A. P.: The end results of the fractured distal tibial epiphysis. J. Bone Joint Surg. *18*:685, 1936.
4. Aitken, A. P., and Magill, H. K.: Fractures involving the distal femoral epiphyseal cartilage. J. Bone Joint Surg. *34-A*:96, 1952.
5. Blount, W. P.: Fractures in Children. Baltimore, Williams & Wilkins Co., 1954.
6. Crock, H. V.: Blood Supply to the Lower Limb Bones in Man. Edinburgh, Livingstone, 1967.
7. Rang, M. C.: Children's Fractures. Philadelphia, J. B. Lippincott Co., 1974.
8. Rockwood, C. A., and Green, D. P.: Fractures. Philadelphia, J. B. Lippincott Co., 1975.
9. Salter, R. B., and Harris, R. W.: Injuries involving the epiphyseal plate. J. Bone Joint Surg. *45-A*:587, 1963.
10. Siffert, R. S.: The growth plate and its affections. J. Bone Joint Surg. *48-A*:546, 1966.
11. Watson-Jones, R.: Fractures and Joint Injuries, 4th ed., 2V. Baltimore, Williams & Wilkins Co., 1952-1955.

3

THE CERVICAL SPINE

The cervical spine serves as the structure upon which the bony skull rests. In addition, it forms a protective wall about the spinal cord and the nerve roots emerging from within this wall. Of all the bony spine, the cervical spine is so constructed as to allow the greatest mobility. For this mobility to exist, the spine must depend upon its attached ligamentous structures and muscles for needed stabilizing effects. The asset of mobility also can be a potential liability. Although the uninjured cervical spine has a stability competence along with this mobility, any injury that causes loss of ligamentous "tethering" or control can easily produce instability. In any treatment program for the injured cervical spine, the real objective must be a stable spine. The stable spine must allow mobility, but only as much as is consistent with stability. Sometimes stability can be achieved with little or no treatment as is seen in the patient with the minimal compression fracture. However, the spine injury in the more complex fracture or fracture-dislocation may require fusion in order to provide the needed stability.

In any discussion of spinal injuries, consideration must be given to the anatomic level of the injury, the causing force or mechanism of injury, and any special factors for the specific injury. In dealing with any injury to the spine, whether it be fracture, dislocation, or soft tissue injury, the potential of neurologic injury also exists. Accordingly, in addition to a general examination for spine injury, an accurate neurologic evaluation must also be performed and an interpretation of any neurologic deficits must be made on the basis of the anatomy of the spinal cord and the nerve roots. The general examination must include palpation for point tenderness as well as a cautious examination of range of motion. Correction of any neurologic deficit is desirable; at the same time further neurologic deficit from inadequate handling at any point must be avoided from the moment of injury until definitive care has been completed.

INJURIES OF THE ATLAS AND AXIS

In the embryologic development of the atlas and the axis, the body portion of the atlas remains in continuity with the axis. That segment is the odontoid process (dens), which extends superiorly from the axis (Fig. 3–1A). The odontoid process maintains a relationship to the ring of the first cervical vertebra anteriorly with a joint between the two bony segments. The stability of this joint is achieved by the cruciform ligament, which embraces the odontoid process and attaches to the ring of the atlas on each side as the transverse or alar ligament of the atlas. This ligamentous structure, which has firm bony attachments into the atlas and furnishes great strength to this joint, allows about 50% of the rotation of the cervical spine and normally 10% of the flexion of the cervical spine.

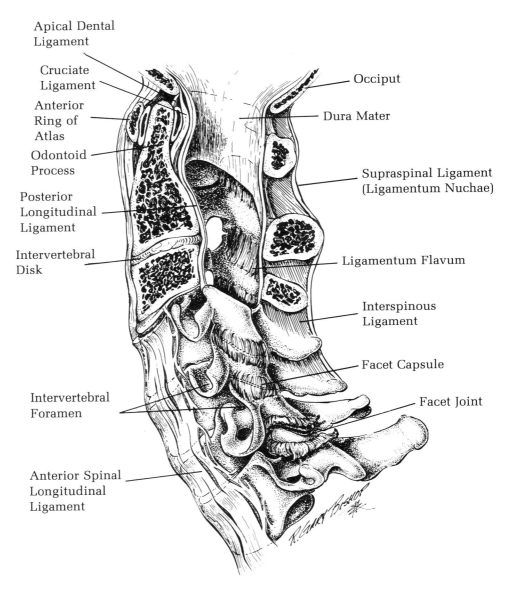

Fig. 3–1A.   Illustration of lateral view of cervical spine. Lateral one half of atlas, axis, and third cervical vertebra have been removed to show the ligaments and internal canal more clearly. Capsule is sectioned at facet joint between sixth and seventh vertebrae to show facets.

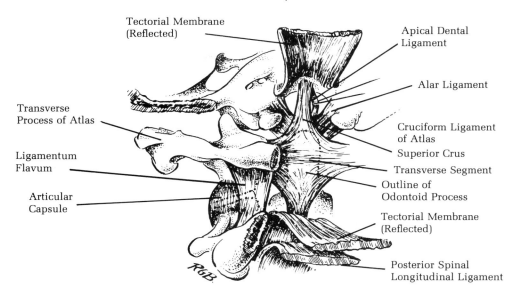

Tectorial Membrane (Reflected)

Apical Dental Ligament

Alar Ligament

Transverse Process of Atlas

Cruciform Ligament of Atlas

Superior Crus

Ligamentum Flavum

Transverse Segment

Outline of Odontoid Process

Articular Capsule

Tectorial Membrane (Reflected)

Posterior Spinal Longitudinal Ligament

Fig. 3–1B. Illustration with posterior ring of atlas and laminae and spinous process of axis removed to reveal contents of spinal canal. Most clearly shown is cruciate ligament holding odontoid process to its relationship with anterior ring of atlas.

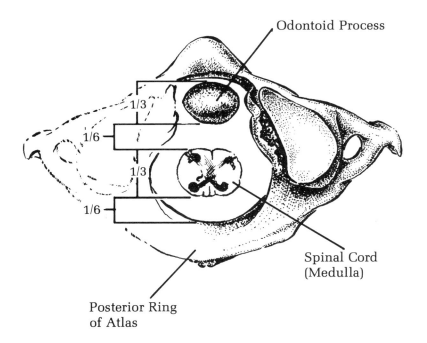

Odontoid Process

1/3

1/6

1/3

1/6

Spinal Cord (Medulla)

Posterior Ring of Atlas

Fig. 3–1C. Superior view of atlas and dens illustrates Steel's rule of thirds. Internal ring of the atlas is occupied equally by odontoid process, spinal cord, and free space. This free space acts as something of a "safety valve" in odontoid fractures and in atlas-axis dislocations, allowing greater mobility of the ring of the atlas before cord damage occurs.

In Steel's rule of thirds, were one to divide the contents of the ring of the atlas into thirds, the odontoid process would fill the anterior third, the spinal cord would fill one-third, and the remaining third would be an empty space (Fig. 3–1C). In the event of fracture or dislocation at this level, this empty space, which allows greater mobility of the ring of the atlas, serves as a protective device for the cord.

Atlantoaxial Dislocations

An atlantoaxial dislocation occurs only by a flexion and/or a rotation force, but is exceedingly rare because of the strength of the cruciate ligament and its attachments. Prior to any rupture of the cruciate ligament, the odontoid process tends to fracture instead. A neurologic deficit from the atlantoaxial dislocation is seldom seen in a *living* person. Should cord compression occur, it is at the level of the medulla and is incompatible with life. This dislocation is occasionally seen following long-standing inflammatory arthritis such as in the rheumatoid process. Spontaneous dislocation at the atlantoaxial joint in children was described by Berkheiser after he had associated several of these dislocations with severe upper respiratory infections. He believed the dislocation to follow laxity of the cruciate ligament and/or its attachment in the bone following inflammation and destruction of either the joint capsule or the bursa between the odontoid process and the atlas.

In the traumatic rupture of the atlantoaxial ligament, it must be assumed from anatomic fact that associated tears of the interlaminar ligaments occur posteriorly, since this injury can occur only with a flexion (posterior to anterior) force or with excessive rotary motion. When significant injury to soft tissue occurs from trauma, stability cannot be achieved by repairing only the rupture. A number of workers, including Badgley, Rogers, and more recently McNab, have noted the tendency for ligamentous tears or ruptures of the cervical spine to fail to reunite with adequate strength for necessary stability.

Because of failure of ligamentous tears to reunite, then, fusion at the atlantoaxial level would be the preferred method for achieving stability following tear of the cruciate (including transverse alar) ligament. A transoral or anterolateral approach is feasible; fixation, however, has not always been satisfactory with these approaches. From the posterior approach stability across this level can be achieved by an occipitoatlantoaxial fusion, by the atlantoaxial fusion or by the fusion of the first through the third cervical laminae. Fusion of the occiput to the atlas abolishes the flexion and extension capability of the occiput on the cervical spine, whereas fusion of the atlas to the axis and to the third cervical vertebra provides stability and removes all flexion, rotation, and lateral bending that can normally occur in these levels. Thus these would be less desirable modes of treatment when other methods can suffice.

Examination. Physical examination will likely reveal tenderness only to palpation at the base of the occiput posteriorly. The patient may feel more secure when holding the head in his hands. Occasionally there are symptoms of pain and burning of the posterior scalp, which is innervated by the greater occipital nerve emerging just posterior to the trapezius muscle attachment at the occipital bone.

Roentgenograms. A lateral roentgenogram of the cervical spine will be the

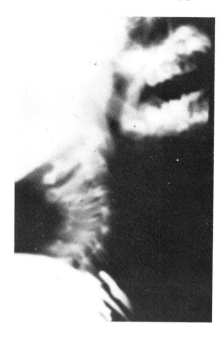

Fig. 3–2. Lateral roentgenogram showing dislocation of atlas (arrow points to anterior ring of the atlas) anteriorly from odontoid process in a seven-year-old child. An atlas-axis fusion was ultimately necessary to achieve stability.

most informative view. When possible, gentle flexion views may show the ring of the atlas riding forward in its relationship to the odontoid process as compared with the same relationship when the neck is in extension (Fig. 3–2). The open mouth odontoid view may show the space between the ring of the atlas and the lateral cortex of the odontoid process to vary between the two sides.

Treatment. Initial treatment of the traumatic dislocation is temporary immobilization of the occiput and cervical spine by head halter traction or sandbags placed along both sides of the head and neck. For more definitive immobilization, the patient should be placed on a turning frame with the turning axis longitudinal rather than transverse. The Stryker frame and the Foster bed are examples of this type of frame. The Circ-O-Letric bed should not be used until internal stability has been achieved.

Once the patient has been placed on the longitudinal axis frame, skeletal skull traction should be instituted via the Vinke tongs, Gardner-Wells tongs, or the halo (Fig. 3–3). The halo can be used as a traction device if some modification is made. Reduction of the atlas on the axis should be accomplished by an extension type of force through the tongs or the halo. When the patient is lying prone on the anterior frame, the pad under the forehead will help maintain this extension. When the patient is on the posterior frame, a pad between the scapulas usually should help in maintaining extension of the atlas on the axis. The minimum amount of weight necessary for the traction device should be used and would generally be about 10 pounds. Operation can be performed with the patient on the turning frame, as it maintains stability of the dislocation and at the same time provides an easy access to the airway for an anesthetic.

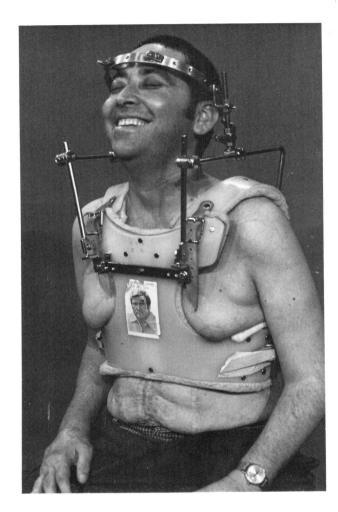

Fig. 3–3. Frontal oblique view of halo vest is seen here immobilizing dislocation of atlas on axis while Gallie fusion is maturing.

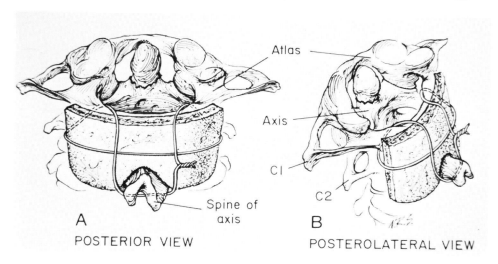

Fig. 3–4. Illustration of Gallie fusion of atlas to axis. This method of wiring laminas of C1 and C2 against bone graft immediately provides good stability between these two vertebrae. (From Hartman, J. T.: Fractures, dislocations, and fracture-dislocations of the spine and pelvis. *In* Practice of Surgery: Orthopedics 2. Hagerstown, MD, Harper & Row, 1971.)

I prefer the Gallie type of fusion for the atlantoaxial dislocation because it provides instant stability by wiring the lamina of the atlas and the spinous process of the axis against the bone graft (Fig. 3–4). In addition, this type of fusion causes the smallest permanent loss of flexion, extension, and rotation of any types discussed. As soon as the patient has passed the major morbidity period of the operative procedure, he may be mobilized wearing a brace such as a Guilford two-poster cervical orthosis (Fig. 3–5). Immobilization should be continued until evidence of bony union between the lamina of C1, the bone graft, and the lamina and spinous process of the axis is seen on a roentgeno-gram.

In treating the spontaneous dislocation that is associated with an infectious process, usually head halter traction can be used until the original reaction subsides and then a Thomas collar can be substituted. In more severe disloca-tions, the Guilford type of orthosis is used (Fig. 3–5). Approximately four to six weeks of immobilization should be sufficient in that circumstance.

Atlas Fractures

The lateral masses of the atlas lie between the cartilaginous joint surfaces of the occipital condyle and the superior facets of the axis. A longitudinal compressive force across this area will trap the lateral masses of the atlas between these two joint surfaces and can result in a shattering of the ring of the atlas. This is an essentially decompressive type of injury, rarely causing neurologic deficit because of the centrifugally directed forces. This type of fracture of the atlas is commonly referred to as the Jefferson fracture. It is unusual for the Jefferson fracture to be associated with atlantoaxial dislocation, although I have a patient with just this combination of injuries. A first year

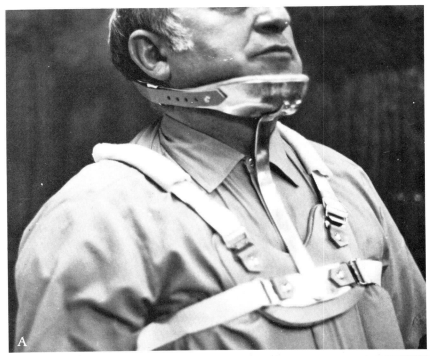

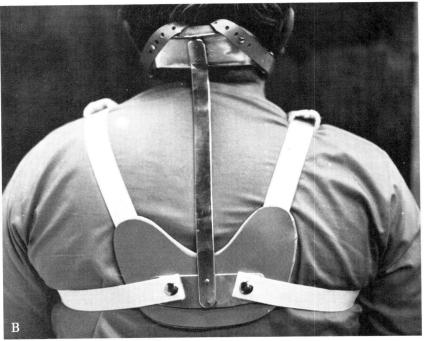

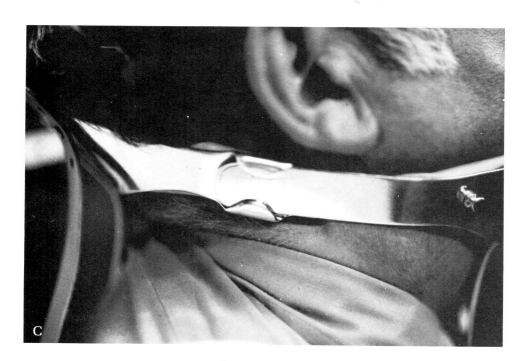

Fig. 3–5. Guilford two-poster cervical orthosis. A, Anterior view. Note flattened metal upright with firm attachment to chest and chin pieces. B, Posterior view. Posterior upright has attachments similar to those anteriorly. Axillary and over-the-shoulder straps attach anterior and posterior chest pieces. C, Enlarged side view showing bilateral metal strut attachments from chin piece to receptacle in occipital piece. Adjustable leather strap from chin piece to occipital piece prevents disengagement. These plus features shown in Fig. 3–4 provide relatively good immobilization. (From Hartman, J. T., Palumbo, F., and Hill, B. J.: Cineradiography of the braced normal cervical spine. Clin. Orthop. *109*:97, 1975.)

house officer noted the onset of apnea in this injured child each time the head was raised from the cart for examination of the fundus. Roentgenograms confirmed the fracture of the ring of the atlas, as well as a dislocation of the atlas on the axis. The fracture of the atlas was treated by placing the child in traction and then in a Minerva jacket until evidence of union was seen on a roentgenogram. Following this, when lateral dynamic roentgenograms showed significant mobility of the anterior atlas from the odontoid process in flexion, an atlantoaxial fusion was performed. Stability was thus achieved.

Examination. The patient with an atlas fracture complains of point tenderness of the superior neck area to palpation. Seldom is there any neurologic deficit. Often, however, the patient holds his head in his hands to provide a sense of stability.

Roentgenograms. Roentgenographic diagnosis of the Jefferson fracture may be difficult. In the open mouth view of the *normal* spine, the lateral margins of the lateral masses of the atlas do not extend laterally beyond the lateral masses of the axis. In a roentgenogram of the Jefferson fracture, however, a separation will be seen between the lateral bony masses and the odontoid process. In lateral roentgenograms in the normal person, the tubercle of the posterior arch of the atlas does not usually rest as far posterior as the spinous process of the axis. The tubercle often lies posterior to the spinous process of the axis in a Jefferson fracture. In addition, the posterior wall of the anterior ring of the atlas should lie against the anterior wall of the odontoid process. With a fracture of the ring of the atlas, there is usually alteration of this relationship (Fig. 3–6). One may see a loss of cortical continuity in the ring of the atlas on the lateral view or in rotational oblique views in this particular injury.

Treatment. Once the diagnosis of atlas fracture is established, it is advisable to utilize skull traction to provide stability. This can be done with tongs and a longitudinal turning frame or with a halo traction device (Fig. 3–3). This latter method provides excellent stability and allows instant mobility. Traction immobilization for this fracture should be continued for two months or until evidence of union is present. The cervical brace as described in atlantoaxial dislocations should be worn for an additional two months for a total of four months' protection.

Fractures of Odontoid Process

When a flexion or an extension force is expended at the atlantoaxial junction, the odontoid process may be fractured. With the extension force, the anterior ring of the atlas forces the odontoid process to fracture at its base, the axis. In flexion, the alar ligament strikes the odontoid process and when the force is sufficient causes a fracture of the odontoid process. Displacement of the fractured odontoid process may occur toward an anterior or a posterior position. The most proximal part of the odontoid process will remain in its usual relationship to the ring of the atlas.

Fig. 3–6. Roentgenograms showing Jefferson fracture of atlas. A, Anteroposterior view. The arrow points to widened surface of lateral atlas joint in relationship to opposing surface of axis. (Compare with normal, Fig. 3–12.) B, Lateral view. The arrow points to fracture in posterior ring of atlas.   →

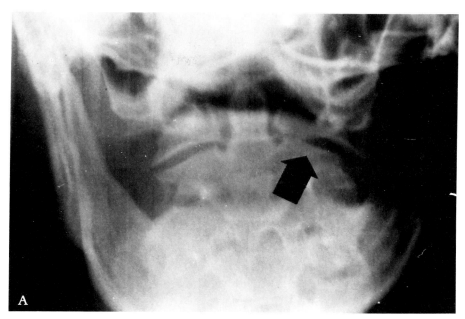

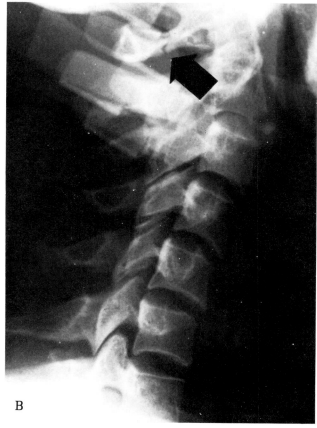

Examination. The patient with an odontoid fracture usually complains of an occipital headache and feels it necessary to stabilize his head with his hands. Although seldom seen, neurologic deficit is possible in this displaced fracture. Because this cord compression would occur at the bulb level, however, it would tend to be incompatible with life. In this area of the spinal canal, the spinal cord occupies one half of the canal, and free space occupies the other half. This allows a considerable margin of safety.

Roentgenograms. Roentgenographic views essential for the accurate diagnosis of the odontoid fracture are the lateral cervical spine and the open mouth views (Fig. 3–7). If no displacement is present, the open mouth view may provide the only evidence of a break in cortical continuity of the odontoid process. Loss of continuity of the lateral margins of the lateral masses of the atlas and the axis is an indication of fracture of the odontoid process with lateral displacement. Anterior or posterior displacement is seen best on the lateral roentgenographic view. The odontoid process may fracture at the isthmus, at the base, or "scooped" down into the body of the axis. Occasionally, laminograms are necessary for accurate identification of the bony injury.

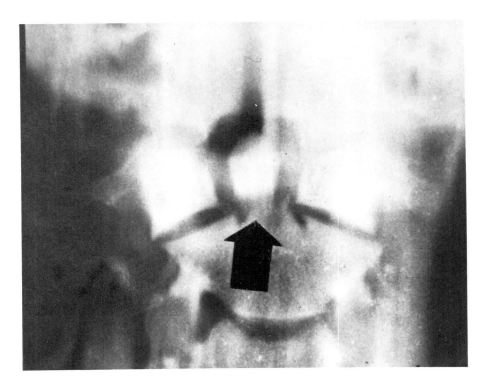

Fig. 3–7. Anteroposterior open mouth view laminagram showing fracture at isthmus of odontoid process. A fracture at this level of odontoid process will not unite as readily as will a fracture at the base. (From Hartman, J. T.: Fractures, dislocations and fracture-dislocations of the spine and pelvis. *In* Practice of Surgery: Orthopedics 2. Hagerstown, Md., Harper & Row, 1971.)

Treatment. Fractures at the base of the odontoid process tend to unite readily with proper immobilization by traction, the halo cast method, or even a Minerva plaster cast. When early evidence of union is seen across the fracture site, the immobilization can be switched to a cervical orthosis as described under atlantoaxial dislocations.

The fracture in the isthmus of the odontoid process has a definite tendency to proceed to nonunion, perhaps because of interposition of the transverse ligament as suggested by Bailey. A period of immobilization should be tried with this fracture, but often an atlantoaxial fusion as described under atlanto-axial dislocation will be needed to achieve adequate stability.

The odontoid process ossifies in two separate segments, one contiguous with the body of the axis and the other at the superior tip of the process. Occasionally, following trauma, separation occurs at the level of the cartilage between these two ossific centers. Adequate immobilization for two months should achieve union of the proximal ossification center to the base. Should such stability not be evident on lateral dynamic films in either the child or the adult, an atlantoaxial fusion is recommended in order to achieve the necessary stability.

INJURIES FROM THE THIRD TO THE SEVENTH CERVICAL VERTEBRAE

Anatomically, the third through the seventh cervical vertebrae have many common features. The particular factor providing stability in this area is primarily soft tissue, although the point at which the facets meet and the shape of the vertebral bodies themselves offer some assistance in this regard.

The longus colli and longus capitis muscle groups anterior to the bodies, as well as the paraspinous muscles posteriorly, provide control of motion and add to the stability of the spine. In the anticipated injury to the neck, these muscles are the first line of defense to resist excessive motion. If the force is not an anticipated one, however, the muscles remain relaxed, and the ligamentous structures must passively accept the force until its energy has been expended.

Posteriorly, strong fibers run from the inferior surface of the spinous process above to the superior surface of the spinous process below to add a distinct element of tethering. These are the interspinous ligaments which prevent excessive widening of the interspinous space. The ligamentum nuchae is a fibrous membrane running from the occipital protuberance posteriorly to the tips of the spinous processes as low as the seventh cervical vertebra. Little if any resistance to excess motion appears to be provided by this structure.

Between the laminae run strong ligamentous fibers that make up the ligamentum flavum. Lateral to these fibers and surrounding the facets at each side lie the capsular ligaments. The posterior spinal longitudinal ligament lies anterior to the cord and runs from the axis above to the sacrum below. Definite fiber attachments go into the posterior bodies within the spinal canal and into the anulus fibrosus of each disk.

The intervertebral disk lies between the opposing cartilaginous surfaces of the vertebral bodies and is composed of the dense fibrous tissue and fibrocartilaginous materials peripherally which surround the softer gelatinous nucleus pulposus. Fibers from the anulus fibrosus attach into the bodies of the vertebrae. These fibers of the anulus form strong bonds between the vertebrae.

Amorphous gelatinous material containing few fibers composes the nucleus pulposus that rests within the center of the anulus fibrosus. The anterior spinal longitudinal ligament lies anterior to the vertebral bodies; it sends fibers into the bodies, as well as interdigitating fibers into each anulus fibrosus from the atlas down through the sacrum.

The type of injury occurring in the cervical spine depends upon the direction from which the force originates and the position of the spine at the time of initiation of the force. The severity of the injury is largely determined by the magnitude of the force.

If the spine is extended at the time of receipt of the longitudinal force, the injury will be an extension type. In contradistinction to this, the flexed cervical spine that receives a longitudinal force will eventuate in a flexion type of injury. In this injury, the anterior body compresses, most commonly along the superior cartilage plate of the vertebral body. Should the force in this type of injury continue, it may cause the teardrop type of fracture described by Schneider and Kahn. In this event, there may be a neurologic deficit caused by a fragment of bone driven posteriorly into the spinal cord at the involved level.

Injuries from a Longitudinal Force

The longitudinal force occurring from a blow on the top of the skull is transmitted across the facets, the intervertebral disks, and bodies. In the spine that is straight, this force, when of sufficient magnitude, will tend to expend itself primarily in the body, shattering it. The body that does fracture is the first one in the line of force to present sufficient resistance to the force to cause this injury.

A centrifugal type of force thus occurs which tends to displace the fragments outward from the centrum of the vertebra. The spinal longitudinal ligaments, both anterior and posterior, and the anulus fibrosus act to restrain displacement. Neurologic deficit can occur from this type of injury but is not common in the purely shatter type of fracture.

Examination. The patients' complaint will be rather nonspecific as to exact location of pain, but palpation at the level of the injury will cause more pain than at other levels. Seldom will one see a neurologic deficit with this injury.

Roentgenograms. The anteroposterior roentgenogram of the vertebral body that has sustained a longitudinal compression will show a decrease in the height of the vertebral body while the height of the adjacent disk spaces remains normal (Fig. 3–8A). The spinous processes are seen at regularly repeating intervals, even at the involved level. The shattered body tends to broaden as viewed on the anteroposterior roentgenogram. The lateral roentgenogram often shows a decreased height of the involved body, but a normal height for disk space above and below (Fig. 3–8B). The diameter of the compressed body is increased from anterior to posterior. The posterior portion of the involved body may lie posterior to a line drawn from the posterior margins of the bodies above and below.

Treatment. Inasmuch as a neurologic deficit is unusual in vertebral injuries from a longitudinal force, the objective of treatment is to prevent further injury while achieving stability. In the most severely crushed vertebrae, skeletal traction should be instituted and may be accomplished on a frame with the

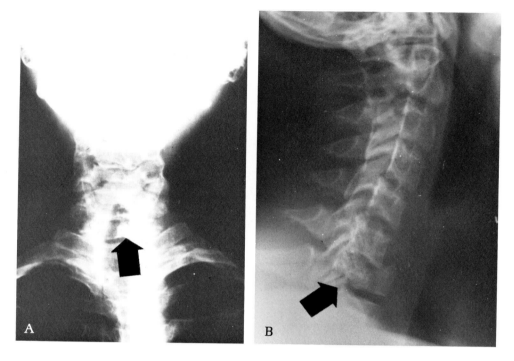

Fig. 3–8. Roentgenograms showing compression fracture of seventh cervical vertebra. A, In anteroposterior view arrow points to spinous process. Note increase between sixth and seventh spinous processes as compared to others. B, In lateral view arrow points to compression fracture.

skull tongs; the more recently popularized halo apparatus may be used so that the patient can be mobilized earlier. Once evidence of early union of the fragments can be seen on the roentgenograms (approximately two months), the patient may be placed in a Guilford cervical orthosis as described previously (Fig. 3–5). An additional three months in this orthosis should be sufficient. When the brace is discontinued, it will be essential for the patient to be instructed in exercises to achieve as great a range of motion of the cervical spine as possible. The similar lesser injury in which apparent stability exists may be treated with a head halter until symptoms subside and then the patient may be placed in the Guilford cervical orthosis.

Injuries Caused by a Flexion Force

When a sudden acute flexion force is applied to the cervical spine, the ligamentous structures will most likely progressively tear from the posterior to the anterior side (Fig. 3–9A). The significant ligaments to tear and the order in which they tear are the interspinous ligaments, ligamentum flavum, the capsular ligaments, and the posterior spinal longitudinal ligament. Tearing is followed by separation of the anulus fibrosus from its attachments to the cartilage plate and the vertebral body (this separation may occur from the body above or the body below). Such a flexion force may rarely tear the anterior

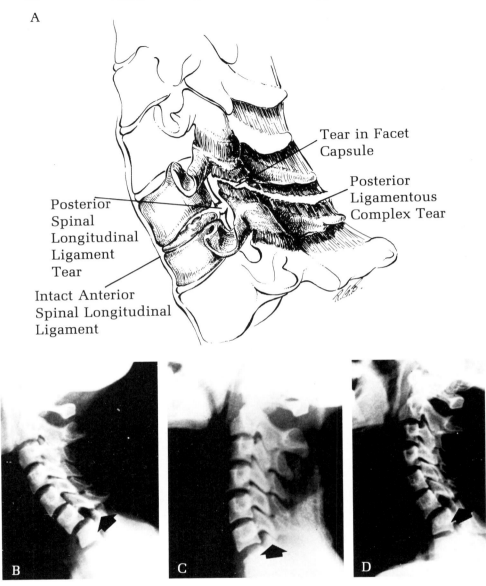

A

Tear in Facet
Capsule

Posterior
Ligamentous
Complex Tear

Posterior
Spinal
Longitudinal
Ligament
Tear

Intact Anterior
Spinal Longitudinal
Ligament

Fig. 3–9. A, Illustration of flexion injury without displacement. As seen here, tear may extend from interspinous ligament through ligamentum flavum and capsular ligaments. As force continues, posterior spinal longitudinal ligament may tear and anulus fibrosus separate from vertebral bodies. Note intact anterior spinal longitudinal ligament, a factor providing stability when spine is extended. B, Lateral roentgenogram following original flexion injury. Sixth vertebrae is subluxed, and its inferior facets are poised ready to dislocate anterior to facets from below (arrow). C, Lateral roentgenogram through plaster reduction of subluxation shown in B. Head and neck were immobilized in Minerva jacket for three months. D, Lateral roentgenogram taken three weeks after removal of Minerva cast. Subluxation of sixth on seventh cervical vertebra has recurred, clearly indicating unstable nature of this injury. (From Hartman, J. T.: Fractures, dislocations, and fracture-dislocations of the spine and pelvis. *In* Practice of Surgery: Orthopedics 2. Hagerstown, Md. Harper & Row, 1971.)

spinal longitudinal ligament and the muscle attachments from the anterior surfaces of the lateral masses.

Should the posterior soft tissues tear as far anterior as the anterior spinal longitudinal ligament, bilateral facet dislocations may occur in which the inferior facets ride up and over and come to rest anterior to the opposing superior facets (Fig. 3–9B, C, D, E). This type of injury is more commonly the end result of a continuation of the flexion force, once all of the posterior structures have been torn. When the posterior soft tissue structures provide greater resistance to tearing than the body has structural strength, then a wedge compression of the body anteriorly will satisfy the energy requirements to expend the force.

Combinations of fractures and dislocations of the bodies can occur, particularly with a fracture of the anterior-inferior margin of the vertebral body. Should the inferior-posterior portion of the body be displaced sufficiently posteriorly into the canal, an anterior cervical cord compression could result. This is the mechanism in the teardrop fracture-dislocation (Fig. 3–10) as described by Schneider and Kahn.

Barnes observed that the flexion injury resulting in fracture or dislocation with forward displacement will not cause sufficient narrowing of the spinal

E

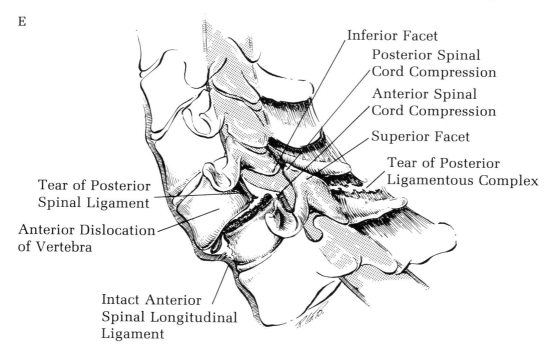

Inferior Facet

Posterior Spinal Cord Compression

Anterior Spinal Cord Compression

Superior Facet

Tear of Posterior Ligamentous Complex

Tear of Posterior Spinal Ligament

Anterior Dislocation of Vertebra

Intact Anterior Spinal Longitudinal Ligament

Fig. 3-9 (Continued). E, Illustration showing final position of flexion injury with ligamentous tearing plus a flexion force unyielding until inferior facet has dislocated anterior to superior facet from below. Note cord compression caused by laminae of dislocated vertebra and posterior superior corner of body below. Once reduced, intact anterior spinal longitudinal ligament will provide stability with spine extended. Posterior fusion and wiring will provide short-term and long-term stability.

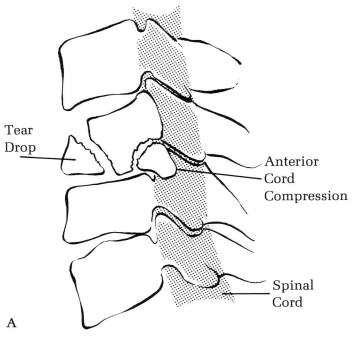

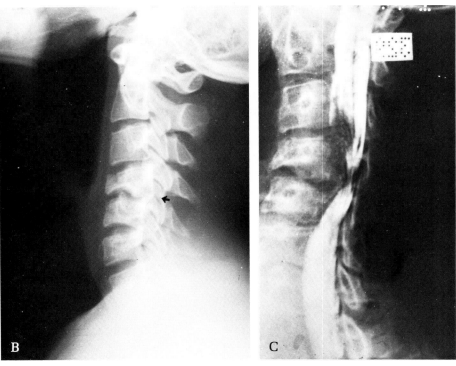

canal to compress the cord unless there is dislocation or locking of at least one pair of articular facets. The only exception to this observation would be the teardrop fracture.

Examination. When an injury to the cervical spine is suspected in a patient, that patient should be handled in the same manner as the patient with known fracture or dislocation. The patient should be maintained on a cart with the neck and head immobilized by sandbags to protect the patient from any further injury. Differentiation between mild and severe cord damage is difficult in the early post-trauma period. Should early evidence of cord damage be present, regardless of roentgenograms, the patient should be placed on a turning frame with a longitudinal turning axis such as the Stryker frame (not Circ-O-Lectric bed) or the Foster bed, and skull traction should be instituted.

The initial examination should include the most thorough possible neurologic assessment. Neurologic sparing distal to the level of the lesion in the paralyzed patient may be looked upon as a hopeful prognostic sign. Visible contraction of the anal sphincter when the perineum is stroked, often referred to as the "anal wink," is consistent with but not an absolute sign of significant neurologic continuity.

One of the most perceptive contemporary observers in spinal cord injuries, Schneider, described an important entity known as the acute central cord compression syndrome (Fig. 3–11A). This must be recognized or ruled out in any patient with neurologic deficit following cervical spine injury. The mechanism of acute central cord compression is the impingement of the spinal cord between the ligamentum flavum posteriorly and spurs or a bulging disk anteriorly (Fig. 3–11B). The neurologic pattern in this lesion is one of more profound paralysis of the arms than of the legs, with the arms becoming weak or paralyzed first and then the legs. The continuation of the lesion will cause loss of bowel and bladder control last. Operative decompression is *contraindicated* in this condition. The recovery occurs spontaneously during simple bed or frame immobilization. The more distal elements (mainly bowel and bladder) regain motor function first followed by improving leg control; the arm functions return last.

As documented by Schneider, the progression and regression of neurologic signs in the acute central cord compression syndrome can be well understood on an anatomic basis. At the cervical level, the most central portion of the cord contains anterior horn cells and fibers to the upper extremity. Peripheral to this, in the pyramidal lateral tracts, lie the fibers to the lower extremities,

Fig. 3-10. A, Illustration of acute teardrop cervical fracture-dislocation as result of acute flexion injury. Anterior part of vertebral body is forcibly squeezed off anteriorly while inferior portion is displaced posteriorly into spinal canal, thus being in position to cause anterior cervical spinal cord compression. (After Schneider, R. C. and Kahn, E. A.: Chronic neurological sequelae of acute trauma to the spine and spinal cord. J. Bone Joint Surg., *38A*:985, 1956.) B, Lateral roentgenogram of cervical spine showing typical acute flexion or teardrop fracture-dislocation (arrow) of fourth cervical vertebra in seventeen-year-old tumbler. C, Lateral myelogram two and one-half years after injury indicates encroachment on spinal canal by bony overgrowth at interspace between fourth and fifth cervical vertebrae. (From Schneider, R. C.: The syndrome of acute anterior spinal cord injury. J. Neurosurg. *12*:95, 1955.)

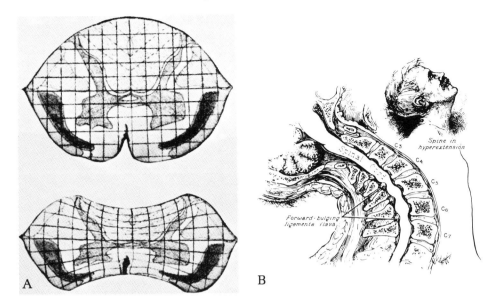

Fig. 3–11. A, Model of cross section of cord with pathways shaded (top). Model compressed by both an anterior and a posterior force, demonstrating distortion of spinal cord fiber tracts (bottom). B, Drawing illustrating impingement of ligamentum flavum on posterior aspect of spinal cord. Counter pressure is exerted anteriorly by hypertrophic spurs on vertebral bodies. (From Schneider, R. C., Cherry, G. L., and Pantek, H.: The syndrome of acute central cervical cord injury. J. Neurosurg. *11*:546, 1954.)

bowels, and bladder. Edema begins in the most central (and severely compressed) portion of the cord and spreads peripherally; it recedes in reverse fashion.

An acute anterior cervical cord compression syndrome may be associated with the flexion injury as described by Schneider and Kahn. This tends to occur specifically with the teardrop type of fracture, in which there is an immediate, complete paralysis associated with hypalgesia from the level of the lesion distally; there is, as well, preservation of motion, position, and vibratory sense (posterior columns). The localized cord compression does not block the canal. Progression of the depth of neurologic deficit is rare in this circumstance. The treatment of choice is relief of the compression through an anterior approach to the cord and anterior fusion. The anterior fusion championed by Bailey provides early relative stability.

Roentgenograms. To initiate a survey of the spine, only the anteroposterior and lateral roentgenograms need be taken (Fig. 3–12). Following evaluation of the more evident injuries, one can proceed with the open mouth, oblique, and pillar views for a more thorough evaluation (Figs. 3–13, 3–14, 3–15). Should it be determined necessary to take lateral dynamic roentgenograms (lateral views with full flexion and full extension), they may at this point be taken with confidence that no further injury will likely occur from necessary positioning.

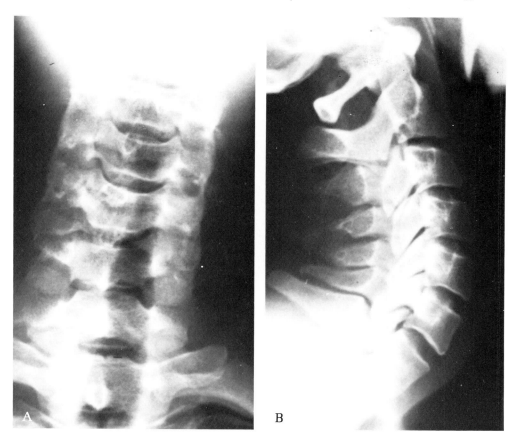

Fig. 3–12. Roentgenograms of normal cervical spine. A, Anteroposterior view. B, Lateral view. These two views are essential for roentgenographic survey of any cervical spine that has been injured. If these views are read as normal, further investigation is pursued as warranted by clinical or other findings.

In assessing the roentgenograms one should note the overall appearance of the spine. Are the heights of vertebral bodies and disk spaces normal? On the anteroposterior view are the spinous processes repeating at regular and equal intervals? Should dislocation of the facets be present in the flexion injury, the spinous processes at the level of dislocation appear usually widely separated as compared to those of the uninjured levels. With the body compression seen in the occasional flexion injury, the lateral masses may be displaced laterally at the affected level. The subchondral bone plate at the superior and inferior margins of the body should be intact in any uninjured vertebra.

In assessing roentgenograms of flexion injury, the lateral views often provide the best diagnostic clues. The posterior margin of the vertebral bodies should form a gentle smooth extension arch in the normal spine. If this arch is angulated or displaced at any point, injury must be suspected. Badgley pointed out that the long axis of the spinous processes, if drawn out, converge at a point

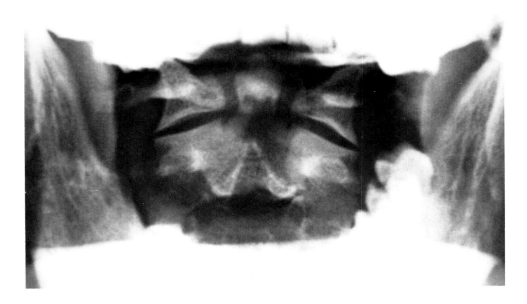

Fig. 3–13.   Open mouth view, an essential roentgenogram in assessing injury to atlas or axis. Note joint surfaces of atlas and axis are equal in width.

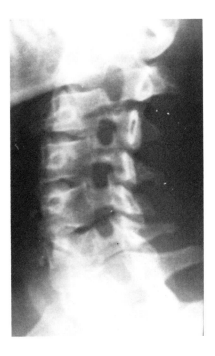

Fig. 3–14.   Oblique roentgenographic view of cervical spine. Such views allow visualization of foramina at 45° obliquity and facet relationships at 60° obliquity off anteroposterior plane.

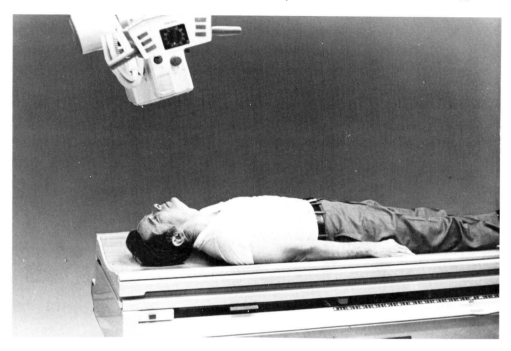

Fig. 3–15. Patient with roentgenogram tube properly positioned for pillar view. Pillar views of the cervical spine give better visualization of the pedicle injuries.

posterior to the neck. A divergence of any two of these lines suggests flexion injury. Invariably this will be noted with dislocated or subluxated facets. The facets must be studied carefully on the lateral view for evidence of lack of usual apposition.

The oblique view more clearly defines the relationship of the opposing facets, as well as any evidence of lack of continuity in the pedicles. The foramina can be viewed at 45 degrees obliquity and the facet relationships at 60 degrees obliquity off the anteroposterior plane (Fig. 3–14).

Most difficult to visualize roentgenographically are the low cervical and cervicodorsal junction levels. Particularly is this so in any short, stocky person. Because some of the more commonly missed injuries in the cervical spine are in the cervicodorsal area, it is incumbent upon the examining physician to confirm that no fracture or dislocation exists at this level.

In the more difficult circumstance of attempting to assess the cervicodorsal junction, one may be able to get satisfactory lateral roentgenograms by simply placing traction on the arms in an inferior direction (Fig. 3–16). If this does not permit a satisfactory lateral view of the spine down to the first dorsal vertebra, then one should try the "swimmer's view," a lateral roentgenogram taken with one arm raised over the shoulder and the other arm down at the side (Fig. 3–17). The tube is placed in the axilla of the raised arm; a slightly lateral oblique view may be necessary.

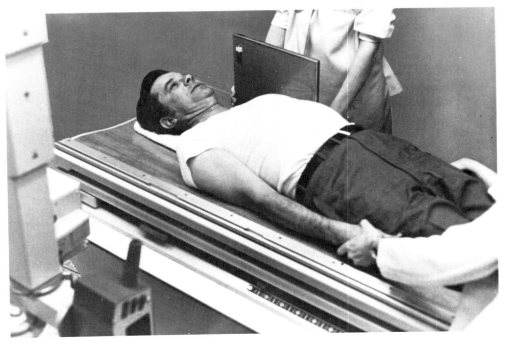

Fig. 3–16. Lateral roentgenograms of cervical spine being taken while inferior traction is applied to arms. This is one method of securing better visualization at cervicodorsal junction, an area difficult to diagnose.

Only when one is convinced that a cervical spine injury exists and no fracture or dislocation has been found on the anteroposterior, lateral, oblique, and the open mouth view roentgenograms, are the lateral dynamic roentgenograms indicated (Fig. 3–18). These will demonstrate presence or absence of ligament integrity in the face of no evident bony injury and can confirm excessive facet opening. One must recognize that the lateral dynamic roentgenograms show only the position of the vertebrae at extremes of flexion and extension but cannot show the motion through which the vertebrae passed to reach those extremes of motion. The source for this latter information lies in the use and interpretation of the cinefluoroscopic examination. Useful guidelines for normal or acceptable movements of the cervical spine under cinefluoroscopic examination are emerging.

Treatment. Having established a diagnosis of flexion injury of the cervical spine, one then should institute plans for appropriate treatment of the spine in order to achieve stability. The first stage of treatment in any flexion injury to the spine with displacement or dislocation is to reduce the fracture or dislocation by use of skull traction and the longitudinal turning frame. This is the *most ideal* method of cord decompression.

In the anterior dislocation of a cervical vertebra without evidence of fracture, the reduction is best achieved by skull traction applied to a moderately flexed cervical spine. The patient is on the longitudinal turning frame, and once

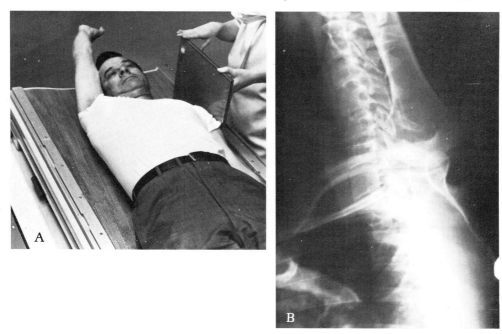

Fig. 3–17. Swimmer's view for accurate cervicodorsal diagnosis. A, Patient in position. B, Lateral roentgenogram giving accurate visualization from the midcervical spine inferiorly to the third dorsal vertebra.

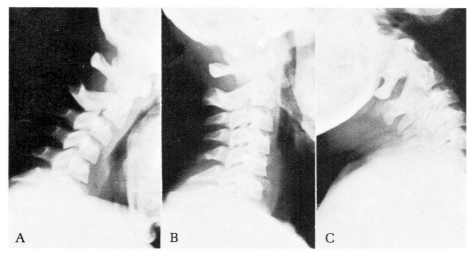

Fig. 3–18. Lateral dynamic roentgenograms of cervical spine. A, In flexion one notes equidistant spinous processes and relatively gentle curve outlining posterior bodies. Spaces between occiput and tubercle of atlas as well as between tubercle of atlas and spinous process of axis widen only slightly when compared to those spaces on neutral film (Fig. 3–17B). B, In neutral position, lines drawn down axis of spinous processes of C4 through C7 should converge at a point posterior to the neck in the normal spine. C, In extension, note spaces between occiput and tubercle of atlas, between tubercle of atlas and spinous process of axis, as well as between spinous processes inferiorly, all decrease. A smooth arc is noted by line connecting the posterior bodies of C2 through C7. (From Fielding, J. W.: Dynamic anatomy and cineradiography of the cervical spine. *In* The Cervical Spine by R. W. Bailey. Philadelphia, Lea & Febiger, 1974.)

length has been achieved (the facet tips separated) by traction, extension of the spine is effected and then the amount of the weights is reduced. Occasionally, traction may need to be increased up to 40 pounds through skull tongs in order to achieve sufficient separation of the facets for reduction. The increase in weights by increments of 5 pounds is the easiest method when accompanied by roentgenographic monitoring of the displacement or dislocation at regular intervals of one to two hours. These weights can be fairly quickly cut back to 15 pounds following reduction of the fracture or dislocation. The more quickly the reduction can be accomplished, the more quickly the decision regarding the need for operative treatment can be established. Such haste with due deliberation is essential to relieve any cord compression and to preserve all potential residual cord function. The easier the reduction is to accomplish, however, the more likely is a redislocation to occur.

If the neurologic deficit persists or deepens following the reduction, a myelogram should be performed with greatest caution to determine the presence and, if so, the level of a block. Reduction of the pure dislocation has been known to scrape the disk into the canal and lead to further cord compression. The skilled radiologist, neurosurgeon, or orthopaedic surgeon can introduce dye into the patient's spinal canal from a lateral point at the occipitocervical junction. In this circumstance, this approach is preferred to the more common introduction at the lumbar level.

Increased pressure at the site of lumbar puncture following jugular compression is not a reliable means of diagnosing complete or incomplete block. A narrow passage no larger than the inner diameter of the spinal needle will allow passage of spinal fluid. Thus, even in the face of a functionally complete block, increased spinal fluid pressure will be noted when the jugular vein is compressed. The myelogram and computerized transaxial tomography are the only accurate means of determining this information.

In the patient with the dislocation or fracture-dislocation without neurologic deficit, posterior fusion and wiring should be accomplished as soon as reasonable following reduction. This procedure utilizes the intact anterior group of ligaments while the wire is tightened around the spinous processes posteriorly to lock the facets together. Relative stability of the cervical spine is achieved as soon as the operation is complete. This patient may be treated in a Guilford cervical brace with thoracic pieces as soon as general recovery warrants it (Fig. 3–5). Immobilization is necessary following the operation until there is roentgenographic evidence of fusion, generally seen in three to four months postoperatively.

In the patient with neurologic deficit and evidence by myelogram of cord compression, the operative approach may need to be anterior in order to relieve the source of pressure against the cord. In this circumstance, this approach is necessary even though one would theoretically prefer to preserve the intact anterior ligaments for stability. I prefer a thrust graft of iliac crest keyed from the normal vertebral body above the level of the lesion down to the normal body below the lesion. As much of the involved body and disk is excised as is necessary to remove the compressing force from the cord. Should the disk alone be the compressing force against the cord, it can be removed, and fusion can be accomplished at this level only. In my experience, the thrust graft as described by Bailey offers greater stability than does the dowel graft. The thrust graft may cross several levels while retaining relative stability. Postoperatively the patient with a multilevel fusion is maintained on the longitudinal turning frame until early evidence of fusion is seen on the roentgenogram. This may well be at six weeks to two months. Following this, the Guilford cervical orthosis as described under atlantoaxial dislocations is my preference for the immobilizing orthosis. Immobilization is continued until there is good evidence of union of the graft to all of the involved bodies (approximately four months).

The experience of many clinicians in the management of patients with cervical spine injuries strongly recommends that the fusion be accomplished even in the flexion injury with little or no neurologic recovery. Fusion protects the nerve root at this level from further deterioration. In some instances, preservation of the one neurologic level may spell the difference between dependence and independence in the activities of daily living (Fig. 3–19).

Repeatedly one hears the suggestion that the flexion injury, once reduced, can be immobilized and its stability can be determined later. This is a potentially dangerous approach in flexion injuries. As pointed out by Badgley, Rogers, and McNab, the posterior ligamentous complex, once torn, is not prone to regain its strength.

Skeletal traction through the skull has generally been accomplished by tongs. The tongs in most common usage are the Crutchfield tongs; resembling an ice tong, they are easy to insert. They do erode the bone of the outer table, however, by pressure, and thus require daily or at least regular tightening. Because of the constant pressure erosion, there is a tendency for the Crutchfield tongs to pull out in long-term usage (two or more months). Vinke tongs are more difficult to insert, but do not have the tendency to pull out or to erode the outer table of the skull. The flange in the bolt of Vinke tongs engages the space between the two tables of the skull and permits application of any amount of weight without pulling out. The more recently developed Gardner-Wells tongs are also easy to use and very effective.

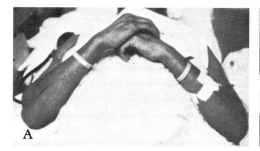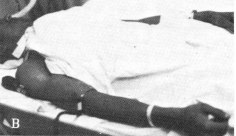

Fig. 3–19. A, Typical position of patient with neurologic deficit caused by injury between fifth and sixth cervical vertebrae. Biceps remains innervated but is unopposed by triceps which has lost its nerve supply. B, Cord injury between sixth and seventh cervical vertebrae leaves both biceps and triceps innervated. Shoulder and elbow remain balanced from muscular standpoint and arms rest at sides. (From Hartman, J. T.: Fractures, dislocations and fracture-dislocations of the spine and pelvis. *In* Practice of Surgery: Orthopedics 2. Hagerstown, Md, Harper & Row, 1971.)

The use of a halo device for traction has become more popular in recent times. This is easily inserted under local anesthetic and has the advantage of being attached to the halo cast outrigger, should that be determined as the treatment of choice, after reduction is accomplished. This is a strong point in favor of its use.

Laminectomy in the acute cord injury must only be utilized by the most experienced persons. There is the distinct potential for increasing the deficit by laminectomy. Inability to decompress the cord by reduction may be an indication for laminectomy, however. Schneider and Kahn have best pointed out the indications for this procedure.

Injuries Caused by an Extension Force

A sudden extension force to the cervical spine can initiate a tearing of the soft tissue anteriorly. This soft tissue injury may include the longus colli and longus cervicis muscles and the anterior spinal longitudinal ligament; it may even separate the anulus fibrosus from its attachment to the cartilaginous plate of the vertebral bodies above or below. The anulus separation may be from the inferior plate of the body above or from the superior plate of the body below. After the anterior anulus has given way in the extension injury, the next structure to separate will be the nucleus pulposus followed by the posterior anulus fibrosus. If the injuring force continues, the posterior spinal longitudinal ligament will then tear. Once this structure is torn, the separation has extended into the spinal canal. Here the obliquity of the facets from anterosuperior to posteroinferior and the fibers of the facet capsules create a mechanical obstruction to further soft tissue tearing. When the extension force continues unabated, it will then fracture along the pedicles at their base or run obliquely posterior and superior. Following this, the fracture line will run transversely across the lamina.

A continuation of the extension force following fracture tends to displace the vertebral column anteriorly above the separation of the anulus fibrosus (Fig. 3–20). In this injury, the fracture at the junction of the pedicle and the body allows spontaneous decompression. However, when a fracture is oblique and leaves laminar rims on either side of the fractured lamina, it is recognized that the displacement will trap the spinal cord between the posterosuperior margin of the vertebral body below and the segment of the lamina superiorly. The acute angulation of the spinal cord thus caused may well create irreversible cord damage. Whereas it was previously thought that anterior displacement could accompany only flexion injuries, Forsyth has documented the definite tendency for a continuation of the extension force to cause anterior displacement in the extension injury.

A continuation of the extension force, particularly with an added superior direction, can tear the ligamentum flavum and the interspinous ligaments. Application of traction greater than 7 to 10 pounds will likely cause a large separation between the bodies and potentially increase any present neurologic deficit. This particular instability is potential in any extension injury and should be borne in mind when the patient from this type of injury is moved about, as well as when he is initially placed in traction.

The "hangman's" fracture is a product of an extension mechanism in which a

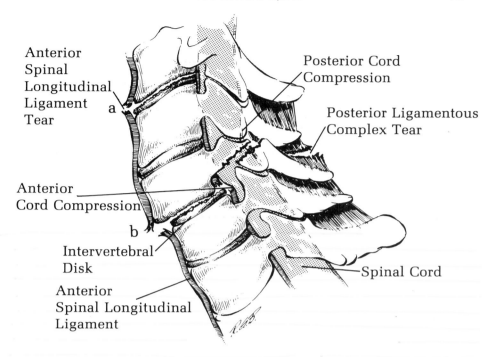

Anterior
Spinal
Longitudinal
Ligament
Tear

a

Posterior Cord
Compression

Posterior Ligamentous
Complex Tear

Anterior
Cord Compression

b

Intervertebral
Disk

Anterior
Spinal Longitudinal
Ligament

Spinal Cord

Fig. 3–20. Illustration indicating type of ligamentous and bony injury seen in extension injury: extension injury without displacement (a). Mechanism of anterior displacement and mode of cord compression which occurs from lamina of displaced body (b).

separation occurs between the second and third vertebral bodies from the anterior to the posterior side. The pedicle fractures at its base bilaterally or obliquely in the laminae while the body of the second cervical vertebra displaces sharply anteriorly. This extension force is caused by a submental knot of the hanging rope striking the inferior mandible in a superior direction. In contemporary America, the most common cause of this type of fracture is the forehead striking the windshield. The force of the anteriorly displacing posterior lamina of the atlas against the bulb of the spinal cord can crush the bulb and thus destroy the respiratory control center. This injury may also occur in people wearing seat belts. There may be evidence of an abdominal injury in this setting also, so the examiner must be on the alert for this. ■

Examination. If the patient with an extension injury has no neurologic deficit, the patient will complain only of a sore neck. On palpation there will be a striking muscular guarding against motion. Pain may be palpated anteriorly along the lateral masses, as well as along the anterior spinal longitudinal ligament at the involved level. (To palpate the anterior spinal ligament, the examiner must gently displace the trachea and esophagus complex slightly laterally and palpate deeply just anterior and medial to the sternocleidomastoid muscle). Should neurologic deficit exist, it can run the gamut from minimal sensory and motor loss to complete paraplegia. Whatever the deficit, it must be documented in every detail. ■

Roentgenograms. The anteroposterior roentgenogram following the extension injury may give no clues as to the existing injury. However, should a complete anterior dislocation occur, there will be overlapping of the margins of the vertebral body. A lateral view roentgenogram will show possible widening of the disk space, as well as the fracture between the vertebral body and the base of the pedicle. A fracture line may run obliquely posterosuperiorly into the laminae from the pedicles. Should this be present with a complete separation, a widening of the interspinous space will be noted superior to the fractured pedicle (one level superior to the disk space separation) (Fig. 3–21).

Displacement of the pharynx anteriorly prior to its transposition with the esophagus (approximately at the level of the fourth cervical vertebra) will be seen as a soft tissue shadow indicating hematoma present in the retropharyngeal space (Fig. 3–21B). This, of course, would imply anterior spinal longitudinal ligament tearing or other anterior soft tissue injury. The allowed space between the anterior vertebral margin and the air column of the pharynx or larynx should not exceed 4 millimeters in the normal spine. Distal to the larynx, the trachea lies anterior to the esophagus, so bleeding from an anterior spinal ligament tear below the fifth or sixth cervical vertebra is not as well

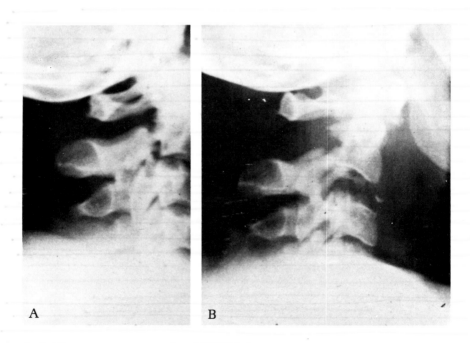

Fig. 3–21. Lateral roentgenograms of extension injury between C2 and C3. A, Note fracture across base of pedicle of second vertebra. B, Two hours after application of 15 pounds of skull traction on Stryker frame, note distraction between bodies of C2 and C3. Also to be noted is distraction between *posterior* elements of C1 and C2 and wide ''hematoma space'' between anterior second and third bodies and posterior pharynx and larynx. Traction was reduced to 7 pounds for two months and followed by Minerva cast and brace. (Hartman, J. T.: Fractures, dislocations and fracture-dislocations of the spine and pelvis. *In* Practice of Surgery: Orthopedics 2. Hagerstown, Md., Harper & Row, 1971.)

recognized on a lateral roentgenogram. Another occasional telltale sign of extension injury is the avulsion chip fracture from the margin of the anterosuperior vertebral body immediately below the level of disk separation.

Once the anteroposterior and lateral roentgenograms have been taken and show appropriate bony relationship, one can be justified in getting lateral dynamic views if one is concerned that a significant cervical spine injury exists. The lateral view in extension in the instance of the extension injury may show an undue amount of opening at the anterior disk space of the involved level.

Treatment. It must be reemphasized that neurologic assessment need be thorough and complete before any treatment of injuries from extension force is begun. Any dislocation should be reduced as promptly as possible consistent with protecting the spinal cord from further injury. Reduction would best be accomplished with skeletal traction onto the skull of a patient who is on a frame that turns on the longitudinal axis. Weights to the extent of 10 pounds should be used initially. Following a lateral roentgenogram one to two hours after initial traction is applied, additional weights and/or change in flexion or extension (pads under the anterior or posterior thorax aid in this control) may need to be applied as determined from this first roentgenogram. Once the dislocation is reduced, its chances of achieving stability through autounion between the two vertebral bodies are excellent. The torn intervertebral disk often ossifies during the year following injury to create this autofusion. Once reduced, the immobilization should be maintained on a frame with skull traction or with the halo cast device for two months. A cervical brace as described under dislocation is also necessary for an additional three months until there is evidence of union and stability. Should any question regarding stability exist following four months of immobilization, lateral dynamic roentgenograms may be taken with caution.

On occasion this type of fracture is treated surgically as the primary procedure, but the requirement for this type of treatment is rare, inasmuch as this fracture and separation will usually unite and achieve stability spontaneously if treated by traction and immobilization. The only occasion for primary operation in this injury is in the event that disk material or bony fragments have been extruded posteriorly into the canal to create cord compression. Should this have occurred, the anterior approach as outlined by Bailey and Badgley is the procedure of choice. However, I have not seen such an occurrence in the extension injury.

Although exceedingly rare, nonunion has been reported following immobilization of this type of injury. Should this occur, a fusion at the level of nonunion is necessary to achieve comfort and stability. Either the anterior or posterior approach is feasible by the time nonunion becomes evident. The posterior fusion must run from the laminae of the body above the fractured vertebra to the laminae of the body below the separation. This means a three-level fusion (across two intervertebral levels). However, with the anterior fusion one can achieve the necessary stability across the single involved disk space in an operation that does not carry as much morbidity as does the posterior fusion. Because of these considerations, the anterior fusion would be considered the preferred approach to this type of nonunion.

Injuries Caused by Rotary Dislocation Forces

Ligamentous structures normally allow approximately 45 degrees of rotation at the atlantoaxial joint. The remaining rotation, totaling approximately 45 degrees, is divided equally between the joints of the second through the seventh cervical vertebra.

As previously noted, the facets of the cervical spine slope from anterosuperior to posteroinferior; with movement of the joint, some flexion of the spine must also occur because of the aforementioned joint obliquity. The stability at this joint level is aided by the facet capsule, the ligamentum flavum, and the anulus fibrosus of the disk. When a rotational force is delivered to the cervical spine through the skull and upper cervical spine, soft tissues will prevent rotation beyond this limit. However, if the force is of such magnitude as to surpass the strength and endurance of the ligaments, a tearing of the fibers of the ligamentum flavum, the facet capsule, and the anulus fibrosus occurs; the facet on the side opposite the direction of the rotation can dislocate (Fig. 3–22A). Some flexion is obligatory as the inferior facet rides up and off of the superior facet from below (Fig. 3–22B, C).

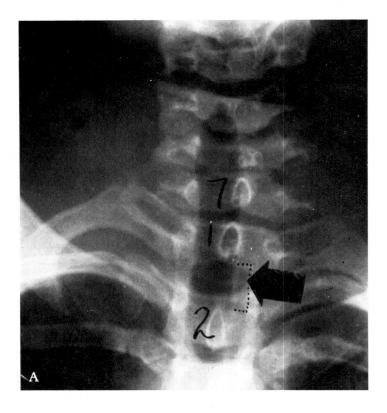

Fig. 3–22. A, Anteroposterior roentgenogram of unilateral dislocation of right facet of first dorsal vertebra on second. Note widened interspinous space between first and second vertebrae (arrow). Oblique laminograms confirmed dislocation. (Courtesy Frank Palumbo, M.D.)

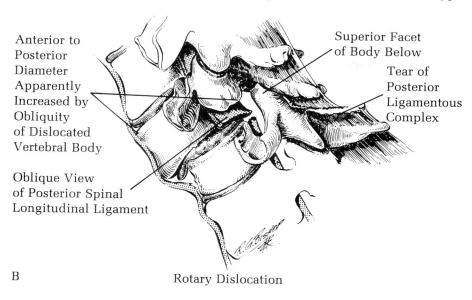

Anterior to
Posterior
Diameter
Apparently
Increased by
Obliquity
of Dislocated
Vertebral Body

Oblique View
of Posterior Spinal
Longitudinal Ligament

Superior Facet
of Body Below

Tear of
Posterior
Ligamentous
Complex

B

Rotary Dislocation

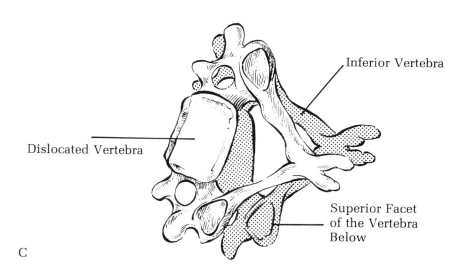

Inferior Vertebra

Dislocated Vertebra

Superior Facet
of the Vertebra
Below

C

Fig. 3–22 (Continued). B, Lateral view of rotary dislocation of cervical spine. Tears in ligamentum flavum and facet capsule are obligatory. Posterior spinal longitudinal ligament may tear as shown in this illustration. Inferior facet on one side has dislocated anterior to its opposing superior facet from below. On a lateral roentgenogram, the anteroposterior diameter of the dislocated body appears to be greater than that of the body immediately below because view of dislocated body is in actuality an oblique one. C, Superior view of rotary dislocation in which inferior facet has dislocated anterior to its opposing superior facet from below. Dislocated vertebra is the unshaded one.

The facet may fracture if the ligamentous structure does not tear when this type of force is excessive. There is often little or no neurologic deficit from this type of injury, but should there be evidence of neurologic symptoms or signs, they will most likely be of a nerve root type involving the level of dislocation only.

Examination. The primary complaint of the patient who has no neurologic deficit is one of a "crick" in the neck. On visualization, the examiner will note an obligatory rotation of the head and that portion of the neck above the injury. Muscle guarding prevents rotation to the neutral position; in fact all motion is guarded.

When neurologic deficit or symptoms exist, they are most likely caused by entrapment of the nerve root from encroachment of the inferior facet into the root canal. Occasionally a Brown-Séquard syndrome is seen due to cord injury at the dislocated level. This causes a loss of sensation, including heat and cold, on the side opposite to and below the cord damage, along with exaggeration of reflexes on the same side as the injured cord.

Roentgenograms. No clear-cut evidence of injury may be seen on the anteroposterior view of the cervical spine when a rotary dislocation is present. However, narrowing of one side of a disk space should create suspicion of this injury. In addition, the spinous processes immediately above such rotary dislocation are displaced toward the side of the injury and separated (Fig. 3–22C).

The lateral view roentgenogram of the cervical spine which has sustained this injury requires careful study. The dislocated facet may be apparent, resting anterior to the superior facet from below. The facet of one side is often dislocated while that on the opposite side is not dislocated, a fact that can create confusion when reading these roentgenograms. Careful observation of the anterior to posterior depth of the vertebral bodies will often show an increase in this depth of the body immediately above a rotary dislocation. This apparent increase in depth is seen because the vertebrae above the dislocation are seen in a semioblique view while the bodies below the dislocation are seen in the true lateral view. The diameter of the vertebral body is greater from side to side than from anterior to posterior; thus one may also see the appearance of an uninterrupted line along the posterior margin of the bodies. At the same time an overhang of the anterior margin of the body just superior to the dislocation is seen.

Treatment. The rotary dislocation of the cervical spine should be reduced by skeletal traction while the patient is on a longitudinal axis turning frame. This should be accomplished whether or not a patient shows neurologic deficit on examination. The most effective reduction of nerve root and/or cord compression is by reduction of the dislocation. The initial weight on the skeletal traction should be about 15 pounds. The unilateral dislocated facet also needs to be flexed at the same time that longitudinal traction is initially applied. Once the response to traction has been determined by a lateral roentgenogram two hours after placing the patient in traction, further changes in weights and positioning can be made. Using roentgenograms for control, one may increase the weights on the skeletal traction system by 5-pound increments to as high as 40 pounds. Should reduction not be accomplished with this amount of weight, it is not likely to occur without operative means.

When neurologic change is present, it is mandatory that reduction be accomplished either by traction or operation, and the sooner the better from the standpoint of the patient's potential recovery. Inasmuch as the locked facets lie posterior, the most logical surgical approach to the involved facets is from the posterior side. This operation can be performed with the patient prone on the turning frame with traction in place. After the patient is intubated, he is turned into the prone position. The approach may be made with a midline excision and stripping of the paraspinous muscles and periosteum from the laminae lateral to the facets. A torn ligamentum flavum and facet capsule may be seen with adequate exposure. It will be noted that the superior facet from the body below the dislocation will present as the most posterior of the facets at the level of dislocation. Anterior to it will lie the inferior facet from the body above the dislocation. Traction, modest flexion, and rotation away from the side of the dislocation may be attempted by the anesthesiologist under the surgeon's direction as he sees the facets under direct vision. If that maneuver is not successful under direct vision, a flat dull periosteal elevator may be used by the surgeon to lift the inferior facet up and over the superior facet. Should these maneuvers not prove successful, it will be necessary to remove the superior tip of the superior (most posterior) dislocated facet by rongeur. Should the dislocation still not be reduced, then the inferior tip of the inferior (anterior) facet also needs to be carefully removed by rongeur. After both tips have been removed, it is almost always possible to reduce the dislocation.

If closed reduction has been effected with the manipulation and there is no persisting neurologic change, a simple immobilization in extension in a Minerva cast or a cervical orthosis (see the description under atlantoaxial dislocation) may be used for three months. Lateral dynamic roentgenograms should be taken at this time to show the extent of the stability. As has been pointed out by Badgley and others, the easily reduced dislocation will tend to easily redislocate; therefore, one must be wary of this entity. Extensive mobility seen on the dynamic roentgenograms at three months postreduction is an indication to treat this type of injury by fusion.

If operation has been necessary to accomplish reduction, then posterior wiring of the two adjacent spinous processes along with posterior fusion of the two laminae is indicated. Particularly is this so when segments of the facet tips have been removed to facilitate reduction. The wiring provides immediate stability, and the posterior fusion provides long-term stability. Following this type of reduction and fusion, immobilization on the frame need be continued no longer than the initial week to ten days. A cervical orthosis is then used to support the spine until roentgenographic evidence of union is seen across the area of fusion.

The rotary dislocation with locked facets tends to be unstable if left untreated. Even without alteration in the neurologic picture, this dislocation should be reduced openly and fused if it cannot be reduced closed.

LESSER FRACTURES OF THE CERVICAL SPINE

Fractures of the cervical vertebrae may occur in the spinous process or in the margin of a vertebral body. Usually these are not accompanied by injury to the soft tissue.

The "Clay Shoveler's" Fracture

A fracture of the tip of the spinous process of the sixth or seventh cervical vertebra (occasionally it occurs at the level of the first dorsal vertebra) is seen most commonly as an avulsion of the tip by an attached muscle. This was first described in clay shovelers who sustained a spontaneous fracture of the spinous process as they lifted a heavy shovel loaded with clay, hence the eponym. It is best seen on the lateral roentgenogram (Fig. 3–23). Symptomatic treatment suffices once the examiner has determined that no injury of significance has occurred to the posterior ligamentous complex. If symptoms persist, a small fragment may be excised. The examiner must be certain this injury does not herald a significant underlying ligament tear accompanied by spinal instability at the level befow the fracture. The history of the injury will tend to rule out a significant lesion. Should any question persist, lateral dynamic roentgenograms will confirm the significance of the injury.

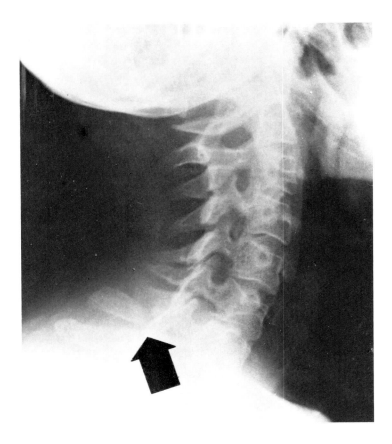

Fig. 3–23. Lateral roentgenogram showing classic "clay shoveler's" fracture of spinous process of seventh cervical vertebra. Symptomatic (arrow) treatment suffices once the examiner has determined that no injury of significance has occurred to posterior ligamentous complex.

Chip Avulsion Fracture of the Anterior-Inferior Margin of the Vertebral Body

Avulsion of the anterior-inferior tip of a vertebral body can occur as an isolated injury from an extension force. In this instance, the anterior spinal longitudinal ligament and the anterior anulus fibrosus provide the anatomic structures to avulse the tip. If examination and the lateral dynamic roentgenogram show stability to be present, the patient with this injury may be treated symptomatically.

CERVICAL SPINE INJURIES IN THE CHILD

The ligamentous structures and the bony spine of the child are considerably more resilient than those of the adult from the time of the predominantly cartilaginous spine up until full growth is achieved. Any of the aforementioned injuries to the cervical spine can occur, and it appears that no one injury type is more common to the child, with the possible exception of the atlantoaxial dislocation following the retropharyngeal abscess. This is distinctly more common in the child than in the adult.

The only variation in method of treatment in the child is in the skeletal traction system which is not easily accomplished, what with the skull not having achieved the outer and inner tables. Should skeletal traction be required prior to the time at which the skull tongs or the halo can be used, Kirschner wires may be run epidurally from anterior to posterior through two bur holes on each side of the midline. This will then allow adequate control of traction in the child prior to the age at which the tables are sufficiently developed to accommodate the adult traction device.

Facet Subluxation

A not uncommon occurrence in the cervical spine of the child is the subluxation of a pair of facets. Particularly might this subluxation be noted between the second and third cervical vertebral bodies with angulation evident posteriorly. Head halter traction is usually effective in relieving the pain and spasm that accompanies this. A simple cervical collar also may be worn and is often sufficient immobilization.

A complete unilateral dislocation does occur in the child, particularly following a known rotation force. This remains in the position of dislocation and can be seen particularly in the anteroposterior roentgenogram at the occiput C1 level and on the lateral roentgenogram at the levels below this. As mentioned before, head halter traction will help relieve the pain and relax the muscles sufficiently to allow for relocation of the dislocated facets. Once this is accomplished, one can use a Queen Anne's collar. If a more intensive immobilization is needed, the Minerva plaster of Paris jacket will be effective.

REFERENCES

1. Adams, J. C.: Outline of Fractures, Including Joint Injuries, 6th ed. Baltimore, Williams & Wilkins Co., 1972.
1a.Badgley, C. E.: Personal Communication. 1957.
2. Bailey, R. W.: The Cervical Spine. Philadelphia, Lea & Febiger, 1974.
3. Bailey, R. W.: Fractures and dislocations of the cervical spine. In Adams, J. P. (ed.): Current Practice in Orthopaedic Surgery. St. Louis: C. V. Mosby Co., 1969.

4. Bailey, R. W., and Badgley, C. E.: Stabilization of the cervical spine by anterior fusion. J. Bone Joint Surg. *42-A*:565, 1960.

5. Barnes, R.: Paraplegia in cervical spine injuries. J. Bone Joint Surg. *30-B*:234, 1948.

5a. Berkheiser, E. J.: Non-traumatic dislocations of atlanto-axial joint. JAMA 96:517, 1931.

6. Blount, W. P.: Fractures in Children. Baltimore, Williams & Wilkins Co., 1954.

7. Buonocore, E., Hartman, J. T., and Nelson, C. L.: Cineradiograms of cervical spine in diagnosis of soft tissue injuries. JAMA *198*:143, 1966.

8. Cone, W., and Turner, W. G.: The treatment of fracture dislocations of the cervical vertebrae by skeletal traction and fusion. J. Bone Joint Surg. *19*:584, 1937.

9. Fielding, J. W.: Normal and selected abnormal motion of the cervical spine from the second cervical vertebra to the seventh cervical vertebra based on cineroentgenography. J. Bone Joint Surg. *46-A*:1779, 1964.

10. Forsyth, H. F.: Extension injuries of cervical spine. J. Bone Joint Surg. *46-A*:1972, 1964.

11. Garber, J. N.: Abnormalities of the atlas and axis vertebrae. J. Bone Joint Surg. *46-A*:1782, 1964.

12. Hartman, J. T.: Fractures, dislocations and fracture-dislocations of the spine and pelvis. *In* Practice of Surgery: Orthopedics 2. Hagerstown, Md., Harper & Row, 1971.

13. Hartman, J. T., Palumbo, F., and Hill, B. Jay: Cineradiography of the braced normal cervical spine. Clin. Orthop. *109*:97, 1975.

14. Hohl, M.: Normal motions in the upper portion of the cervical spine. J. Bone Joint Surg. *46-A*:1777, 1964.

15. Holdsworth, F. W.: Fractures, dislocations and fracture-dislocations of the spine. J. Bone Joint Surg. *45-B*:6, 1963.

16. MacNab, I.: Acceleration injuries of the cervical spine. J. Bone Joint Surg. *46-A*:1797, 1964.

17. Rockwood, C. A., and Green, D. P.: Fractures. Philadelphia, J. B. Lippincott Co., 1975.

18. Rogers, W. A.: Fractures and dislocations of the cervical spine: An end result study. J. Bone Joint Surg. *39-A*:341, 1957.

19. Rothman, R. H., and Simeone, F. A.: The Spine. Philadelphia: Saunders, 1975.

20. Schneider, R. C.: Chronic neurologic sequelae of acute trauma to the spine and spinal cord: V. The syndrome of acute central cervical spinal-cord injury followed by chronic anterior cervical-cord injury (or compression) syndrome. J. Bone Joint Surg. *42-A*:253, 1960.

20a. Schneider, R. C., Cherry, G. L., and Pantek, H.: Syndrome of acute central cervical spinal cord injury with special reference to mechanisms involved in hyperextension injuries of cervical spine. J. Neurosurg. *11*:546, 1954.

21. Schneider, R. C., and Kahn, E. A.: Chronic neurological sequelae of acute trauma to the spine and spinal cord: I. The significance of the acute-flexion or teardrop fracture-dislocation of the cervical spine. J. Bone Joint Surg. *38A*:985, 1956.

22. Watson-Jones, R.: Fractures and Joint Injuries, 4th ed., 2V. Baltimore, Williams & Wilkins Co., 1952-1955.

4

THE DORSAL AND LUMBAR SPINE

The anatomic features of the cervical spine permit great mobility at the expense of bony stability, but the dorsal and lumbar vertebrae are shaped to enhance stability. Although some mobility is provided, it is distinctly more restricted by the bony structure than by soft tissue or ligamentous complexes such as those that characterize cervical spine stability.

ANATOMY

Not only are the vertebrae of the thoracic spine intermediate in size, between the cervical and lumbar vertebrae, but there is also a gradual increase in size from superior to inferior. Facets in the lateral body just anterior to the pedicle on each side articulate with the heads of the ribs. Facets on the transverse processes of all but the lowest two of the dorsal vertebrae articulate with the tubercles of the ribs. In the transverse, as well as in the anteroposterior direction, the bodies of the thoracic vertebrae are equally broad. The pedicles on each side arise from the superior part of the posterior vertebral body. The superior articular processes arise at the junction of the pedicle and the body, and the cartilaginous surfaces in the superior facets face posteriorly. The inferior articular processes arise from the pedicle and their cartilaginous surfaces face anteriorly to meet the superior articular process from the vertebra below (Fig. 4–1).

Extra stability is added to the dorsal spine by the ligamentous structures. These are from posterior to anterior (1) the ligamentum flavum, (2) the anterior costotransverse ligaments. (3) the facet capsules, (4) the posterior spinal longitudinal ligament, (5) the anulus fibrosus, and (6) the anterior spinal longitudinal ligament. Because of its anatomic structure, the ligamentous reinforcement, and the attached rib cage, stability in the normal dorsal spine is remarkably good.

The lumbar vertebral body is wider from side to side, than it is from anterior to posterior. The pedicles in the lumbar spine are relatively large bony structures arising from the superior lateral part of the posterior body margins. The pedicles attach posteriorly to the laminae, which are also broad and strong. The right and left laminae join to form the spinous process, a rather large bony prominence which projects posteriorly and inferiorly. In a superior-inferior orientation, the laminae and spine of a vertebra lie at the level of the disk space below and at the superior margin of that body immediately inferior (Fig. 4–2).

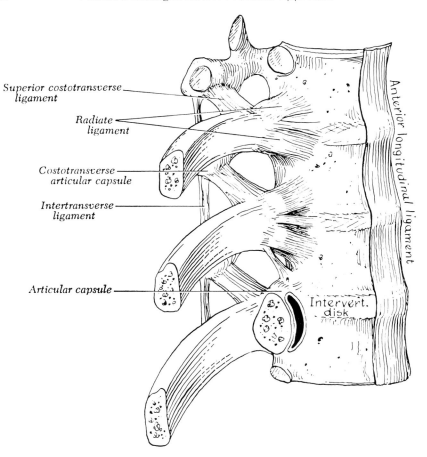

Superior costotransverse ligament

Radiate ligament

Costotransverse articular capsule

Intertransverse ligament

Articular capsule

Anterior longitudinal ligament

Intervert. disk

Fig. 4–1. Illustration of midthoracic vertebrae and their relationships with the ribs. At superiormost vertebra, note pedicle, facet direction and intervertebral foramina. (From Goss, C.M.: Gray's Anatomy, 29th Edition. Philadelphia. Lea & Febiger, 1973.)

The articular facets arise at the junction of the pedicles with the laminae. A superior articular process extends cephalad from this junction to meet the inferior process from above. The inferior process extends caudad from the inferior side of the pedicle-laminar junction to articulate with the superior process from below. The articular surface of the superior facet faces medially and has a gentle concavity. The articular surface from the inferior facet will face laterally and has a matching convexity. The arrangement of these structures and their anatomy allow freedom for flexion, extension, rotation, and lateral bending.

The transverse processes arise from the lateral surface of the body at the base of each pedicle and serve as the anterior origins for the psoas major muscles. The tendons of the quadratus lumborum also insert into the lumbar transverse processes.

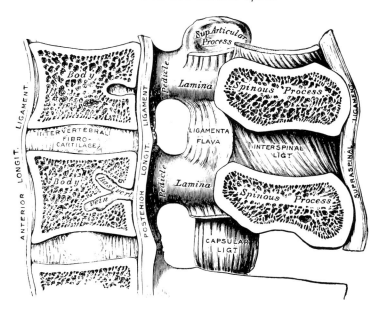

Fig. 4–2. Median parasagittal section of two lumbar vetebrae and their ligamentous attachments. Note superior articular facet facing toward midline and that only inferiormost part of intervertebral foramen lies near anulus fibrosus and that emerging nerve root would have more intimate relationship to the disk above. (From Goss, C. M.: Gray's Anatomy, 29th Edition, Philadelphia, Lea & Febiger, 1973.)

The spinal canal is triangular-shaped in this area, being surrounded by the posterior body in front, both pedicles at the sides, and both laminae posteriorly. The nerve roots emerge from this canal through the intervertebral foramina; this foramen is bounded by the anterior margin of the inferior articular facet and a notch into the inferior margin of the pedicle. Just anterior and inferior to the foramen is the intervertebral disk.

Holdsworth has attributed to the posterior ligament complex of the lumbar spine the function providing the needed stability against excessive motion of the spine. This ligamentous complex includes the interspinous ligaments, the supraspinous ligaments, the ligamenta flava, and the facet capsules. He believes that so long as the posterior complex remains intact, the spine will retain its stability. I believe that the posterior spinal longitudinal ligament, the anulus fibrosus, and the anterior spinal longitudinal ligament also share in maintaining this stability, although perhaps not to the same extent as do the strictly posterior complex.

MECHANISMS OF INJURY

A force which results in injury to the dorsal or lumbar spine can cause longitudinal compression, flexion, rotation, extension, or a combination of any of these. The most common injury to the dorsal or lumbar spine, however, results from the vertical force acting along the long axis of the spinal column. This force may act from superior to inferior or vice versa.

Wedge Compression Fracture

Inasmuch as the resting position of the dorsal spine is a modest gentle kyphosis, the vertical force acting across the kyphosis tends to cause the flexion compression effect on the vertebral body. To this mechanism of injury may be attributed the most common of the dorsal spine injuries—the wedge compression fracture of the vertebral body. In this injury, one or more vertebral bodies collapse anteriorly, become wedge-shaped, and create a prominence of the spinous processes posteriorly; this prominence is the commonly seen dorsal kyphosis. If the force has entirely dissipated in the compressing of the vertebral body(ies) anteriorly, the posterior ligamentous complex will not be compromised; hence the fracture is a stable one.

The lumbar spine, on the other hand, is in some lordosis in the resting position; in the longitudinal force which effects a lumbar wedge compression, there must also exist an element of flexion. This flexion may be produced by the longitudinal force passing from superior to inferior along the kyphos of the dorsal spine into the lumbar spine.

Examination. When the vertical force is violent, there are localizing signs or symptoms related to the spine. However, they may be so few as to allow this injury to be missed, particularly when other more evident injuries are present. Palpation will elicit localized tenderness at the level of injury; percussion of the spinous processes recreates the same distress. Prominence of the spinous processes of the involved vertebra should be looked for when this injury is suspected. There is an unusual amount of paraspinous muscle guarding in this fracture; coincident with this is a distinct limitation of motion at the involved level(s). Pain in this patient may be referred to the intercostal space or the abdomen. Neurologic deficit is rare in this type of injury. The patient with a compression fracture, particularly in the lower dorsal spine, may develop a profound ileus.

Roentgenograms. In the anteroposterior view the height of the vertebral body often appears unchanged, but with careful observation one may note the distance between the spinous process of the involved vertebra and that of the vertebra above to be increased. On the lateral view (Fig. 4–3, 4–4) the involved vertebral body is compressed anteriorly to a wedge shape, the wedge pointing anteriorly. The superior body margin compresses into the body substance below it, often leaving the margin of the inferior vertebral body intact. The facets maintain their normal relationship. In the absence of facet dislocation, the margin of the posterior body should remain in line with the margins of the bodies above and below.

Treatment. The initial treatment with the compression fracture is bed rest with the aim of early mobilization. As soon as the patient is relatively asymptomatic, he is started on a progressive muscle-strengthening program for the entire spine. Many patients are more comfortable when a reinforced lumbar garment (corset) or orthosis is used in the initial six-to-eight-week period. However, the use of the orthosis is seldom essential.

Prior to the second World War, it was common to treat the compression fracture by a forced hyperextension maneuver followed by a hyperextension body cast. It has since been shown, however, that the vertebral body rarely retains reduction but gradually returns to the immediate postinjury compres-

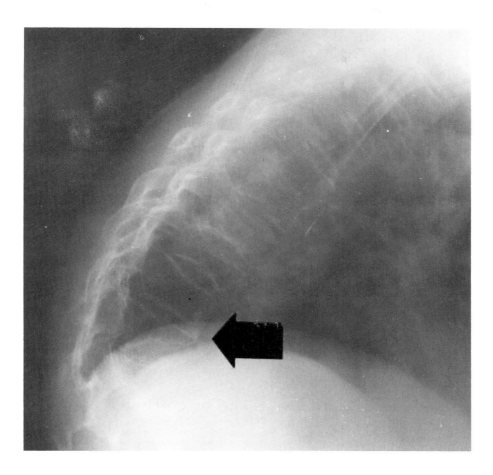

Fig. 4–3. Lateral roentgenogram revealing profound osteoporosis and compression fractures in dorsal spine. Arrow points to vertebral body which shows greatest wedge compression. However, careful observation of the spine above and below this reveals multiple compression fractures. In such osteoporotic bone, these often occur with minimal trauma and do tend to stretch the posterior ligamentous complex without disrupting it.

sion configuration. Occasionally the patient with this injury may have such severe symptoms that a body cast must be applied with the spine in traction to provide relief of pain. The cast in this instance may be discarded at six weeks, and a reinforced garment may be substituted for an additional month to six weeks. During any period of immobilization by plaster or brace, an exercise program to strengthen the muscles is necessary to provide sufficient muscle competence to allow later discontinuation of the external support.

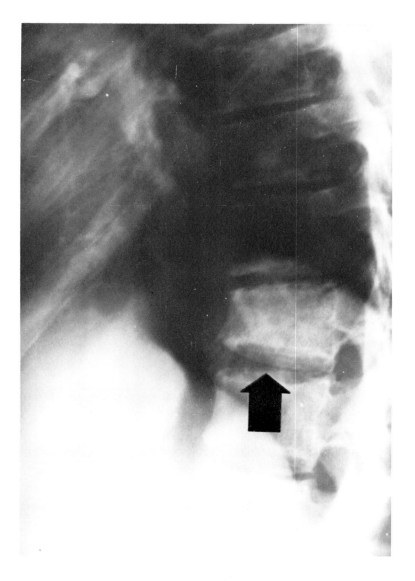

Fig. 4-4. Lateral roentgenogram. Arrow points to compression fracture of body of twelfth dorsal vertebra. This vertebral body appears to be increased in density and could be a pathologic fracture in bone of less structural strength.

Explosion Fracture

When the spine is sufficiently extended at the time a vertical force is applied, the resulting injury can be the typical bursting or explosion type of fracture. There is little stress on the ligamentous structures, since this is a compression type of injury. The ligaments seldom tear, and the spine is basically stable, once the injury has healed.

Examination. On examination a localized tenderness at the spinous process of the involved vertebra is noted on palpation or percussion. Since there has been no wedge compression in this type of fracture, a dorsal prominence of the spinous process is not noted. With the bursting nature of this injury, some body fragments can be displaced posteriorly against the cord, creating a neurologic deficit. However, neurologic deficit is uncommon in the explosion fracture.

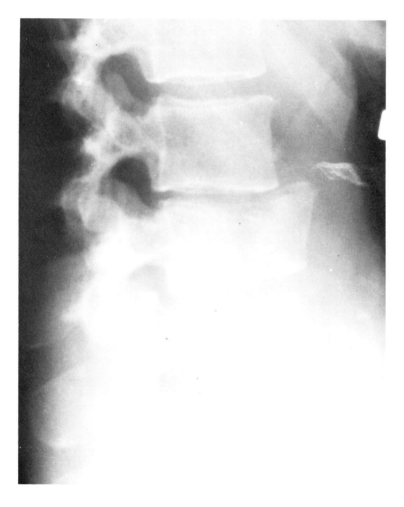

Fig. 4–5. Explosion or "burst" fractures of two lumbar vertebral bodies. Lateral view shows typical shattering. Spinous processes are not separated. (From Holdsworth, F. W.: Fractures, dislocations and fracture-dislocations of the spine. J. Bone Joint Surg. *45-B*:6, 1963.)

Roentgenograms. In the anteroposterior view there is a definite decrease in the height of the vertebral body while at the same time there is an increase in the width of this body. In the lateral roentgenogram, one may see a decreased height with an increased anteroposterior diameter. The posterior margin of the body may intrude into the spinal canal, particularly if neurologic deficit is present. The major body displacement, however, is usually anterior and lateral (Fig. 4–5).

Treatment. In the absence of neurologic deficit, bed rest is recommended until symptoms subside. The patient is then progressively mobilized while wearing a reinforced garment or orthosis that is sufficiently extensive to give adequate support across the injured vertebral body(ies). At the same time, progressive strengthening exercises are begun. In this injury, the spine usually needs orthotic support for approximately three months. Usually stability and comfort occur with union of the fracture(s).

Occasionally the more rigid immobilization of a plaster of Paris body jacket is necessary for relief of pain. If this is used, it may usually be discarded at three

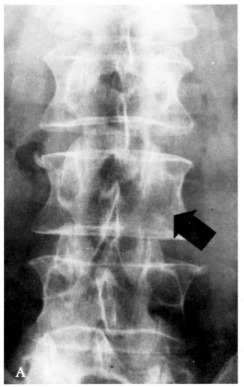
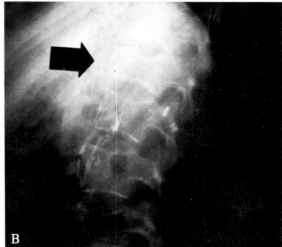

Fig. 4–6. Roentgenograms of pathologic fractures. A, Note absence of left pedicle outline (arrow at lumbar vertebra). This was due to metastatic thyroid carcinoma and is specific to neoplastic invasion. B, On lateral roentgenogram arrow points to pathologic compression fracture of body of first lumbar vertebra in young man with Ewing's sarcoma involving several vertebrae. Although not well demonstrated here, loss of both pedicle outlines at first lumbar vertebra could be seen on anteroposterior roentgenogram.

months, and an adequate garment or orthosis may be substituted for an additional two to three months. During any immobilization period, the progressive resistance exercise program is vital in order to provide sufficient muscle competence for later discontinuation of the external support.

Pathologic Fractures

Pathologic fractures often appear as explosion fractures or wedge compression fractures. A profound osteoporosis may lead to sufficient loss of osseous substance to allow the compression fracture to occur with little or no recognizable trauma and the posterior ligamentous complex may be stretched without being disrupted. The vertebral bodies not involved in the injury will appear to have an almost "chalked-in" outline of the body. The loss of osseous structure occurs throughout the entire vertebra.

Roentgenograms. The pathologic fracture occurring when neoplasm invades the vertebral body may be wedge-shaped, but in this circumstance the inferior vertebral body margin often wedges superiorly into the upper body (as opposed to the superior margin of a normal vertebra wedging into its body below). Loss of pedicle outline of the vertebra is often apparent on the anteroposterior roentgenogram when the vertebra is invaded by neoplasm (Fig. 4–6).

Treatment. In treating the patient with the vertebral fracture complicating neoplastic invasion, the spine should be supported to prevent neurologic deficit and to provide the greatest comfort to the patient. Should the type of neoplasm be unknown, a biopsy of the vertebral body can be done with a Craig needle (the upper limit for a safe biopsy by this technique is D–6). Specific indicated treatment can then be pursued. Many pathologic fractures have healed following radiation therapy; and many patients with myeloma or a blood dyscrasia have been maintained in lengthy periods of remission with chemotherapy.

FRACTURE-DISLOCATIONS

The Flexion Injury

When a flexion force is the injuring agent, it may expend itself in the creation of a dislocation or of a fracture-dislocation in the lumbar and dorsal spine. Particularly is this true at the dorsolumbar junction and in the lumbar spine. Dislocations and fracture-dislocations of the dorsal and lumbar spine are almost all unstable (Fig. 4–7). With this instability goes the concomitant potential of inducing primary nerve deficit where none existed or increasing the deficit in a previously incomplete lesion should an inadequate treatment plan be followed. The neurologic deficit in lumbar dislocations or fracture-dislocations is often pure nerve root (i.e., peripheral nerve) damage. Thus it is that patients with this type of lesion may show a considerable return of function even following profound neurologic deficit. The inferiormost segment of the spinal cord is the conus medullaris lying at approximately the junction of the first and second lumbar vertebra. Injuries at the dorsolumbar junction may involve the adjacent conus.

The pure soft tissue injury allowing dislocation of the dorsal and lumbar spine rarely occurs. The more common occurrence is a tearing of the posterior

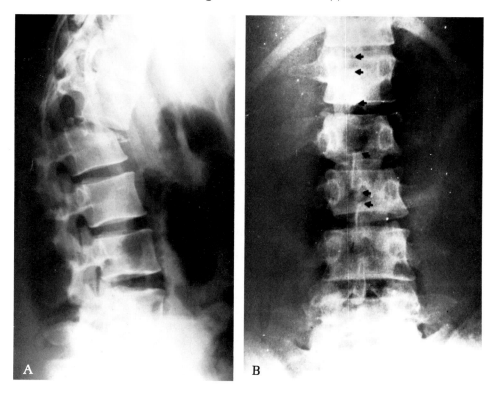

Fig. 4–7. A, Lateral roentgenogram of dorsolumbar spine showing complete dislocation of both posterior articular processes as well as dislocation of twelfth thoracic on first lumbar vertebra (see step-off at posterior body margins). In addition, note crush fracture of body immediately inferior to level of dislocation. B, Anteroposterior roentgenogram with widened central pair of arrows indicating widened interspinous space at level of injury. (From Kaufer, H., and Hayes, J. T.: J. Bone Joint Surg., *48-A*:712, 1966.)

ligamentous complex, allowing the facets to dislocate. Combined with this is a modest anterior compression of the superior vertebral margin at the level immediately below the dislocated facets (Fig. 4–8).

In injuries associated with lap seat belts worn without a shoulder strap a tension or traction force is applied to that portion of the vertebra posterior to the axis of flexion at the same time a compressive force occurs to that portion of the vertebra anterior to the axis of flexion. Facet dislocation may be seen with separation of the spinous processes at the involved level or may be seen with the Chance fracture that transversely splits the spinous process, laminae, and pedicles. In the typical lumbar spine injury associated with the use of the seat belt, one seldom sees any neurologic deficit because little if any vertebral displacement occurs. Should significant displacement of the injured vertebra occur, however, such as in the rotation or flexion injury, the likelihood of a lesion of the spinal cord or cauda equina root occurring is greatly increased.

Examination. In examining the patient with a fracture or fracture-dislocation in the dorsal or lumbar spine, one may sometimes see gross neurologic deficits,

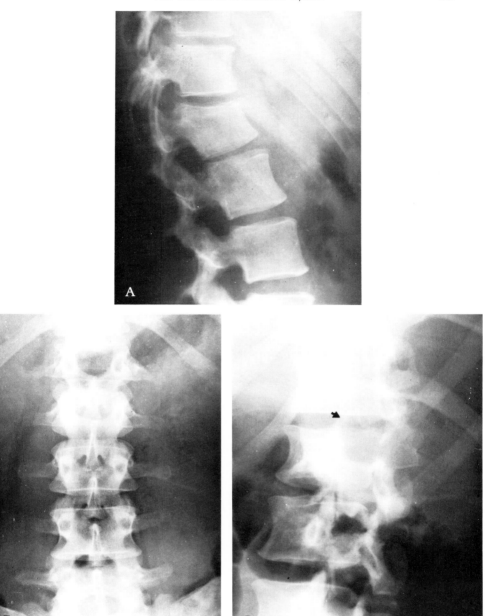

Fig. 4–8. A, Lateral roentgenogram demonstrating dislocation of both posterior articular processes without dislocation of body of twelfth dorsal on first lumbar vertebrae. Spinous processes open at level of injury, indicating tearing of posterior ligamentous complex. Modest compression of anterior-superior body of first lumbar vertebra has occurred. B, Anteroposterior roentgenogram demonstrating excellent alignment but note spread of laminae and spinous processes between twelfth thoracic and first lumbar vertebrae. C, Right oblique view showing dislocation of articular processes (see arrow) to best advantage. (From Kaufer, H., and Hayes, J. T.: J. Bone Joint Surg., *48-A:* 712, 1966.)

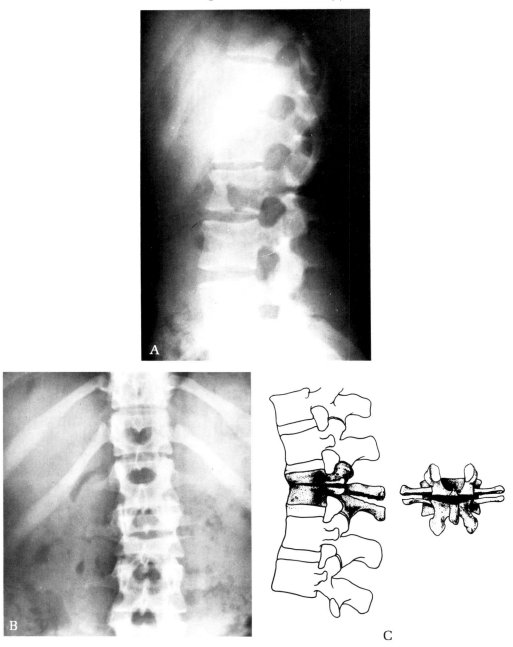

Fig. 4–9.   Chance fracture. A, Lateral roentgenogram shows no separation of spinous processes and no enlargement of the intervertebral foramina but horizontal fracture can be seen extending anteroposteriorly through centrum, pedicles, laminae, and spinous process of second lumbar vertebra. There is no ligamentous separation, and intervertebral disks are intact. B, Anteroposterior roentgenogram shows fracture line passing through transverse processes, pedicles, laminae, and spinous process of second lumbar vertebra. C, Drawing of lateral and anteroposterior roentgenograms showing its characteristic features. (From Smith, W. S. and Kaufer, H.: Lumbar injuries associated with lap seat belts. J. Bone Joint Surg., *51-A*:239, 1969.)

but at other times the deficit may be so slight as to escape recognition by all but the most careful of neurologic examinations. It has been estimated that some neurologic deficit will be present in about 60% of the patients with *dislocation* injuries at these levels.

When the vertebral body is compressed anteriorly, one usually notes an obvious gibbus posteriorly. A history of pain or finding of pain on palpation at the involved level is a feature most commonly present in these patients. One may be able to palpate a gap between the segments of the spinous processes at the level of the dislocation. With the seat belt injury, one may see evidence of ecchymosis anteriorly across the abdomen.

Roentgenograms. Without careful study of the spinous processes and their intervals, the anteroposterior roentgenogram may be deceptively innocent in appearance. When the fracture has occurred through the spinous process, laminae, and pedicles, one will see evidence on the roentgenograms of a spread between the bone fragments at the level of the fracture. This is the Chance fracture (Fig. 4–9).

When the posterior ligamentous complex tears and a dislocation results, the spinous processes at this level are found to be separated more widely than are the spinous processes above or below (Fig. 4–10B). On the lateral roentgenographic view, a widened gap between the spinous processes should be evident in association with dislocation of the posterior articular facets in the flexion injury (Fig. 4–10A). The posterior margin of the vertebral bodies superior to the dislocation will lie anterior to the posterior margin of the body immediately inferior. Often, a crush fracture is noted in the superior surface of the body immediately inferior to the dislocation. An oblique roentgenogram may be necessary to visualize the dislocated facet(s) (Fig. 4–10C). When fracture of the pedicle or pars interarticularis is present, it can be best visualized on the oblique view.

Lateral roentgenograms of the spine in the injury associated with the use of the seat belt may show separation of the spinous processes and subluxation or dislocation of the facet joint; fractures across the spinous process, laminae, pedicles, and body may exist. However, anterior compression of the body immediately inferior to the injured level is seldom seen because this is a traction type of injury. The tomogram can be especially helpful in fully assessing the bony injury to the spine.

Treatment. See section on Flexion and Rotation Force.

Flexion and Rotation Force

When the dorsal or lumbar spine is subjected to sufficient rotational force, the posterior ligamentous complex may give way, separating the spinous processes and expending the energy of the force by shearing across the vertebral body. This type of force creates the slice rotation fracture dislocation described by Holdsworth. In this injury the articular processes are often fractured by the rotation force of one facet against its opposing facet. The anulus fibrosus remains intact at the injured level while the shear force fractures a "slice" of the proximal part of the vertebral body below. This type of fracture dislocation occurs most commonly from the midthoracic level down to the thoracolumbar junction; neurologic deficit is often seen with this injury.

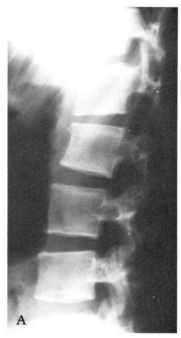

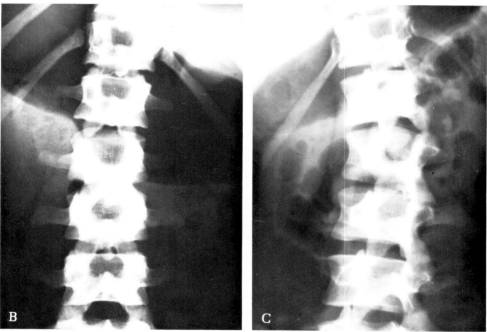

Fig. 4–10. A, Lateral roentgenogram shows widening of intervertebral foramina and wedging of disk space between first and second vertebrae. Minimum compression of anterior body of second lumbar vetebra is also noted. B, Anteroposterior roentgenogram shows widening of interspinous processes and dislocation of articular processes between first and second lumbar body. Posterior ligamentous complex is separated in this injury. C, Oblique roentgenogram showing complete dislocation of articular processes between first and second lumbar vertebrae. Note normal relationship of articular processes at interspaces above and below. (From Smith, W. S., and Kaufer, H.: Lumbar injuries associated with lap seat belts. J. Bone Joint Surg., *51-A*:239, 1969.)

Inasmuch as the integrity of the posterior ligamentous complex has been violated by this injury, this fracture dislocation is unstable and will not achieve stability short of internal fixation with fusion.

Examination. Signs much like those in the flexion fracture-dislocation with the addition of possibly a gibbus or a prominence of the spinous process below the dislocation level may be noted during the examination. A painful "gap" also exists between the spinous processes at the level of the dislocation. The spinous process superior to the dislocation level is often lateral to the midline, having rotated there as part of the effect from the rotation force.

Roentgenograms. The anteroposterior roentgenogram may show little if any evidence of abnormality. Fracture of the facets and fracture across the superior vertebral body can sometimes be seen in this view. Should displacement be present one notes a shift of the relationships of the vertebral body and also a shift of the spinous process immediately above the level of injury to an eccentric position. The interspinous space may appear to be increased.

In the lateral roentgenogram one will note fracture of the facet and a relative shortening of the spinous process above the level of injury (because of its obliquity). The rotation obliquity of the vertebral body immediately above the

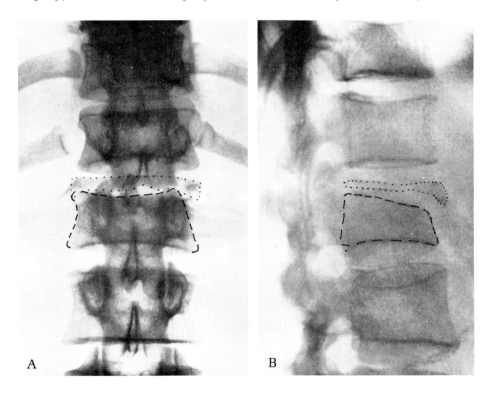

Fig. 4–11. "Slice" fracture in a rotational fracture-dislocation of the twelfth thoracic vertebra on the first lumbar vertebra. A, Anteroposterior roentgenogram. Note displacement of spinous processes above fracture level. B, Lateral roentgenogram. Note slight increase in anteroposterior width of bodies above fracture as compared to those below. (From Holdsworth, F. W.: Fractures, dislocations and fracture-dislocations of the spine. J. Bone Joint Surg., *45-B*:6, 1963.)

level of injury causes an apparent increase in the anteroposterior diameter of that vertebral body. The disk space at the level of injury appears intact; attached to it on the inferior side is a small segment from the vertebral body below, it having been separated from the body in its superior portion (Fig. 4–11).

The full extent of bony damage in the lumbar fracture-dislocation may become more evident on visualization of oblique roentgenograms. These views do show to better advantage the facets and the pars interarticulares between the facets. When taking oblique films, one must recognize the potential instability of a fracture-dislocation and guard against any rotary movement that could increase a neurologic deficit.

Treatment. Since all of the injuries composing the dislocations and fracture-dislocations of the dorsal and lumbar spine are inherently unstable situations, the first step in treatment after the general and neurologic assessment is to place the patient on a longitudinal turning frame such as the Stryker wedge frame or the Foster bed. Such a longitudinal turning frame prevents position change of the unstable injured vertebrae, whereas the Circ-O-Lectric bed does not eliminate the effect of gravity on the weight of the trunk when the patient is changed from the anterior to the posterior (or vice versa) frame. Once stability of the spine has been achieved, the Circ-O-Lectric bed is an excellent means of nursing a patient and is generally preferred by the patient to the narrower longitudinal turning frame. A thorough neurologic as well as general examination must be completed prior to initiation of any treatment program. A myelogram could be helpful in determining whether a block exists: if present, the likely causative structure may be determined from the configuration of the radiopaque column (Fig. 4–12).

Once information as to the extent of deficit is complete, or should no neurologic deficit be present, and examination plus roentgenograms confirm a dislocation or fracture-dislocation as described in the preceding paragraphs, then open reduction with internal fixation and fusion is indicated. The operation should be performed with the patient lying prone on the anterior longitudinal turning frame. After anesthetization and intubation have been established, the patient may be easily turned to the anterior frame without fear of creating greater neurologic deficit. Once open reduction is accomplished, it is followed by a posterior spinal fusion utilizing autogenous iliac bone. Fixation to provide instant stability until fusion is firm is best achieved by the use of the Harrington rods, the Williams spinal plates, or even heavy wire. If the surgical approach is made within two to three weeks of the injury, the surgeon will find a complete disruption of the posterior ligamentous complex. A hematoma is often encountered in the subcutaneous tissue; this hematoma will extend down to the dura through a gap in the ligaments. Careful evacuation of the hematoma usually effects visualization of the dura in the depth of the wound. Caution must be exercised in this particular exposure not to penetrate the neural canal.

A modest amount of the laminae may be removed at the involved level should this aid exposure. Most of the time, however, visualization is sufficient because of the existing ligamentous and bony injury. Laminectomy with removal of large amounts of bone from the posterior elements must be condemned in these types of injuries. A ridge of bone is often present anterior

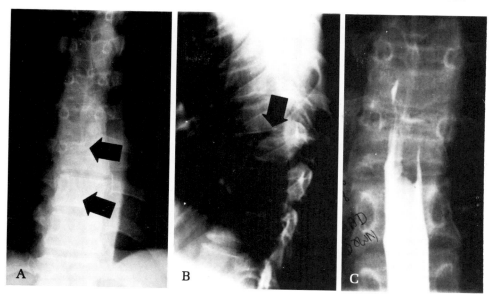

Fig. 4–12. Compression fracture of eighth dorsal vertebra that was sustained from a significant flexion force. A, Anteroposterior roentgenogram. Note divergence of spinous processes between eighth and ninth dorsal vertebrae (arrows). B, Partial posterior displacement is noted on the lateral view. C, Myelogram is posteroanterior view showing complete block of spinal canal at eighth dorsal vertebra.

to the dura. This is the posterior margin of the inferior body participating in this injury and will diminish in prominence or even disappear once reduction of the displacement is accomplished. The intervertebral disk can be extruded into the canal in these injuries and if present in the canal must be removed.

In order to assure that no block is present within the spinal canal, Kaufer and Hayes pass a No. 8 Robinson catheter epidurally both proximal and distal to the injury level. Each nerve root emerging at the level of injury should be visualized at its exit from the root canal; both intervertebral foramina should also be probed with a small double-ended dural probe for patency. Occasionally one finds a bony block from collapse of the foramen by a fracture across the pars interarticularis. Persistent peripheral nerve deficit would follow failure to decompress such a lesion.

If the dura is torn, it must be repaired prior to attempted fusion, inasmuch as a rent in the dura may lead to spurious meningocele and, at times, a pseudarthrosis in the fusion. Reduction of the displacement can usually be accomplished by extending the spine while it is under direct vision. The hinge mechanism of the frame upon which the patient is lying may be used to accomplish this, or previously positioned padding may be removed to allow extension.

Once reduction is accomplished, the laminae over the planned fusion area must be decorticated, facet joints must be excised, and, depending upon the necessity, the transverse processes are decorticated. Spinal stabilization by the use of Harrington rods, Williams plates, or wiring of spinous processes (with 18 or 20 gauge stainless steel wire) is next accomplished. Finally, autogenous iliac bone may be placed in the facet defects, and strips may be placed along the decorticated laminae and, when indicated, the transverse processes. An old axiom dictates fixation and fusion from two vertebrae above the level of dislocation to two vertebrae below that level. Most importantly, however, the surgeon must be sure that stability, both immediate and long-term, has been provided for at the site of injury.

Since spine stabilization has been accomplished at the operation, the patient may be treated postoperatively on the original frame or may be transferred to a Circ-O-Lectric bed. Should no neurologic deficit be present or should recovery ensue rapidly, the patient may be ambulated in a well-fitting high chair back orthosis or a snug body cast. External support should be continued for four to six months or even longer if necessary until one notes roentgenographic evidence of bony fusion.

At the conclusion of immobilization, it is important to instruct the patient in range of motion exercises to improve the mobility and strength in the involved area. This is an often overlooked but important part of the rehabilitation of any patient who has had a spinal injury or operation.

LESSER FRACTURES OF THE SPINE

As in the cervical spine, fractures may occur in the spinous processes of the dorsal and lumbar spine. A more common minor fracture in this area, however, is that of the transverse processes.

The Transverse Processes

The lumbar spine is the site of most fractures of the transverse processes of the vertebrae. The injury may be caused by an unusually strong contraction of the psoas muscles.

Examination. Flank pain and tenderness to palpation associated with paraspinous muscle guarding are the dominant features seen on examination of the patient with fracture(s) of the transverse processes.

Roentgenograms. The most important roentgenogram in injury of the transverse processes is the anteroposterior view (the transverse processes are seen protruding laterally at the midbody of each lumbar spine) (Fig. 4–13). A break in continuity of the cortices of the transverse process will be seen when a fracture exists. The lateral fragment is often displaced and most commonly inferiorly.

Treatment. The treatment for injury to the transverse processes is symptomatic. Initial bed rest may be necessary in the patient with severe symptoms. Mobilization should be begun as soon as symptoms begin to subside. If recovery is not sufficient, a reinforced dorsolumbar garment may be helpful in getting the patient ambulated. In any event, a program on range of motion exercises followed by the progressive strengthening program will be essential for quickest rehabilitation.

Spinous Processes

Occasional isolated fracture(s) of the spinous process(es) may occur. It is usually caused by an acute forceful flexion of the dorsal or lumbar spine.

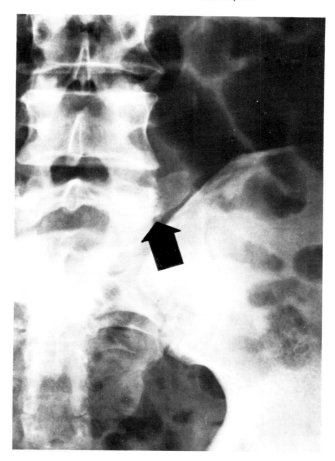

Fig. 4–13. Fracture at base of left transverse process of fifth lumbar vertebra (arrow). Symptomatic treatment usually suffices for this injury.

Examination reveals point tenderness to palpation at the involved level associated with guarded flexion.

Examination. On the lateral roentgenogram, one will see a fracture of the spinous process, with usually slight separation of the fragments.

Treatment. The patient with a fracture of the spinous processes may be treated symptomatically. Often this can be by studied neglect followed by a range of motion exercise program. Occasionally the symptoms are sufficiently severe and lasting to warrant use of a reinforced corset for about six weeks of immobilization. When this method of treatment is followed, the patient must be placed on an exercise program to regain mobility and strength prior to discarding the corset.

FRACTURES OF THE DORSAL AND LUMBAR SPINE IN THE CHILD

The same types of injuries to the dorsal and lumbar spine occur in the child as in the adult. It is important to emphasize again that the immature spine is more resilient and has a greater potential for mobility than the adult spine. In this regard one may find an achievement of stability with a purely ligamentous injury in the child that might not be possible in the adult. A trial period of immobilization followed by dynamic roentgenograms to stress the area of injury at approximately two months is definitely in order. Should instability

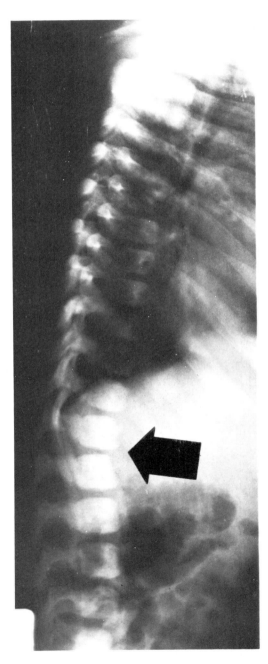

Fig. 4–14. Traumatic compression fractures of bodies of first and second lumbar vertebrae (arrow) in eight-year-old child are shown in this lateral roentgenogram. Treatment is similar to that for adult (see text).

still be present, one can then proceed to fusion. One tries to fuse as few vertebrae as possible in the child in order to alter the normal growth of the spine no more than necessary. A compression fracture of any body through the dorsal and lumbar spines is possible, particularly after the vertebral bodies have more fully ossified and become less resilient (Fig. 4–14). The ligamentous structures in the child over the age of eight years are sufficiently strong to rarely separate. In this setting, then, a compression force can cause a modest compression fracture without creating instability, inasmuch as the posterior ligamentous complex is intact. The compression fracture in the child does require immobilization in a cast in the hyperextended position in order to maintain the height of the vertebral body anteriorly. This type of injury usually requires immobilization for a period of eight to twelve weeks.

The pathologic entity of eosinophilic granuloma (vertebra plana) may be seen in the spine of the child. This neoplastic process (nonmalignant) may invade the vertebral body sufficiently to leave it structurally weak and subject to compression fracture in the absence of significant violence. The lateral roentgenogram will show a markedly flattened vertebral body (usually in the dorsal spine) (Fig. 4–15). Treatment is symptomatic.

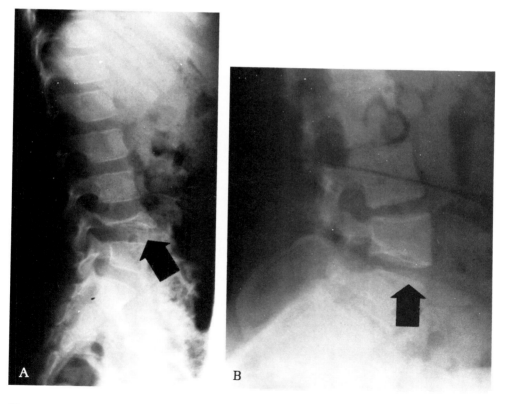

Fig. 4–15. A, Compressed fourth lumbar vertebra in eight-year-old child (arrow). This appearance is typical of vertebra plana—invasion of body by eosinophilic granuloma. Symptomatic treatment is sufficient. B, Lateral roentgenogram of same patient taken after he reached adulthood. Reconstitution of first lumbar body is well demonstrated.

Another entity to be considered in the painful spine seen in the wake of little or no known injury is that of Scheuermann's disease (juvenile apophysitis). In this process, the ring apophysis of the vertebral body becomes involved in an inflammatory process which causes loss of significant growth of the anterior vertebral body. This results in the juvenile round back and is not to be confused with the back problem in the face of known significant trauma.

REFERENCES

1. Blount, W. P.: Fractures in Children. Baltimore, Williams & Wilkins Co., 1955.
2. Hartman, J. T.: Fractures, dislocations and fracture-dislocations of the spine and pelvis. *In* Practice of Surgery: Orthopedics 2. Hagerstown, Md., Harper & Row, 1971.
3. Holdsworth, F. W.: Fractures, dislocations and fracture-dislocations of the spine. J. Bone Joint Surg. *45-B*:6, 1963.
4. Kaufer, H., and Hayes, J. T.: Lumbar fracture-dislocation. J. Bone Joint Surg. *48-A*:712, 1966.
5. Rockwood, C. A., and Green, D. P.: Fractures. Philadelphia, J. B. Lippincott Co., 1975.
6. Rothman, R. H.. and Simeone, F. A.: The Spine. Philadelphia, W. B. Saunders Co., 1975.
7. Smith, W. S., and Kaufer, H.: Patterns and mechanisms of lumbar injuries associated with lap seat belts. J. Bone Joint Surg. *51-A*:239, 1969.
8. Watson-Jones, R.: Fractures and Joint Injuries, 4th ed., 2V. Baltimore, Williams & Wilkins Co., 1952-1955.

5

THE RIBS AND STERNUM

The thorax, or chest, lies between the neck and the diaphragm and is enclosed by the ribs, which extend from the thoracic vertebrae. The first seven ribs are attached to the sternum, which forms the middle of the anterior wall of the thorax. Fractures of the other two bony landmarks of the thorax, the scapula and the clavicle, will be discussed in Chapter 6.

RIB FRACTURES

The twelve ribs on each side of the thorax are encased in their own soft tissue structures. Immediately surrounding each rib is the periosteum of that rib. On the underside of each rib lies a groove that runs the entire course of the rib from posterior to anterior and in which lie the intercostal artery and veins and the intercostal nerve. Between each two ribs lie the external and internal intercostal muscles which provide the major control of the mobility of the rib cage. These muscles are innervated from the intercostal nerve at each level. The ribs are attached at their posterior margin to the base of the transverse process of the appropriate vertebra. This attachment is an intimate one with ligamentous fibers maintaining a strong attachment. Anteriorly ribs one through ten attach to the sternum through the costochondral cartilage. The twelfth rib and occasionally the eleventh rib have no attachment to the sternum. The ribs have an unusual amount of plasticity allowing considerable distortion in shape before reaching the limit of tolerance of this elasticity and fracturing (Fig. 5–1A).

The mechanism of injury in rib fracture(s) in a nonpathologic situation is invariably one of direct blow. The direct blow will fracture one or more ribs but usually leave them within their soft tissue case. If the force of injury is not expended at this point, however, the fractured rib ends may be forced internally through the parietal pleura and possibly even into the lung tissue itself. Although occurring, it would be most unusual for the fractured ends to penetrate skin and communicate with air.

Simple and Multiple Fractures

Little if any significant bleeding occurs with the simple rib fracture(s) contained within the soft tissue structure of the thoracic cage. Occasionally a rib or several ribs are fractured at two different points. Because of the negative pressure within the pleural cavity, this circumstance creates the flail chest that has the paradoxical motion of moving inward when inspiration occurs.

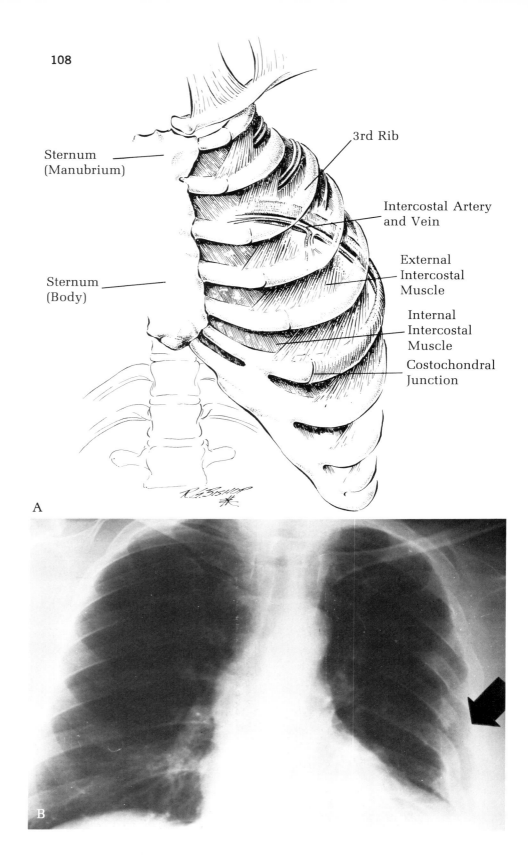

Sternum
(Manubrium)

3rd Rib

Intercostal Artery
and Vein

Sternum
(Body)

External
Intercostal
Muscle

Internal
Intercostal
Muscle

Costochondral
Junction

A

B

Examination. In the true fractured rib, pain should be created when the examiner compresses the sternum toward the spine with countercompression against the spine. The patient can usually point to the site of the fracture.

Roentgenograms. The definite interruption of the cortices of the fractured rib(s) may or may not show on the roentgenograms (Fig. 5–1B). Rotational views are often helpful in visualizing the fracture(s).

Treatment. Elastofoam, an elastic bandage coated on one side with polyurethane foam, is useful to maintain some type of immobilization when ribs are fractured. Strapping of the involved side of the thorax with tape may be helpful, but if this is done, the tape must extend past the midline anteriorly and posteriorly. Intercostal nerve blocks proximal to the fracture also may be beneficial and sometimes will completely break up the pain pattern caused by the fracture. The Elastofoam wrapping aids in diminishing pain which occurs with inspiration and expiration to the extent that the distress is tolerable within several days to a week. There is a distinct tendency to shallow breathing by the patient in an attempt to splint the fracture and prevent pain. However, this is conducive to atelectasis, and the treating surgeon must be alert to prevent this complication. The patient should be encouraged to breathe deeply at intervals during this time in order to maintain adequate aeration of the lungs.

The most effective means of managing the flail chest is to use endotracheal intubation with positive pressure breathing. An older but effective method of treatment was to place a towel clip through a bony portion of the flail segment and place a modest amount of traction on this towel clip. This allows the negative pressure of the chest to be maintained and more adequate aeration to occur. However, the positive pressure of the endotracheal system provides an even better gas exchange.

Tearing of the Pleura and Puncture of the Lung

In the event of a tearing of the pleura, a distinct likelihood exists for bleeding into the pleural cavity. Should the lung itself have been impaled upon the rib fragment, there may also be escape of air into the pleural cavity.

Roentgenograms. A fluid level will be seen on the chest plate if there has been bleeding into the pleural cavity. When air has escaped into the cavity, one may see a fluid and free air level on the roentgenogram.

Treatment. The patient with a hemothorax and fractured rib(s) may be treated by wrapping the thorax with elastic bandage. If the fluid level is too high, it may be aspirated following use of local anesthetic. However, this procedure should be performed only after there is considerable evidence of increased pressure within this portion of the thorax from hemorrhage. In the event of the pneumothorax it is quite possible that the patient may require the insertion of tubes through a suction seal in order to accomplish adequate reexpansion of the lungs.

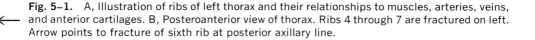

Fig. 5–1. A, Illustration of ribs of left thorax and their relationships to muscles, arteries, veins, and anterior cartilages. B, Posteroanterior view of thorax. Ribs 4 through 7 are fractured on left. Arrow points to fracture of sixth rib at posterior axillary line.

Costochondral Separation

Another injury to ribs is the costochondral separation. This is a separation of the bony end of the rib from the cartilage structure joining it to the sternum. The costochondral separation occurs from a direct blow just as does the rib fracture. It tends to occur in the "weekend athlete" who infrequently engages in contact sports. It is a painful process, with the pain being more severe with inspiration and expiration.

Roentgenograms. Since the cartilages are radiolucent, it is almost impossible to identify this injury on roentgenograms.

Treatment. The treatment most effective has been the use of Elastofoam. Several days of rather intense pain give way to tolerable discomfort, usually within a week, and by two weeks the patient is generally comfortable without external support.

FRACTURES OF THE STERNUM

The sternum consists of three segments. Superiormost is the manubrium to which is attached the clavicle at a notch on each side. The manubrium of the sternum attaches to the body of the sternum at the second rib level by a synostosis (synchondrosis). The lower extension of the body of the sternum has attached to it a small arrow-shaped segment of cartilage and/or bone which is called the xiphoid process. Any injury to the sternum occurs by direct blow. The sternum is primarily of cancellous bone with broad surfaces so that significant displacement seldom occurs. Just posterior to the superior sternum lies the arch of the aorta. Behind the lateral margin of the sternum at its junction with the rib cartilages lie the internal mammary vessels. These maintain a close relationship to the sternum so must be reckoned with in any significant displacement injury (Fig. 5–2).

Examination. The patient may or may not be able to give an adequate history. When he does, it is usually one of being struck on the anterior thorax by an object such as a steering wheel. To palpation one notes pain or tenderness at the area of fracture. There may or may not be palpable displacement or angulation. In any sternal injury a closed heart or aortic arch injury is possible. Auscultation of the heart may reveal harsh murmur(s) at the aortic and pulmonary valve areas with the loudest sound usually in systole. Murmurs over the arch away from the aortic and pulmonary valve areas are distinctly abnormal and must be explained. Careful review of roentgenograms and possibly angiography are in order when this is suspected. If tear of the aorta is shown to be present on angiography, surgical repair of the tear is immediately indicated. One patient died suddenly when an aortic arch tear completed itself at ten days postinjury and was only recognized at the postmortem table.

Roentgenograms. Adequate visualization of the aortic arch is essential in any injury to the sternum. On the plain chest plate (Fig. 5–3A) one may see some haziness of the arch either at its cardiac origin or as it starts its descent at the origins of the intercostal arteries (Fig. 5–3B). Angiography can reveal the ragged edges of the tear either at the origin of the aorta or in its course and is mandatory if clinical suspicion and signs of a tear are present.

A fracture of the sternum may or may not show on roentgenograms. The true lateral view in which one may see an interruption of the anterior and posterior

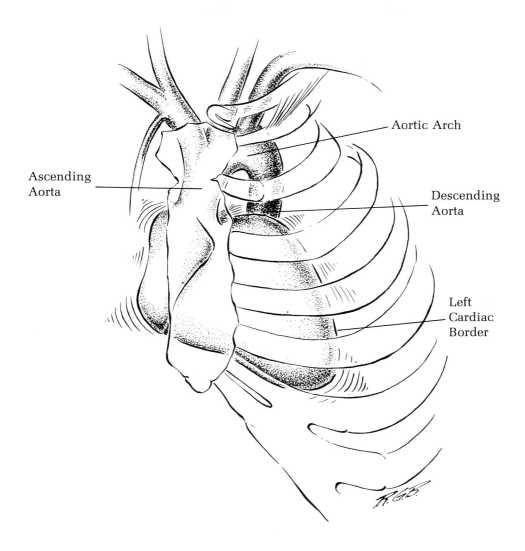

Fig. 5–2. Illustration of relationship of heart and aortic arch to thoracic cage. Note heart is moderately mobile within pericardial sac while aorta is relatively fixed.

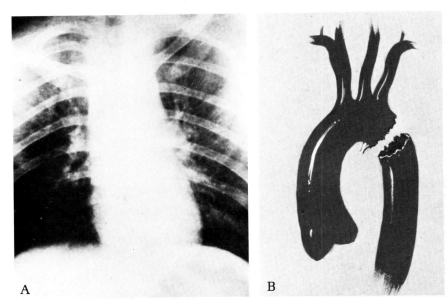

A   B

Fig. 5–3. A, Posteroanterior roentgenogram showing haziness of aortic arch area and widening of superior cardiac shadow. B, Illustration of tear in aortic arch of patient whose chest plate is seen in A. Prompt surgical correction is necessary upon recognition of this entity. (Courtesy Donald L. Bricker, M.D.)

cortex is most likely to give indication of a fracture. Direct injury to the xiphoid process also occurs, and the tip of it may be seen to be displaced toward a posterior direction.

Treatment. The uncomplicated fracture of the body or manubrium of the sternum seldom requires treatment, although the patient may be more comfortable if the chest is wrapped in a bandage such as the Elastofoam dressing. Even though direct injury to the xiphoid process is symptomatic, it is of no long-term consequence and requires only symptomatic treatment.

STERNOCLAVICULAR DISLOCATION

The clavicle serves as a strut on which the scapula may rotate and maintain its position at the lateral margin of the thoracic cage. The head of the clavicle articulates with the sternum into a notch at its superior margin on each side. A detailed group of ligaments anchor the head of the clavicle to the sternum with a meniscus inserted between the two bones (Fig. 5–4). Just posterior to this joint lies the origin of the internal mammary vessel for that side. Along the inferior margin of the clavicle runs the subclavius muscle, and crossing it at the junction of the middle and lateral thirds is the subclavian artery. The articulation of the first rib to the sternum lies immediately inferior to the sternoclavicular articulation, and these share some common ligament binding structures.

The mechanism of injury in the sternoclavicular dislocation may be a direct blow to the medial clavicle which forces this head posterior in its relationship to the sternum. This, however, is the uncommon injury. The sternoclavicular

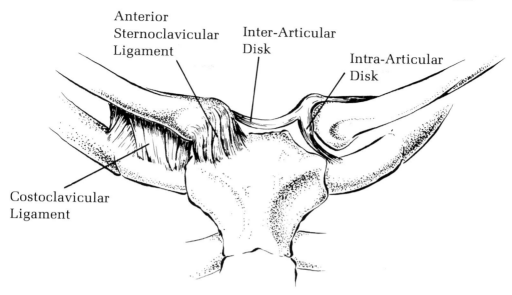

Fig. 5–4. Illustration showing ligamentous capsule of sternoclavicular joint on left and intra-articular disk within this joint on right.

dislocation is not a common injury, but when it does occur, it usually results from a force driving the shoulder posteriorly and levering the head of the clavicle anteriorly and usually a little superiorly. In order for this to occur, there must be a tearing of a portion of these detailed ligamentous attachments.

Examination. On examination, when a sternoclavicular dislocation has occurred, one may note by comparison to the uninjured side a variation in position of the clavicle. In the more typical type of injury, one may palpate the superior margin of the clavicular head more anterior and superior than is its fellow of the opposite side. In addition, there is often ecchymosis overlying this joint area. To palpation there is local tenderness. One must be suspicious that this injury exists or the diagnosis is not likely to be made.

Roentgenograms. Roentgenograms to show the sternoclavicular dislocation (Fig. 5–5A) are difficult to obtain, but in general rotational views are necessary, including oblique views toward each joint from anterior to posterolateral. Similar roentgenographic views of the opposite side are essential for comparison and accurate evaluation of this injury. Dislocation of the sternoclavicular joint is often not recognized because of the difficulty in obtaining adequate x-ray views. Limited experience with sternoclavicular joint arthrography in the anterosuperior dislocation reveals a significant escape of contrast media from either side of the meniscus into the retrosternal space. This confirms a tear of the restraining ligaments at the sternoclavicular joint (Fig. 5–5B).

Treatment. Following analgesia it may be possible to direct the head of the clavicle back into its normal relationship with the sternum. This maneuver usually is done by first increasing the anterior-to-posterior force against the outer shoulder with one hand while directing the head of the clavicle with the

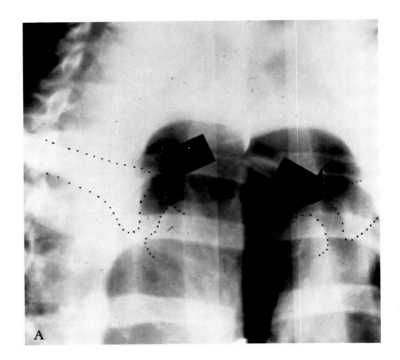

A

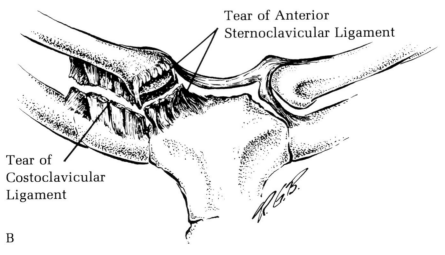

Tear of Anterior
Sternoclavicular Ligament

Tear of
Costoclavicular
Ligament

B

Fig. 5–5. A, Oblique roentgenograms to show right and left sternoclavicular joints. Arrows point to superomedial corner of each clavicle. Note elevation of right one from sternal angle when compared to normal one on left (reader's right). B, Illustration of ligamentous interruption of right sternoclavicular joint that allowed sternoclavicular dislocation to occur.

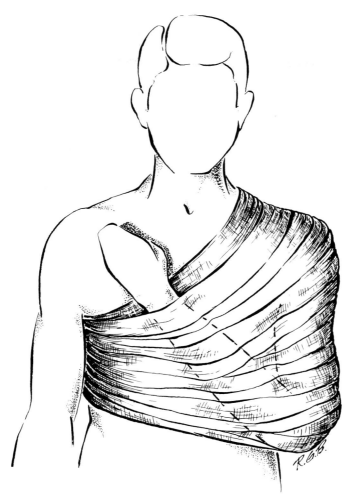

Fig. 5–6. Illustration of Velpeau bandage used to immobilize shoulder girdle.

other hand. As soon as the clavicle begins to fit into its relationship with the sternum, the shoulder is brought forward. Should reduction occur and stability ensue, one should keep this arm bandaged in a Velpeau type of fixation (Fig. 5–6). Elastic wrapping is often used for this dressing, but I prefer a single roll of 6-inch plaster to be wrapped over the softer material of the padding to keep the bandage from shifting. It may be possible that the same maneuver can be accomplished following the use of local anesthetic into the sternoclavicular joint after a surgical preparation of the area. So often, maintenance of the reduction of the head of the clavicle into its normal relationship with the sternum is not possible, and fixation of the clavicle to the sternum with a threaded Kirschner wire is in order, bearing in mind the vital structures lying just posterior to the area of injury. Although some surgeons treat this injury by studied neglect, it has been my experience that too many of these injuries are painful several months or years later and thus require some type of appropriate early attention. Reconstruction has not been nearly so satisfactory as appropriate management at the outset.

Schafer tells of one patient with a posterior dislocation of the sternoclavicular joint in whom cardiac arrest ensued secondary to anoxia. In treating the posterior sternoclavicular dislocation, reduction can often be achieved by simple lateral traction on the shoulder girdle.

FRACTURES OF RIBS AND STERNUM IN CHILDREN

Rib fractures occur in children and are generally from a crushing injury. Because the elasticity of the child's rib is so much greater than is the recognized elasticity in the adult rib, the usual fracture in the child is a greenstick type. It may be difficult to see a fractured rib on a roentgenogram (Fig. 5–7), but oblique films of the thorax with bony detail are of greatest help in this regard. The use of the Elastofoam wrap may be helpful in providing greater comfort to the patient during the early days following rib injury. Many children with rib fractures are never treated, however, because the rib fracture has been an event about which the child complains little.

Blount notes that *fractures of the sternum* occur rarely in older children, but if fresh and displaced, the fracture can be reduced by a hyperextension mechanism with traction cephalad and caudad combined with gentle digital pressure. Local or general anesthetic may be necessary before reduction. The reduction can be maintained by application of a simple body jacket.

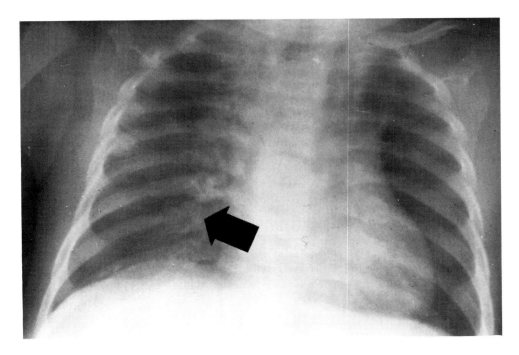

Fig. 5–7.   Multiple healing fractures of ribs 3 through 8 posteriorly on right side. Arrow points to rib that has been refractured. This child was victim of parental child abuse.

REFERENCES

1. Adams, J. C.: Outline of Fractures, Including Joint Injuries, 6th ed. Baltimore, Williams & Wilkins Co., 1972.
2. Blount, W. P.: Fractures in Children. Baltimore, Williams & Wilkins Co., 1954.
3. Kirsch, M. M., et al.: Repair of acute traumatic rupture of the aorta without extracorporeal circulation. Ann. Thorac. Surg. *10*:227, 1970.
4. Ralston, E. L.: Handbook of Fractures. St. Louis, C. V. Mosby Co., 1967.
5. Rang, M. C.: Children's Fractures. Philadelphia, J. B. Lippincott Co., 1974.
6. Rockwood, C. A., and Green, D. P.: Fractures. Philadelphia, J. B. Lippincott Co., 1975.
7. Schafer, M. F.: Personal Communication.
8. Watson-Jones, R.: Fractures and Joint Injuries, 4th ed., 2V. Baltimore, Williams & Wilkins Co., 1952-1955.

6

THE SHOULDER GIRDLE

The shoulder girdle includes the bony structure that supports the upper limb. Its main components are the scapula and the clavicle. Because mobility is required for its complex articulation, the shoulder is easily injured.

THE SCAPULA

The body of the scapula is encased in and serves as the origin for a number of muscles that control the relationship of the scapula to the thorax and of the humerus to the scapula. Along its medial border lie the rhomboid muscles, and at its medial superior border is the levator muscle of the scapula. Along the anterior surface of its vertebral border inserts the serratus anterior muscle which will maintain the close relationship of the scapula to the thoracic cage. The rhomboid and levator scapulae muscles prevent the winging of the scapula and help control its rotation. On the anterior surface of the scapula lies the origin of the subscapularis whose action is to internally rotate the humerus. On the posterior surface superior to the spine of the scapula lies the supraspinatus muscle, and inferior to the spine is the infraspinatus muscle. These insert on the greater tuberosity of the humerus along with the tendon of the teres minor muscle and serve to externally rotate the humeral head, as well as to draw it into the glenoid process for stability so that the deltoid muscle may then abduct the arm in relationship to the shoulder girdle. From the lateral inferior margin of the scapula arises the teres major muscle to insert its tendon along the proximal shaft of the humerus for adduction of the upper arm. The anterior adduction force for the humerus is furnished by the pectoralis major muscle, which arises from the anterior rib cage and inserts in a tendon lateral to the bicipital groove of the humerus. A tendon of the long head of the biceps glides through the bicipital groove of the humerus to insert on the superior rim of the glenoid fossa. The tendon of the short head of the biceps comes directly to a tip of the coracoid process in a conjoined tendon with the coracobrachialis muscle. The pectoralis minor tendon inserts onto this coracoid process also. Deep to this pectoralis minor tendon lie the brachial artery and veins and the brachial plexus.

Coracoclavicular ligaments, the conoid and trapezoid, so named because of their anatomic shapes, run from the clavicle to the coracoid process and assist in providing stability of the relationship of the clavicle to the scapula (Fig.

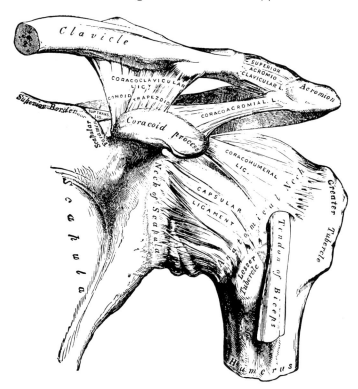

Fig. 6–1. Illustration of left shoulder, with acromioclavicular joint and multiple ligaments about the scapula. (From Goss, C. M.: Gray's Anatomy, 29th Edition. Philadelphia, Lea & Febiger, 1973.)

6–1). The remainder of the stability from the clavicle to the scapula is provided at the acromioclavicular joint by the acromioclavicular ligament. A meniscus lying between the two cartilage surfaces at this joint aids in providing a snug joint and yet one with considerable mobility, particularly of a rotational character.

The acromion process arises from the superior surface of the neck of the scapula and provides the superior margin of the shoulder joint, as well as a source for a part of the origin of the deltoid muscle. The glenoid process is the articular surface of the scapula that receives the articular surface of the humerus. The glenoid process lies at the lateral margin of the neck of the scapula and is rimmed by a fibrocartilaginous ligament called the glenoid labrum which increases the breadth of contact with the humeral articular surface.

The capsule of the shoulder joint arises from the neck of the scapula and inserts circumferentially about the humerus just distal to the articular surface of the head. Along the posterior-superior margin of this capsule lie the conjoined tendons of the supraspinatus, infraspinatus, and teres minor muscles, also called the rotator cuff.

Fractures of the Body of the Scapula

Varied shatter-type fractures of the body of the scapula occur and are invariably due to a direct force driving the body against the thoracic cage. Little if any displacement occurs with these injuries because the body is encased in the periosteum and muscle structures.

Examination. On examination of the patient with fractures of the scapular body, one notes guarded movement of the shoulder, particularly movement that requires any motion of the scapula itself. This would be specifically a lateral abduction force beyond 90 degrees which would create a rotational effect on the scapula.

Roentgenograms. Roentgenograms of the thoracic cage with bony detail would usually show fractures of the body of the scapula (Fig. 6–2). One must suspect them, however, before they would usually be noticed.

Treatment. The treatment for a fracture of the scapular body is a sling for the involved side to remove any rotary forces. The patient is usually comfortable within a week to ten days and may regain using this extremity as soon as comfortable. Full union of the fracture fragments will require about two months.

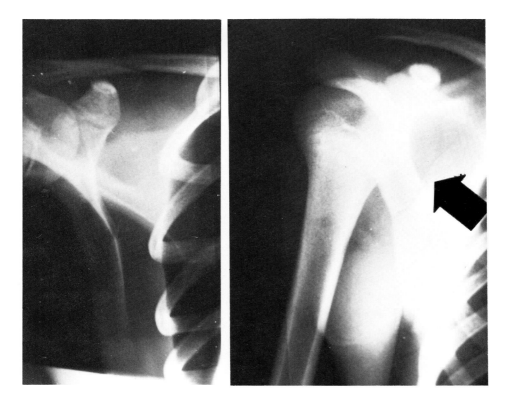

Fig. 6–2. Fracture of body of scapula (arrow)—best visualized at lateralmost cortex to left of arrow.

Fractures of the Scapula Neck

Although a rare injury, the fracture of the neck of the scapula does occur, particularly with a direct force from anterior or posterior creating displacement in the direction of the force. More commonly, the glenoid process stays with the humerus and is displaced anteriorly. No particular complication from an anatomic standpoint occurs with this injury except for the shortening of the distance from the tip of the acromion to the neck.

Examination. Examination reveals a guarded and painful shoulder. The distance from the greater tuberosity to the sternal notch is shortened on the injured side as compared to the normal. The patient is unable to actively flex or abduct the injured shoulder.

Roentgenograms. The roentgenograms (Fig. 6–3) must include not only the regular anteroposterior views, which should show some overlying shadows of scapular neck on scapular neck, but should also include an axillary view in order to adequately assess the fracture and its displacement.

Treatment. Because of the shortening of the shoulder that does occur with fractures of the scapular neck, it is well to attempt to reduce the fracture, particularly if it is an isolated injury. However, reduction failing, lateral sidearm traction should be applied to maintain as great a length as possible until stability occurs. The traction can be applied most effectively by a pin through the olecranon process. This method will allow the patient to have some mobility between the humerus and the glenoid fossa. This fracture requires between three and four weeks of immobilization before stability ensues. The patient should then still utilize a sling for this shoulder and work on a program of exercises to improve range of motion. The most common complications from this injury are a decreased range of motion of the shoulder and, as mentioned previously, a narrowing of the breadth of the shoulder as compared to the opposite side.

Fractures of the Glenoid Process

Occasional fractures of the glenoid process occur with some displacement. These have usually been accompanied by a dislocation of the humerus toward the direction in which the lip of the glenoid process has fractured. If the glenoid rim fracture has occurred with a dislocation, the dislocation is the primary problem and must be treated as described under dislocation.

Examination. The patient with an injured shoulder may present with pain only on active or passive motion. If a significant fracture of the glenoid process is present along with displacement of the humeral head, an undue prominence will be palpated where the head lies associated with an empty glenoid process.

Roentgenograms. For most effective evaluation, roentgenograms of the shoulder in which a glenoid fracture has occurred should be taken in the anteroposterior as well as the axillary views.

Treatment. Any shoulder dislocation, if present, is reduced. If more than one third of the articular surface of the glenoid process is fractured, and the fragment remains significantly displaced, then operative replacement may be necessary to prevent recurring dislocation of the humeral head. However, it would be uncommon to require operation in most fractures of the glenoid process. Trreatment, once the shoulder is in adequate position, can be ac-

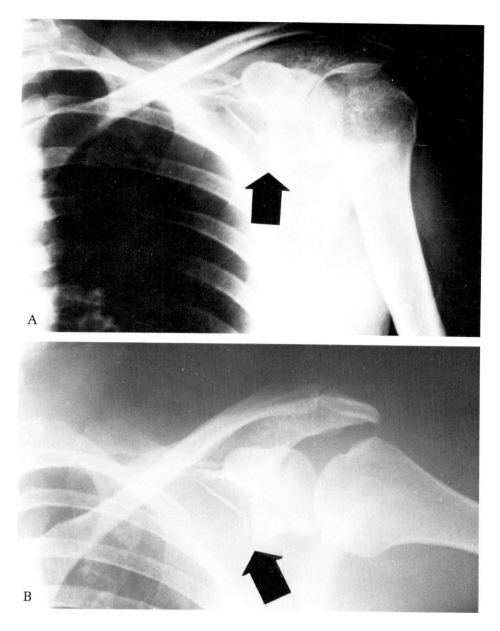

Fig. 6–3. A, Anteroposterior roentgenograms showing fracture of neck of scapula. A, Medial and anterior displacement of glenoid cavity (arrow). B, Shoulder abducted showing fracture (arrow).

complished by a sling and swathe for three to four weeks followed by exercises to increase range of motion.

Fractures of the Clavicle

The clavicle may fracture at almost any portion throughout its extent. Fracture may occur from a direct blow to the clavicle or from an indirect force created by a blow to the shoulder. A force from anterior to posterior on the shoulder usually creates a single fracture, whereas a force from posterior to anterior may create a comminuted fracture. Injury to the brachial plexus can occur with a fracture of the clavicle, and examination should establish presence or absence of such injury.

Examination. There is likely a deformity seen on observation of the patient's shoulder. Since the clavicle is subcutaneous throughout its entire course, on palpation one may feel the fracture, and there will be point tenderness at the fracture site. Probably crepitation will be present.

Roentgenograms. On an anteroposterior view of the superior thorax, roentgenograms will confirm an interruption of the cortices of the clavicle, with or without significant displacement (Fig. 6–4).

Treatment. The figure-of-8 technique is especially effective for treatment of the clavicle fracture. This draws the scapulae posteriorly and tightens the periosteal tube in which the clavicle lies, thus reducing the fracture fragments (Fig. 6–5). The principle of the figure-of-8 is embodied in a number of clavicle

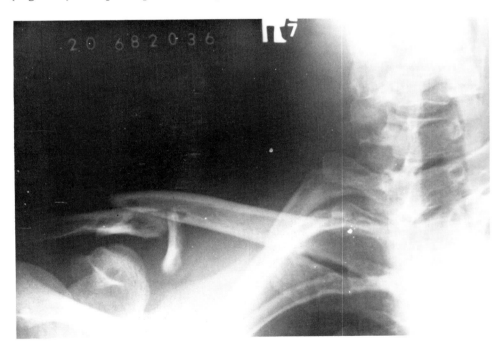

Fig. 6–4. Anteroposterior roentgenogram showing comminuted fracture of clavicle at junction of middle and lateral thirds. A figure-of-8 dressing to draw scapulae back gives excellent results if maintained six to eight weeks.

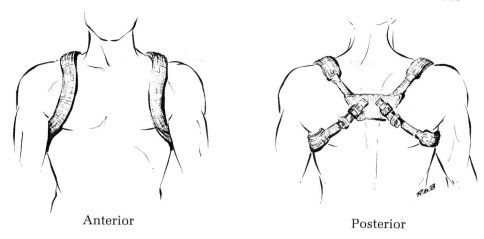

Anterior   Posterior

Fig. 6–5. Figure-of-8 immobilizer used to treat fractured clavicle. Commercially available straps are effective and easy to use. A well-padded plaster of Paris figure-of-8 dressing may be used when greater rigidity is required and/or when the patient cannot cooperate.

straps which in effect draw the shoulders posteriorly and reduce the clavicle fracture. A well-padded plaster of Paris figure-of-8 immobilizer may be used when greater rigidity is required and/or when the patient cannot cooperate. The patient in this type of fixation should be checked by roentgenograms after the first week to determine satisfactory maintenance of position. It will likely be necessary for the patient to wear this device about six weeks before any evidence of early bony union is seen. When effectively used, figure-of-8 immobilization provides comfort to the patient within a matter of hours or days. It can be anticipated that the fracture will unite with this mode of treatment. Treatment of these fractures by operation is not advised unless specifically indicated for reason of inability to maintain contact of fragments or of a developing neurologic deficit. The only nonunion of a clavicle fracture I have seen was one in which the fracture was treated by open reduction.

Acromioclavicular Separations

Separation of the acromioclavicular joint occurs when a major force strikes against the shoulder or the acromion process of the shoulder in an inferior or inferoposterior direction. For a full separation to occur, the acromioclavicular ligament must tear at the joint. In addition, the coracoclavicular ligaments about one and one-half inches medial to the joint must also tear.

Examination. On palpation the patient with acromioclavicular separation has point tenderness directly over the acromioclavicular joint and superior to the coracoid process. The lateral margin of the clavicle can be palpated at a level superior to the superior surface of the acromion process.

Roentgenograms. The roentgenograms of a shoulder with acromioclavicular separation may show obvious elevation of the lateral clavicle in relationship to the acromion. There may also be noted an increase in the distance between the coracoid process and the clavicle. In order to adequately assess the injury, comparison views should be obtained of the opposite shoulder. Occasionally the injury is difficult to document. If one suspects the separation, usually it can be shown conclusively by having the patient hold a 10-pound weight in each hand while an anteroposterior view across the shoulders is taken (Fig. 6–6). If these roentgenograms show the elevation of the lateral clavicle away from its relationship to the acromion be no greater than one-fourth inch, this can be considered a subluxation. Elevation of the clavicle of more than one-fourth inch from the acromion is a frank separation.

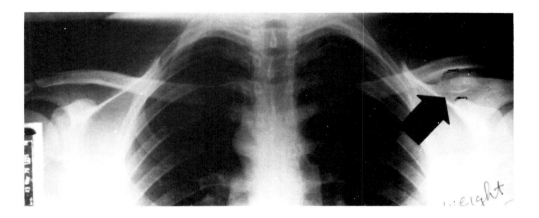

Fig. 6–6. Anteroposterior roentgenogram with patient holding weights (10 pounds) in both hands. Note increased distance between left clavicle and coracoid process (arrow) in comparison to distance on opposite side. This increased space indicates complete tear of coracoclavicular ligaments.

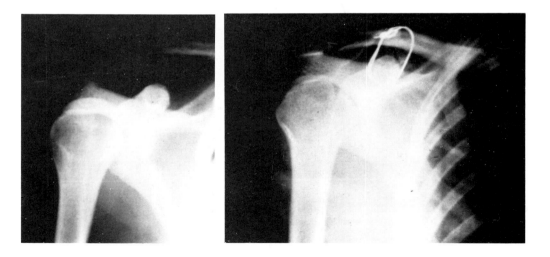

Fig. 6–7. Roentgenogram showing fixation of clavicle to coracoid process by wire, which will have to be removed or allowed to break prior to initiation of activity. This method is used to repair the coracoclavicular ligaments, as well as the capsule of acromioclavicular joint.

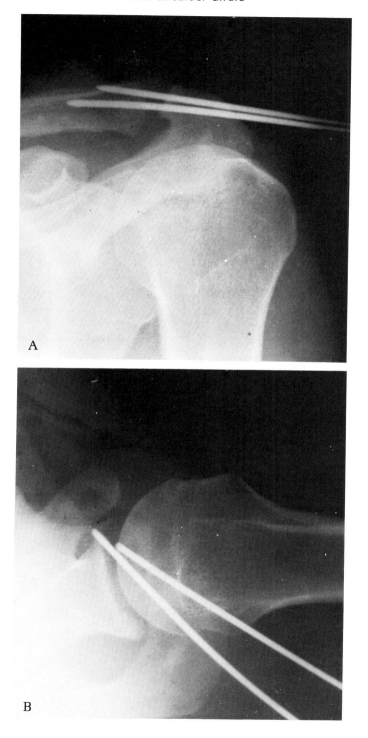

A

B

Fig. 6–8.   Roentgenograms showing acromioclavicular separation has been reduced and fixed by use of threaded Kirschner wires. A, Anteroposterior view. B, Axillary view.

Treatment. The subluxed acromioclavicular joint may be treated by an elevating sling for the arm. The effect of this elevating sling is to bring the scapula superiorly to meet the clavicle. A number of variations of this method have been used, but the basic principle is the same. In the frank and complete acromioclavicular separation, however, the best long-term results have followed internal fixation of the distal clavicle into an anatomic relationship with the acromion. The author prefers the figure-of-8 wire method as recommended by Alldredge. This fixes the clavicle to the coracoid process by a loop of wire over the clavicle and under the coracoid process (Fig. 6–7). At the same time the conoid and trapezoid ligaments and the capsule of the acromioclavicular joint are repaired. The patient must understand that the wire is to be removed at six weeks, or else it needs to break in order to allow the mobility necessary for normal shoulder motion. An alternative to this method is the fixation of the clavicle to the acromion by Kirschner wires inserted from the tip of the acromion process (Fig. 6–8). If the latter method of fixation is used, the lateral tips of the Kirschner wires should be bent to prevent migration. These wires also need to be removed after six to eight weeks. Nonoperative treatment of this severe injury in the adult has not provided sufficiently good results to warrant its lengthy consideration.

SHOULDER DISLOCATIONS

The object of this book is to discuss acute fractures and dislocations. Since these conditions cannot be totally separated from the recurrent dislocations in the shoulder, there will also be some consideration of the recurrent shoulder dislocation. Both acute and recurrent dislocations of the shoulder share common mechanisms of injury as well as methods of reduction. The point of divergence is that the acute dislocation, once properly immobilized, will not tend to recur, whereas the chronic dislocation of the shoulder will likely recur unless operated upon.

Anterior Dislocation

The anterior dislocation of the shoulder occurs by an external rotation force. In this circumstance the posterior humeral neck at the cartilage margin catches on the anterior rim of the glenoid process. As an internal rotation or neutralizing motion then follows, the head levers completely out of its joint relationship with the glenoid process. This injury may be associated with a fracture of the greater tuberosity, particularly when the injury has been caused by a more violent force. Specific other complications that may occur with this type of injury are axillary nerve palsy and tear of the rotator cuff.

Examination. On examination of the patient with the anterior dislocation of the shoulder, there will be noted to observation and palpation a fullness in the anterior portion of the shoulder. To firm palpation there will be loss of fullness over the lateral aspect of the shoulder as one palpates toward the glenoid process. Once dislocated, the shoulder is usually guarded but is in a neutral position. Fracture of the greater tuberosity may be noted by evidence of crepitation on palpation. Certainly the examination should include a sensory check peripheral to the injury and in the quarter-sized area of skin innervated by the axillary nerve at the apex of the deltoid muscle. Occasional axillary and

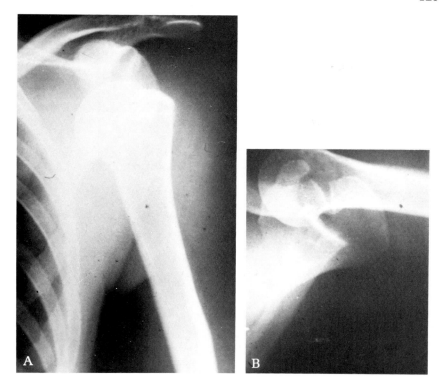

Fig. 6–9. Roentgenogram of dislocated humeral head. A, In anteroposterior view humeral head is inferior and medial to its usual relationship with glenoid cavity. B, In axillary view humeral head can be seen lying anterior to glenoid cavity.

other nerve palsies occur as a complication to this injury. A rotator cuff tear may be sustained with the dislocation, but this is usually not diagnosed at the time of the acute injury.

Roentgenograms. Roentgenograms of the shoulder with an anterior dislocation will show the head overlying the neck of the scapula and the glenoid process (Fig. 6–9A). An axillary or transthoracic view will be necessary to show the exact position of the humeral head in relationship to the glenoid (Fig. 6–9B). The pain experienced by the patient is often severe enough to preclude the axillary view so that the transthoracic view can be acceptable if properly performed. Fracture of the greater tuberosity can occur with this injury and if present should be shown clearly on the roentgenograms (Fig. 6–10).

Treatment. Reduction of the anterior dislocation of the shoulder should be accomplished as soon as is reasonable. In most instances a combination of meperidine (Demerol) and diazepam (Valium) provides sufficient relaxation to allow reduction. The "talking" Kocher maneuver, in my opinion, is the method of choice in reduction of the dislocated shoulder (Fig. 6–11A). A constant stream of discussion and explanation to the patient accompanies the gradual external rotation of the involved limb while maintaining the humerus adducted to the thorax as much as possible (Fig. 6–11B). Once a full 90 degrees of external rotation has been accomplished, the patient is advised to expect a fairly quick movement in which the elbow is brought medially along the anterior thoracic wall (Fig. 6–11C) approximately 30 degrees followed by a quick internal rotation maneuver to bring the hand to the opposite shoulder (Fig. 6–11D). It is during this part of the maneuver that the humeral head is felt to drop back into its relationship with the glenoid process.

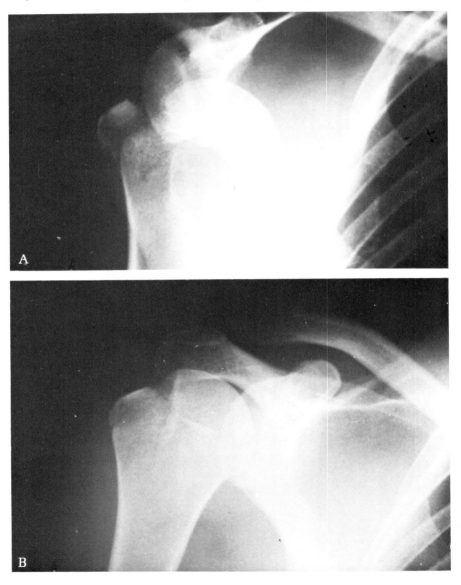

Fig. 6–10. Anterior dislocation of shoulder accompanied by displaced fracture of greater tuberosity. A, Anteroposterior view before treatment. B, Following reduction of dislocation. Note normal relationship of humeral head to glenoid cavity. In addition, fractured greater tuberosity has fallen into place.

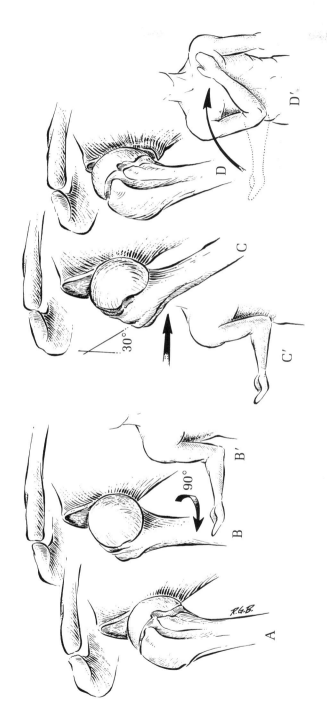

Fig. 6–11. Illustrations showing reduction of anterior dislocation of shoulder by Kocher maneuver. A, Anteriorly dislocated shoulder and its abnormal relationships. B, Adduction accompanied by external rotation of shoulder is shown. C, While external rotation is maintained, adduction with elbow anterior to thorax is accomplished. D, Final maneuver is internal rotation quickly brought about while adduction is maintained. During this part of maneuver humeral head is felt to drop back into its relationship with glenoid process.

131

Other methods for reduction of the dislocation include the Hippocratic method by which the stockinged foot is placed into the axilla of the dislocated shoulder and longitudinal traction accomplishes the reduction. In the Stimson method of reduction the patient is placed prone on a table and a weight of about 15 pounds is attached to the arm of the dislocated shoulder as it hangs anteriorly over the side of the table. This is a lengthier procedure from the standpoint of time but is an effective method of reduction.

Once reduced, the shoulder should be maintained in an internal rotation position with a Velpeau dressing (Fig. 6–12) for three weeks. I prefer a padded Velpeau bandage with one or two rolls of plaster of Paris wrapped on to provide stability for the dressing. At three weeks, the arm is then placed in a double

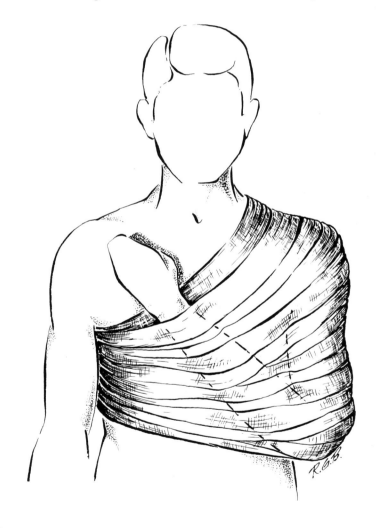

Fig. 6–12. Velpeau dressing to maintain adduction and internal rotation. Soft rolls of elastic bandage may be used. I prefer bias cut stockinette covered by two six-inch rolls of plaster of Paris.

sling system so that the circumferential sling may be removed several times daily for active exercising. The patient is warned against external rotation for the first six weeks. Attention must be directed toward achieving a full range of motion eventually. The lack of adequate immobilization of the dislocation of the shoulder may well presage the recurrent dislocation of the shoulder, inasmuch as the anterior ligament and capsule have insufficient chance to heal their torn or separated fibers.

Posterior Dislocation

The posterior dislocation occurs through an internal rotation force that tears the capsule posteriorly and allows the head to escape into the space posterior to the glenoid rim. This is not a common injury but one requiring attention. Because the axillary nerve approaches the deltoid muscles posteriorly, it stands a greater chance of injury with this type of dislocation.

Examination. The most notable feature in the examination of the patient with a posterior dislocation is that there is an *internal* rotation position of the arm which the patient cannot actively correct. In addition, there is an absence of fullness to the lateral shoulder and an increased fullness posteriorly. Should

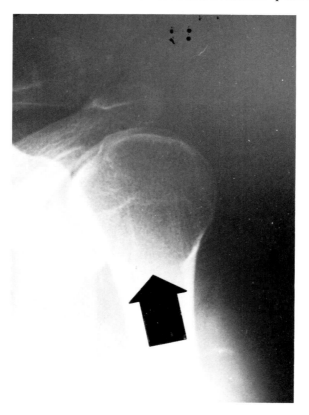

Fig. 6–13. Anteroposterior view showing posterior dislocation of shoulder. Arrow points to "pseudocyst" of humeral head which should alert examining physician to possibility of this diagnosis.

the axillary nerve receive injury, there would of course be a decrease or loss of sensation over the quarter-sized area of skin innervated at the apex of the deltoid muscle. The anteroposterior roentgenograms may confirm this diagnosis (Fig. 6–13), but most likely one will need to view a roentgenogram taken at a plane of 90 degrees from the anteroposterior view. Either the axillary or the transthoracic view could provide this information. Because of the distress of the patient, the transthoracic view is likely the most easily obtainable.

Treatment. Once the diagnosis of posterior dislocation of the shoulder has been established, one should reduce the shoulder as soon as is reasonable. The earlier a reduction can be accomplished, the less intense is the spasm of the muscles about the shoulder. A combination of meperidine and diazepam is usually sufficiently relaxing to allow reduction of this dislocation. This reduction can be accomplished by slightly increasing the internal rotation and adduction of the upper arm, placing a force from the posterior side of the shoulder anteriorly, and slowly rotating externally. The humeral head should

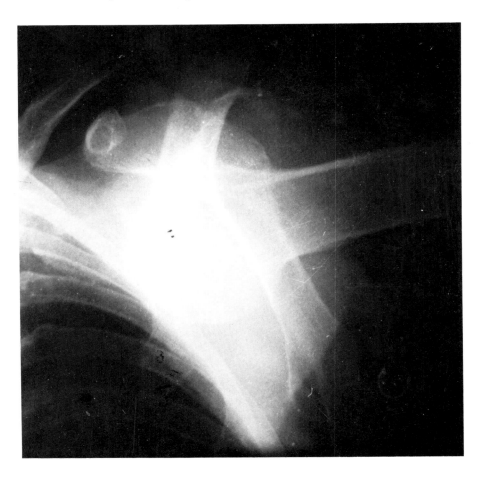

Fig. 6–14. Anteroposterior roentgenograms showing inferior dislocation of humeral head, which is called luxatio erecta. It can be reduced by superolateral traction.

slip into position with this maneuver. A simple sling is generally adequate immobilization for this type of injury. At one time it was thought that an external rotation casting system must be accomplished in order to allow healing of the capsule, but this has not proved essential and is an unnecessary burden to the patient. The simple sling will hold a sufficient position for healing of the fibers of the capsule.

Luxatio Erecta

Luxatio erecta is caused by a pure abduction mechanism which forces the humeral head inferiorly. The humeral head catches under the rim of the glenoid process at its inferior margin and comes to rest against the inferior neck of the scapula. Although rare, this does occur but usually without complicating factors.

Examination. On examination of the patient with the luxatio erecta, one notes that any attempts to bring the arm from the abducted position are accompanied by a rotation of the scapula only.

Roentgenograms. The anteroposterior roentgenogram shows the position of the humeral head inferior to the scapular neck and rim of the glenoid process (Fig. 6–14). The axillary view shows the head overlying the glenoid process.

Treatment. A combination of meperidine and diazepam usually allows sufficient relaxation for reduction. Reduction of luxatio erecta is most easily accomplished by superolateral longitudinal traction on the arm with some gentle rotary movements during the superolateral traction. Countertraction against the acromion process by an assistant is necessary to immobilize the scapula and achieve reduction. Occasionally an extra force against the humeral head by the heel of the hand from inferior to superior position will help relocate the reluctant dislocation. Only rarely has it proved necessary to attempt to convert this dislocation to an anterior dislocation in order to achieve reduction. The postreduction treatment for this patient should be a simple sling for approximately three weeks followed by active exercises to improve range of motion.

FRACTURES OF THE SCAPULA AND CLAVICLE IN CHILDREN

Fractures of the scapula in children may occur from falls onto the shoulder. These are generally undisplaced and create no question of treatment, it being symptomatic such as use of the sling. Considerable displacement of a fractured scapula can occur in the child following major injury and may be treated also with the double sling method (Fig. 6–15) or with a Velpeau bandage (Fig. 5–6) if this is more comfortable to the patient. Little concern should be given to the displaced fragment inasmuch as a remodeling of the scapula will occur in the ensuing months and years following the injury.

Fracture of the clavicle may occur at the time of delivery and occasionally occurs when an infant is dropped onto his shoulder. The alerting symptom to this injury is an *apparent* paralysis which Blount refers to as a pseudoparalysis of the arm. With examination one may palpate crepitus and the area of pain over the clavicle. In the newborn, the use of a figure-of-8 bandage is difficult, but a rolled towel may be placed between the scapulae, and the infant should be kept on his back. In the little older infant, the figure-of-8 bandage made from

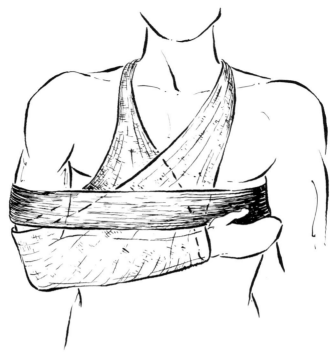

Fig. 6–15. Illustration of double sling method of immobilization used in treating certain shoulder injuries.

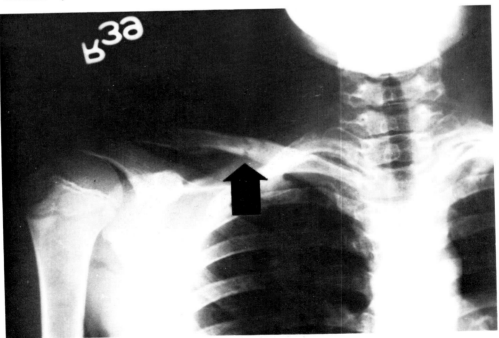

Fig. 6–16. Undisplaced clavicle fracture (arrow) in ten-year-old child. A figure-8 immobilizer will provide adequate immobilization for excellent union in six to eight weeks.

stockinette and padding may be placed on the shoulder to provide comfort and support.

Whereas in the infant a fracture of the clavicle is more often a greenstick type of fracture, the older child sustains a complete fracture with some overriding. A figure-of-8 dressing can be used in the youngster for four to six weeks, depending upon evidence of need. Difficulty in maintaining the figure-of-8 bandage may be encountered, and if so, plaster of Paris may be used to increase firmness and stability of the dressing.

Roentgenograms will often show a small "kink" in the clavicle of the infant or the smaller child and will show the fracture with some overriding in the older child (Fig. 6–16). No special complications would be anticipated from the clavicle fractures, since these invariably heal with a good long-term result.

REFERENCES

1. Adams, J. C.: Outline of Fractures, Including Joint Injuries, 6th ed. Baltimore, Williams & Wilkins Co., 1972.
1a. Alldredge, R. H.: Surgical treatment of acromioclavicular dislocations. J. Bone Joint Surg. 47-A:1278, 1965.
2. Blount, W. P.: Fractures in children. Baltimore, Williams & Wilkins Co., 1954.
3. Bost, F. C., and Inman, V. T.: The pathologic changes in recurrent dislocation of the shoulder, a report of Bankart's operative procedure. J. Bone Joint Surg. 24:595, 1942.
4. Ralston, E. L.: Handbook of Fractures. St. Louis, C. V. Mosby Co., 1967.
5. Rang, M. C.: Children's Fractures. Philadelphia, J. B. Lippincott Co., 1974.
6. Rockwood, C. A., Jr.: The diagnosis of acute posterior dislocation of the shoulder. J. Bone Joint Surg. 42A:235, 1960.
7. Rockwood, C. A., and Green, D. P.: Fractures. Philadelphia, J. B. Lippincott Co., 1975.
8. Watson-Jones, R.: Fractures and Joint Injuries, 4th ed., 2V. Baltimore, Williams & Wilkins Co., 1952-1955.

7

THE HUMERUS

The proximal humerus is composed of a hemispherical cartilage surface which articulates with the cartilage covering the glenoid process of the scapula. Distal to the cartilaginous surface of the humeral head, the circumferential depressed area is referred to as the humeral neck. Reference is made to this portion of the humerus as the anatomic neck. At its lateral margin is a bony elevation, the tuberosity, into which the tendons of the supraspinatus, infraspinatus, and teres minor muscles insert. Just inferior to this tuberosity is an area referred to in fracture texts as the surgical neck of (Fig. 7–1) the humerus. Distal to this is the shaft of the humerus leading down to the medial and lateral flare, the condyles, just proximal to the elbow. The brachial artery and veins, as well as the radial, musculocutaneous, median, and ulnar nerves, enter the arm along the medial side just deep to the deltopectoral groove (Fig. 7–2). The radial nerve leaves this grouping and moves posterior to the humerus at midshaft, running in a groove in the humeral shaft. It reaches the lateral intermuscular septum and lies immediately posterior to it along its insertion into the lateral humerus (Fig. 7–1). The musculocutaneous nerve leaves the grouping at midshaft to pass into the anterior compartment, sending branches into the biceps and to the brachial muscles and then providing the sensory nerve for the lateral aspect of the anterior forearm. The brachial artery and veins, as well as the median and ulnar nerves, continue anterior to the intermuscular septum to a point just proximal to the flare of the medial condyle of the humerus. At this position, the ulnar nerve passes posterior to the septum to seek its position in the ulnar groove of the medial epicondyle of the humerus.

FRACTURES OF HUMERAL NECK

Although the anatomic and surgical necks of the humerus have been separated in much of the writing regarding fractures, fractures of the neck area are treated essentially the same, and this relatively nonfunctional distinction will not be made in this text. Fractures of the neck of the humerus tend to occur by abduction or adduction force.

Examination. In visualization of the shoulder in which a fracture of the humeral head has occurred, one may see much swelling and ecchymosis. The upper arm may have lost significant active range of motion, either because of

139

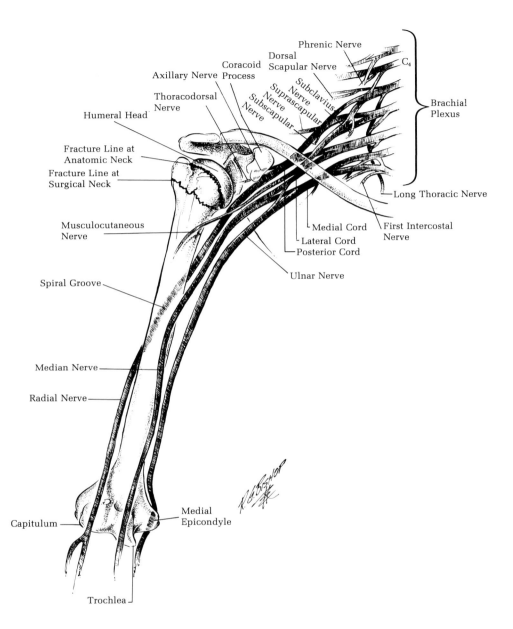

Fig. 7–1. Illustration of relationships of humerus. Fracture lines are shown at the anatomic neck and at the surgical neck. Note lateral brachial plexus and peripheral nerve relationships upon entering upper arm.

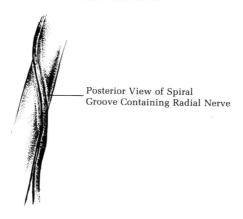

Posterior View of Spiral
Groove Containing Radial Nerve

Fig. 7–2. Location of spiral groove in humerus. Through it runs the radial nerve. Being relatively fixed, the radial nerve is more subject to injury in a displaced fracture at this level.

pain or because of loss of continuity of the humeral head into the glenoid process. If impaction is present, an active (though often painful) and incomplete range of motion is present. Seldom is there any neurologic deficit associated with shoulder fractures.

Roentgenograms. Roentgenograms required for evaluation of a fracture of the humeral neck include the anteroposterior (Fig. 7–3A) as well as the lateral views (Fig. 7–3B). The lateral view in this instance can often be the transthoracic view if taken with proper technique. The roentgenogram will confirm the amount of comminution. Comminution of fragments is not uncommon in fractures of the humeral neck, particularly in the elderly. The roentgenograms may also indicate the mechanism of injury. In the adduction injury, more common in the young adult and seldom comminuted, one notes the humeral shaft to be shifted into an adducted position in relationship to the head. The abduction force, on the other hand, creates an abducted angulation of the humeral head and neck (Fig. 7–3C). This information may be useful in treatment, the treatment of choice tending to utilize a force in the direction opposite to that of the causative force. The humeral neck fracture in the elderly is often impacted as can be identified on the roentgenogram with a line of increased density across the fracture site (Fig. 7–4).

Treatment. If the fracture is deemed stable, then a sling or a collar and cuff device should be sufficient for management until the symptoms of injury to the shoulder itself have subsided. This may well take three to four weeks; following this period, an intensive, active program of range of motion exercises should be pursued. For most humeral neck fractures, including the comminuted, but not impacted ones, a light hanging arm cast is often the most effective treatment (Fig. 7–5). This cast should be applied from the base of the metacarpals to a point just proximal to the elbow. One and one-half rolls of 4-inch plaster should provide sufficient weight to this cast. A loop is then attached at the wrist, and a sling is placed around the neck and through the loop (Fig. 7–6). In this particular method of treatment the patient must stay in a

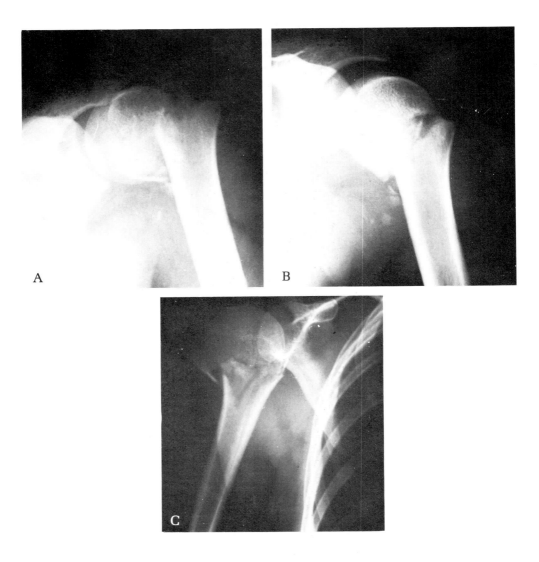

Fig. 7–3. Roentgenograms for evaluating fracture of humeral neck. A, Anteroposterior view showing an adduction fracture. B, Attempted lateral view. Note shaft is adducted in relationship to head. This fracture can be treated effectively by collar and cuff traction or by hanging arm cast. My preference is for the latter under well-controlled circumstances. C, Anteroposterior view. As compared to A, humeral shaft is abducted in relation to head. However, treatment can be the same for either type of fracture.

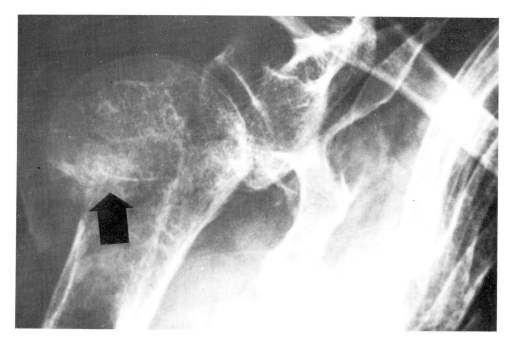

Fig. 7–4. Anteroposterior roentgenogram showing impacted abducted fracture (arrow) of neck of humerus. Note profound osteoporosis of all bones shown here. A sling to relieve symptoms for brief period will allow early mobilization and use of arm following this fracture.

relatively upright position for the hanging cast (a device for applying traction) to be effective. This means that the patient should not recline more than 45 degrees during the early phase of treatment in which the bones are becoming "sticky." At approximately six weeks, the patient may be able to progress from the hanging cast to a sling or a collar and cuff (Fig. 7–7), depending upon the preference of the treating doctor. Prior to this change in treatment, roentgenograms must show maintenance of position of the fragments and early union.

The displaced proximal humeral fracture can often be treated by the hanging arm cast method, also. Occasionally, a spike of the long fragment impales muscle tissue and will not allow reduction by this method. In this instance, operation may be necessary in order to achieve reduction. Once this is reduced, a single long oblique screw through the cortex of the distal fragment up into the head of the humerus serves as an excellent means of maintaining the longitudinal position postoperatively.

In the abduction injury, the proximal fragment may move into a position of flexion and external rotation. If this occurs, traction in an overhead position with external rotation while the patient is supine may move the distal fragment into such a position as to be adequately reduced to the proximal (or head) fragment. Maintenance of this position in traction until stability is present (often three weeks) can be followed by a shoulder spica cast in which the arm is maintained in this position (Fig. 7–11E). It is probable that six weeks in this

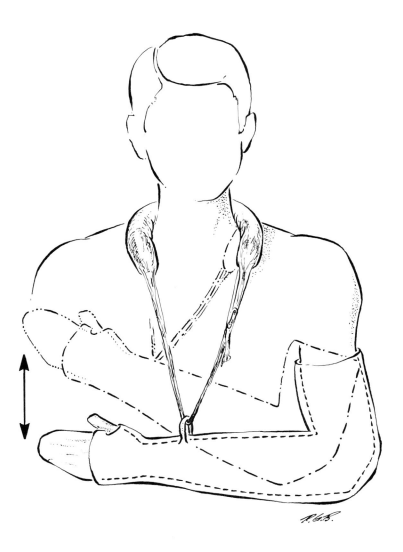

Fig. 7–5. Hanging cast. To correct anterior angulation of distal fragment, sling may be lengthened. Shortening sling will correct posterior angulation of distal fragment.

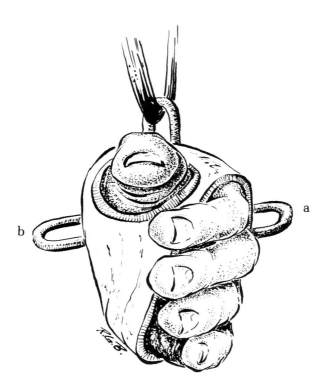

Fig. 7–6. Loop attached to wrist of hanging cast. Angulation of distal fragment laterally would be corrected by placing wrist loop on dorsal side (a). Angulation of distal fragment medially is corrected by placing loop on volar side of wrist (b). It must be emphasized that this type of cast is a traction device.

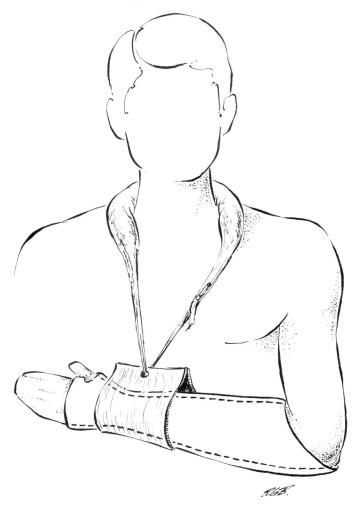

Fig. 7–7.   Collar and cuff. Indications for its use are given in the sections on treatment.

position would be sufficient before bringing the arm back down to a neutral position. The attractive alternative to traction management of this particular fracture would be open reduction and internal fixation.

FRACTURES OF HUMERAL SHAFT

Fractures may occur in any portion of the shaft of the humerus and may be caused by direct injury or by indirect force. The direct force tends to create a transverse or oblique fracture, whereas the indirect force tends to create the spiral type of fracture. Of particular concern with the midshaft humeral fracture is the possibility of injury to the radial nerve, as it lies in the spiral groove of the humerus.

Examination. The examination of the patient with a fracture through the shaft of the humerus reveals most typically an angulation deformity, caused by contraction of the deltoid muscle, associated with abduction of the proximal fragment. There is also loss of stability of the arm. In the examination, one should make certain that there is no loss of motor control or sensation peripheral to the injury. Most specifically, the question exists regarding possible injury to the radial nerve and its points of distribution. Such loss would lead to decreased or absent sensation on the dorsum of the wrist to the radial side as well as the dorsal thumb, index, and middle fingers. The accompanying muscle weakness would involve all wrist, thumb, and finger dorsiflexors.

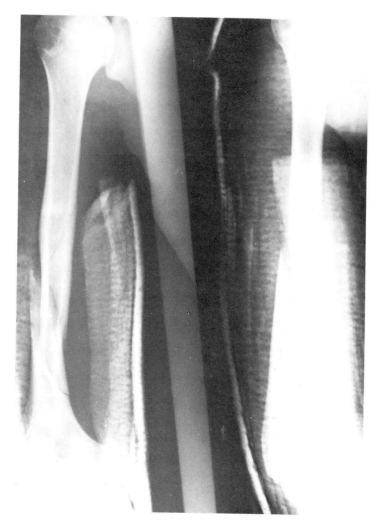

Fig. 7–8. Anteroposterior and lateral roentgenograms showing spiral fracture in middle and distal one third of humerus. Of special concern is possibility of injury to radial nerve in groove. This particular fracture was treated by a plaster of Paris cap over the shoulder and under the elbow with the arm placed in a sling. (See outline of the plaster on the lateral, or right hand, view.)

Roentgenograms. Two roentgenographic views (Fig. 7–8) must be taken at 90 degree planes from each other in order to allow as full an assessment of the humeral shaft fracture as possible. These must include the shoulder and elbow joints.

Treatment. Many fractures of the humeral shaft can be treated by use of the hanging cast technique. It is important to understand, however, that in the hanging cast technique the cast must not be placed higher on the arm than the lowest point of the fracture. Medial and lateral angulation can be managed in the hanging cast by positioning the loop for the sling on the volar side to correct lateral bowing (Fig. 7–6) and on the dorsal side to correct medial bowing. Anterior and posterior angulation can be corrected by changing the length of the sling around the neck appropriately.

Shaft fractures require approximately ten to twelve weeks in order to achieve adequate union, but the hanging cast may be removed at two months, and the

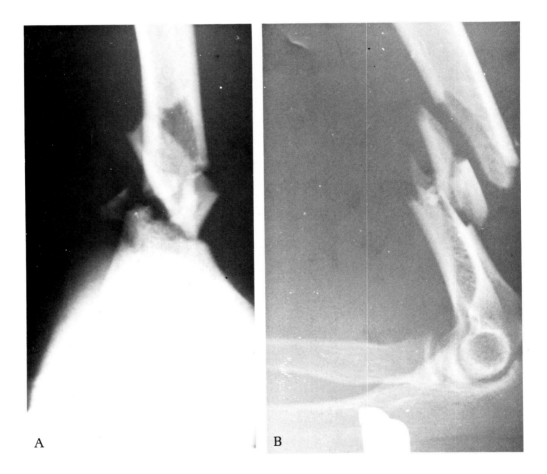

A   B

Fig. 7–9.   Roentgenograms of a comminuted fracture of the distal humerus. This was treated by sidearm skeletal traction (Kirschner wire through the proximal ulna) until "sticky," at which time a snug-fitting long arm cast was applied.

arm may be placed in a collar and cuff so that motion at the elbow and the shoulder may be begun. Again, the necessity for an intensive, active program of range of motion exercises for the shoulder and the elbow of this involved side cannot be overemphasized. Seldom does nonunion occur in this area if the fracture has not been operated upon and if the patient follows closely the recommendations of the physician. Nonunion can occur in the shaft fracture, however, and may require a bone graft along with internal fixation.

Occasionally, immobilization can be accomplished by use of plaster splints wrapped over the shoulder cap and under the elbow while the elbow is maintained at a 90-degree position (Fig. 7–8). This entire device then needs to be placed in a sling or strapped to the body. The hanging cast has proved much easier for patient to tolerate. Sidearm traction can also be used to treat humeral shaft fractures (Fig. 7–9).

When a radial nerve palsy accompanies the midhumeral fracture and there is a deepening radial deficit, surgical nerve decompression (and probably internal fixation of the humerus) should be performed within the first few days to a week. Lack of significant return or change at six weeks postinjury is indication for nerve exploration and lysis from the bone of any impaled segments of nerve.

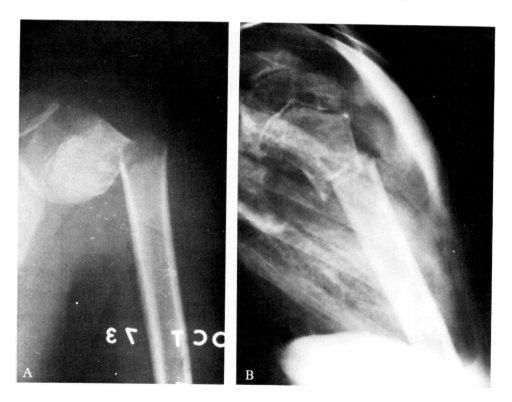

Fig. 7–10. A, Anteroposterior view. Fracture in proximal shaft of nine-year-old male. Note proximal fragment is abducted and externally rotated by unopposed attachments of supraspinatus, infraspinatus, and teres minor muscles. B, Transthoracic view. Displacement was treated by hanging cast method.

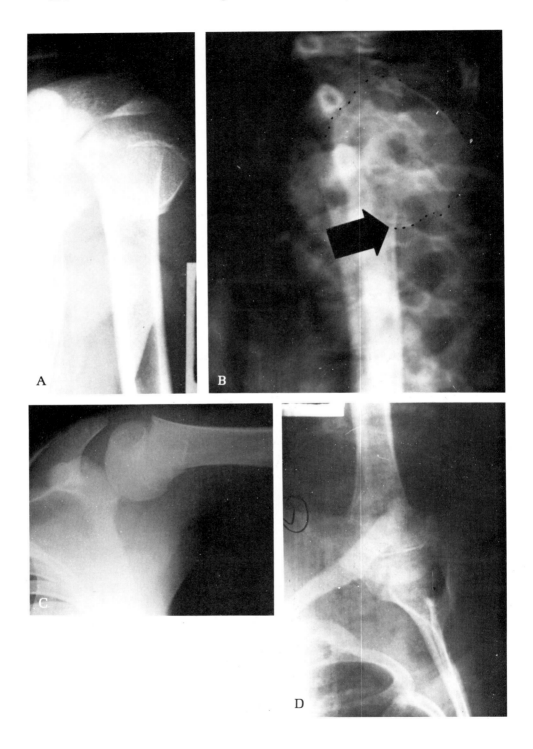

FRACTURES OF THE HUMERUS IN CHILDREN

Although dislocations of the humerus rarely occur in the infant or child, the injury that does occur in the child from two to seven years of age is a *transverse fracture of the proximal humerus* at the subtubercular level (Fig. 7–10). This may be greenstick fracture with a modest angulation of up to 15 degrees and may be treated with a collar and cuff. If significant displacement has occurred, the fracture is best treated with a hanging arm cast. A circumferential sling may provide comfort at night for the first several days.

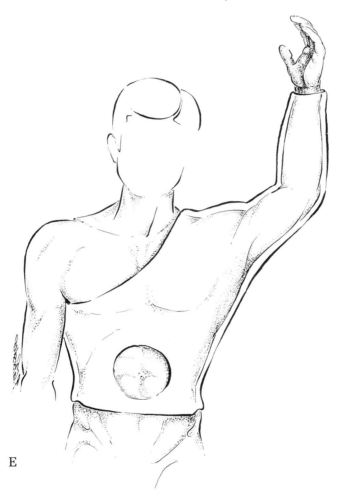

E

Fig. 7–11. Type II injury to proximal humeral epiphysis in fourteen-year-old male. A, Anteroposterior roentgenogram. B, Transthoracic roentgenogram showing flexed head and partial neck fragment. Arrow points to lower margin of fractured humeral metaphysis. C, Overhead (flexion and external rotation) traction has almost reduced displacement of distal fragment in relationship to proximal fragment. D, Following reduction and early healing the patient was placed in single shoulder spica cast with arm in "Statue of Liberty" position. Six weeks total immobilization was followed by active exercises to retrieve full range of motion. E, Illustration of shoulder spica cast used to maintain position seen in D.

The child over eight years of age tends to sustain epiphyseal slip at the proximal humeral epiphysis (Fig. 7–11). The motor pull of the rotator cuff may tend to flex and externally rotate the proximal fragment. The roentgenograms must include anteroposterior as well as lateral views in order to determine the treatment plan. The hanging cast may provide adequate reduction. However, should the hanging arm cast not succeed in reducing the epiphyseal separation within two to four days, then traction must be applied with the arm in an overhead position and the patient supine (Fig. 7–11D) in order to bring the distal fragment to meet the proximal fragment. Following reduction, a shoulder spica may be applied with the arm in adduction and external rotation for approximately six weeks (Fig. 7–11E).

Fracture of the midshaft of the humerus is not common in children. In the infant, overface traction after the fashion of Smith (see treatment of supracondylar fractures in Chapter 8) or sidearm traction may be utilized to treat this fracture until stability ensues; in the relatively short period of seven to ten days, the arm may then be placed in a sling and swathe or in a Velpeau bandage. Blount points out that up to 15 degrees of angulation can be accepted in the midshaft fracture of the humerus in the younger child. Older children from ambulatory age on can be treated with the hanging cast with which good union is anticipated. The bayonet apposition of the humeral fragments resting side to side is ideal in the growing child, inasmuch as the increased vascularity following injury will cause some stimulation to epiphyseal growth. Bayonet apposition has thus accommodated for any overgrowth that will occur from the epiphyseal plate at either end. Only if the child has other injuries that preclude his being ambulatory would traction treatment be used in a patient of this age. Immobilization with traction or cast generally requires no greater a time than six weeks at the maximum.

REFERENCES

1. Adams, J. C.: Outline of Fractures, Including Joint Injuries, 6th ed. Baltimore, Williams & Wilkins Co., 1972.
2. Blount, W. P.: Fractures in Children. Baltimore, Williams & Wilkins, 1954.
3. Charnley, J.: Closed Treatment of Common Fractures, 3rd ed., 1961 (Fourth Reprint) 1972. Edinburgh & London, Churchill Livingstone, 1972.
4. Ralston, E. L.: Handbook of Fractures. St. Louis, C. V. Mosby, 1967.
5. Rang, M. C.: Children's Fractures. Philadelphia, J. B. Lippincott, 1974.
6. Rockwood, C. A., and Green, D. P.: Fractures. Philadelphia, J. B. Lippincott, 1975.
7. Salter, R. B., and Harris, R. W.: Injuries Involving the Epiphyseal Plate. J Bone Joint Surg. 45-A:587, 1963.
8. Watson-Jones, R.: Fractures and Joint Injuries, 4th ed., 2V. Baltimore, Williams & Wilkins, 1952-1955.

8

THE ELBOW

The human elbow is formed with a close tolerance for the normal movements expected between the distal humerus, the proximal ulna, and the proximal radius. The distal humerus flares at its lower end to form the condyles for articulation and the epicondyles for origin of muscles. The cartilaginous surface on the ulna between the coronoid process anteriorly and the olecranon process posteriorly is gently curved to allow for the flexion of the elbow that does occur between it and the trochlea of the distal humerus. The radial head nestles against the lateral margin of the ulna in just such a position as to allow it to flex and extend against the capitulum of the humerus and at the same time to allow rotation motion to provide supination and pronation in the forearm (Fig. 8–1). At the lower end of the upper arm, the brachial artery and veins and the median nerve continue into the antecubital space from a medial position just anterior to the intermuscular septum (Fig. 8–2). About an inch proximal to the elbow the ulnar nerve turns posteriorly through a notch in the intermuscular septum and runs in the ulnar notch on the posterior aspect of the medial humeral condyle. Just distal to the elbow, the ulnar nerve returns to the anterior aspect of the forearm through the two heads of origin of the flexor carpi ulnaris. The radial nerve, which had gone posterior and lateral in the midhumerus, pierces the lateral intermuscular septum at its distal end and passes into the anterior muscular compartment between the brachialis and the brachioradialis near the lateral epicondyle. Here it divides into a superficial and a deep branch. The deep branch dips through the fibers of the spinator some three finger breadths distal to the elbow joint and descends down the forearm as the dorsal interosseous nerve (Fig. 8–2).

Supracondylar and Intercondylar Fractures of Humerus

The mechanisms of injury by which the supracondylar and intercondylar fractures of the humerus occur appear to be varied. The most significant mode of injury is thought to be a longitudinal force from a fall that tends to hyperextend the elbow and create a compressive force at the same time. The proximal ulna and radius, being well fitted to the distal humerus, maintain their relationship, and the bony continuity of the distal humerus gives way to the injuring force.

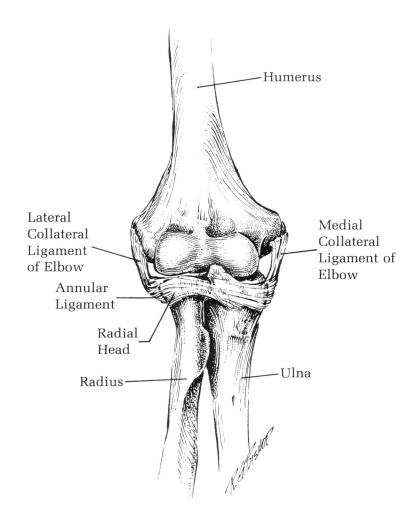

Fig. 8–1. Illustration of articulations at elbow between humerus, radius, and ulna. The stabilizing collateral and annular ligaments are shown in relief.

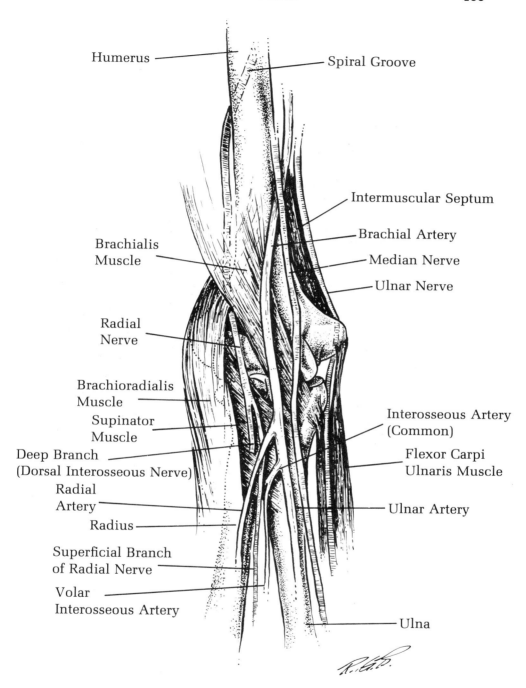

Fig. 8–2. Anterior view of elbow with its complex of brachial vessels. Study of the detailed relationships of median, ulnar, and radial nerves to elbow joint will give a clearer understanding of complications with which elbow injuries are fraught.

Examination. On examination of the involved limb, there is often an extension deformity at the elbow. It is difficult to assess the extent of damage by observation and palpation alone. Although injury to the median nerve, as well as to the brachial artery, is possible, it is not common with this injury in the adult.

Roentgenograms. Roentgenographic examination must include the anteroposterior and lateral views which will show the fracture(s) to have occurred transversely across the humerus just proximal to the condyles and through the thinnest part at the olecranon notch (Fig. 8–3). The fracture may be comminuted through the supracondylar area and may include some comminution into the trochlea. Fracture through the condyle may have also occurred, causing separation of the trochlea and the capitulum.

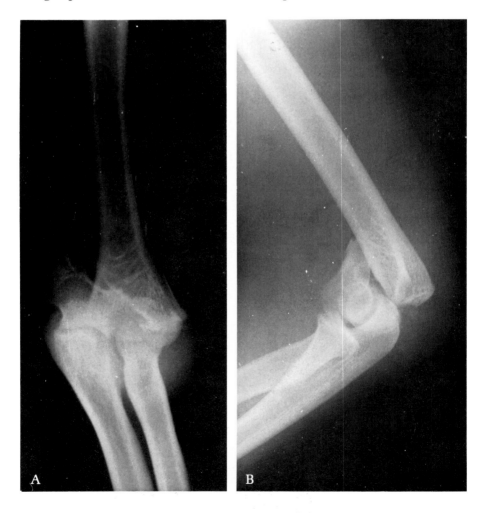

Fig. 8–3. Roentgenograms showing supracondylar fracture of humerus in an adult. A, Anteroposterior view. B, Lateral view. Note anterior displacement of distal fragments. This fracture was treated by traction reduction and maintenance followed by a long arm cast at three weeks.

Treatment. The simple supracondylar fracture that is undisplaced can be treated in a long arm plaster of Paris cast for six weeks followed by early mobilization. Such a fracture, however, is the exception and more commonly one is dealing with a comminuted fracture which requires either overface or sidearm traction from a Kirschner wire placed through the olecranon process. Each of these two methods of treatment requires approximately three to four weeks in traction followed by immobilization in a cast until evidence of bony stability is seen (about eight weeks). Mobilization must be begun as soon as fracture stability is present in order to obtain the optimum result. Occasionally the fracture fragments are sufficiently large to allow open reduction and internal fixation with Kirschner wires, screws, or a blade plate device. The

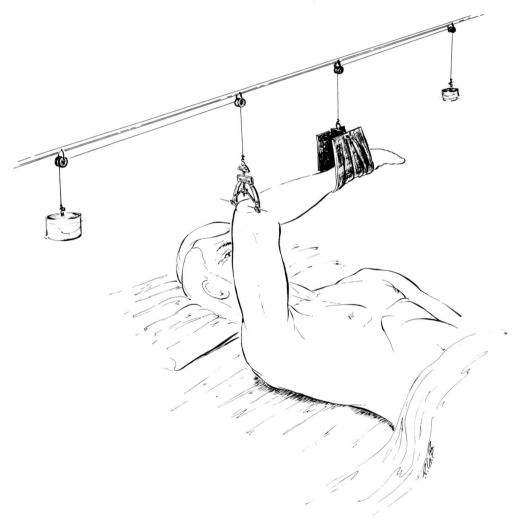

Fig. 8-4. Overface skeletal traction. Of particular value with the supracondylar humeral fracture in adult or child.

proponents of open reduction and internal fixation point out the necessity for as accurate a reduction as possible for the greatest ultimate range of motion in the elbow. The overface method of traction (Fig. 8–4) followed by immobilization in a cast and then by an intensive program of range of motion exercises has given as good a result as any single system of treatment.

Posterior Dislocation of Elbow

Posterior dislocation of the elbow without fracture of the coronoid process can only occur with the elbow flexed at approximately 45 degrees. With the elbow flexed at this position, a longitudinal force along the shaft of the radius and ulna can cause this dislocation. The olecranon process seems to catch in the olecranon fossa and lever the anterior ulna and radius off the joint surface of the distal humerus, allowing both bones to slip posterior to the humerus. Often there may be some temporary occlusion of the brachial artery and occasionally temporary injury to the ulnar or median nerve because of their anatomic location and their compromise by the posterior position of the forearm at the elbow.

In order for a posterior dislocation to occur, there must be a tearing of the medial and lateral collateral ligamentous structures at the elbow. In addition, some separation of fibers must occur in the anterior and posterior capsules of the elbow joint. Should these separations and fiber tears occur at the points of insertion into bone, likely there will be an effort on the part of the body to repair these areas by new bone growth. Because of this, the timing of mobilization is crucial. It must be started sufficiently early to regain adequate motion and yet not too early to foster lack of stability.

Examination. Examination of the dislocated elbow shows the olecranon process to be posterior to its usual relationship. The elbow cannot flex and extend through its usual range of motion. Supination and pronation of the forearm are often unimpaired. Neurologic deficit may or may not be present; this information must be documented prior to any treatment.

Roentgenograms. Anteroposterior and lateral roentgenographic views confirm the positioning of the proximal radius and ulna posterior to the distal humerus (Fig. 8–5). On the anteroposterior view, the radial head and the coronoid process and olecranon are superimposed directly over the joint surface of the distal humerus. On the lateral view the roentgenogram will show the radius and the ulna lying directly posterior to the joint surface of the distal humerus.

Treatment. The treatment for a posterior dislocation of the elbow is reduction of the dislocation as soon as possible. A combination of meperidine and diazepam may provide sufficient relaxation and analgesia in the period immediately following dislocation to allow manipulative relocation. If not, then a general anesthetic is indicated. The relocation can be accomplished with the forearm supinated, the elbow flexed to 45 degrees from full extension, and a longitudinal traction applied to the forearm while countertraction is placed against the upper arm. As soon as the radius and ulna slip back into their normal relationship with the humerus, the arm is immobilized in a long arm plaster of Paris cast with the elbow flexed to 90 degrees. For comfort, the forearm is placed in a neutral pronation-supination position. The arm should

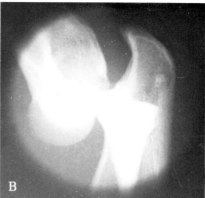

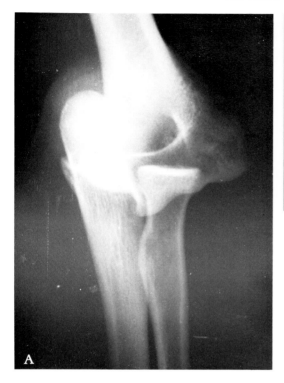

Fig. 8–5. Roentgenograms of elbow dislocated by excessive supination coupled with a distal to proximal force. A, Anteroposterior view. B, Lateral view confirming posterior position of proximal ulna and radius.

be kept in this position approximately four weeks. Careful postreduction monitoring is necessary to assure no complication ensues from swelling. The cast is then removed, the arm is placed in a collar and cuff or a sling, and gradual range of motion exercises are begun.

Anterior Dislocation of Elbow

Although not as common an injury as the other types of dislocations of the elbow, the anterior dislocation does occur and tearing of muscle must be accompanied by a fracture of the olecranon process. The mechanism is a posterior to anterior force to the flexed proximal forearm.

Examination. An evident anterior position of the forearm is noted in relationship to the elbow and upper arm. There is significant instability and crepitus on examination. Since the displacement is toward the major neurovascular bundle, there is seldom a neurologic or a vascular deficit.

Roentgenograms. On anteroposterior roentgenograms the proximal radius and coronoid process of the ulna are seen to overlie the distal humerus (Fig. 8–6A). Fracture fragments from the olecranon process are in evidence. On the lateral view the distal humeral condyles are seen to lie posterior to the proximal radius and coronoid process of the ulna. The olecranon process is fractured (Fig. 8–6B).

Treatment. An anterior dislocation of the elbow is unstable until reduced and the olecranon process fixed surgically. For further treatment of olecranon fractures see the section on fractures of the olecranon process.

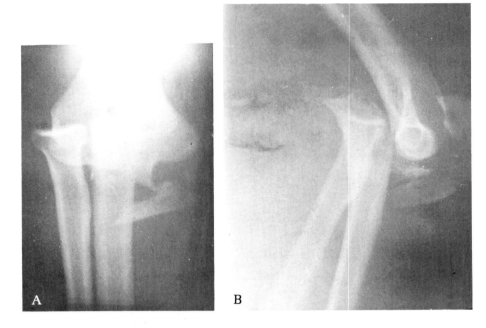

Fig. 8–6. Roentgenograms of fracture dislocation of elbow. A, Anteroposterior view. B, Lateral view confirming anterior dislocation of radius and ulna on humerus with obligatory fracture of olecranon process. Open reduction and fixation of olecranon will be necessary to secure adequate elbow control.

Posteromedial Rotary Dislocation of Elbow

The mechanism of injury for the posteromedial dislocation of the elbow is a hypersupination force to an arm flexed to approximately 45 degrees. At the same time a longitudinal force passes proximally along the axis of the radius and ulna. The effect is to rotate the entire radius and ulna into the medial aspect of the distal upper arm.

Posteromedial rotary dislocation is not typically associated with nerve or vascular injury, inasmuch as the shift of the bones is toward the vital structures. Just as in the pure posterior dislocation, there must be separation of fibers of the collateral ligaments, medial and lateral, as well as some tearing of the anterior and posterior elbow joint capsule for this injury to occur.

Examination. On examination of the arm with a posteromedial rotary dislocation, the prominence of the olecranon process will be medial. The forearm can be pronated less than the anticipated normal amount, but supination can be performed to a greater than normal extent. There is definite guarding against flexion and extension of the elbow following this injury.

Roentgenograms. On the anteroposterior roentgenogram the radius and ulna will be seen to lie medial to their normal relationship with the distal humerus (Fig. 8–17A). When the distal humerus appears to be in its anteroposterior position, the view of the proximal radius and ulna will be an oblique one. On the lateral roentgenogram of the elbow, there will be superimposition of the proximal radius and ulna over the distal humerus (Fig. 8-17B). Whereas the distal humerus will show typical features of a lateral view, the proximal radius and ulna will show some features of the anterior view.

Treatment. The treatment of the posteromedial rotary dislocation is to reduce the dislocation as promptly as possible. A combination of meperidine and diazepam often provides sufficient relaxation and analgesia to allow a reduction of the radius and the ulna into their normal relationship with the humerus. Should this not be easily possible, there should be no hesitancy in utilizing a general anesthetic for this purpose. Once relaxation is obtained, the reduction is accomplished by flexing the elbow at approximately 45 degrees while longitudinal traction is applied to the forearm. A pronation rotary type of motion is accomplished with the opposite hand on the proximal forearm. During the manipulation, countertraction and a counterforce are applied to the distal upper arm by an assistant. Once reduced, the arm is immobilized in a long arm cast with the elbow at a right angle and with the forearm pronated slightly more than neutral. This position should be maintained for three to four weeks, and if stability is present at this point, then a collar and cuff or a sling may be used for an additional three weeks while the patient initiates an active exercise program to regain range of motion.

Posterolateral Rotary Dislocation of Elbow

The posterolateral rotary dislocation of the elbow is the least common of the dislocations of the elbow. It occurs when a predominantly longitudinal force passing from distal to proximal along the axis of the radius and ulna is accompanied by a hyperpronation force. The elbow is flexed about 45 degrees when this dislocation occurs. The direction of this dislocation may put an unusual stress on the brachial vessels, the median nerve, or the ulnar nerve, causing a deficit in the distribution of any one of them.

Examination. In the posterolateral rotary dislocation the olecranon process is prominent and the radial head is lateral to its usual relationship with the distal humerus. A medial defect will be palpated at the point of usual contact between the proximal ulna and the distal humerus. Supination is limited in the forearm, and pronation is excessive. Flexion and extension are guarded.

Roentgenograms. The anteroposterior roentgenographic view shows the proximal radius and ulna lying lateral to the usual articular process of the distal humerus (Fig. 8–7A). Some of the features seen in an anteroposterior view of the distal humerus will be combined with features seen in a lateral view of the proximal radius and ulna. There will be on the lateral view superimposition of portions of a typical anteroposterior view of the proximal radius and ulna (Fig. 8–7B).

Treatment. The posterolateral rotary dislocation should be reduced as soon as is practical. A combination of meperidine and diazepam will often provide sufficient analgesia and relaxation to allow the reduction of this dislocation. However, should relaxation be insufficient with this combination, a general anesthetic should be used for reduction of this dislocation. The reduction of the dislocation is accomplished with the elbow flexed to 45 degrees; longitudinal traction is applied, and simultaneously a supination force is added to the proximal forearm. At the same time, an assistant will provide countertraction

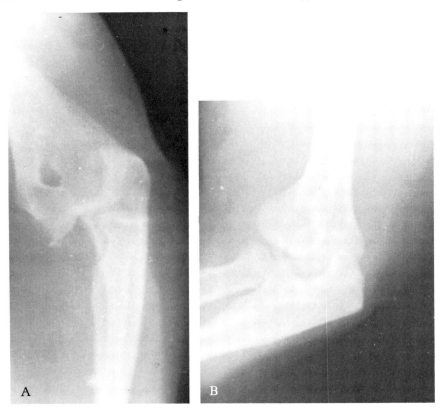

Fig. 8–7. Roentgenograms showing pronation dislocation of elbow in young adult. A, Anteroposterior view. The distal humerus is seen in a relative anteroposterior view while the proximal radius and ulna are seen in the relief expected in the lateral roentgenogram. B, Visualization in a plane 90 degrees from that seen in A, not a true lateral view. The distal humerus is seen more toward a lateral view while the proximal radius and ulna are seen more toward an anteroposterior configuration.

and a counterforce to the distal upper arm. As soon as this dislocation is reduced, a long arm plaster of Paris cast is applied with the elbow flexed to 90 degrees and the forearm supinated approximately 20 degrees from midrotation neutral. This position should be maintained for three to four weeks and followed by use of a collar and cuff or a sling. At this point, the patient should begin early range of motion exercises in an effort to ultimately regain full flexion and extension as well as supination and pronation.

Fracture of Radial Head or Neck

Fractures of the radial head or neck in the adult usually occur by application of a longitudinal force along the axis of the radius with the elbow either fully or almost fully extended. If the elbow is fully extended, the neck of the radius tends to fracture and may well impact. If the elbow is slightly flexed, a shear fracture may occur along one side of the radial head, or the radial head may be tipped by a fracture occurring at its neck.

Examination. On examination, the elbow is extremely tender to any movements of flexion and extension or supination and pronation. There often is a bulge posteriorly in the small synovial space between the ulna and the radial neck.

Roentgenograms. Anteroposterior and lateral roentgenographic views should confirm the exact nature of the fracture (Fig. 8–8).

Treatment. If there is no significant displacement and/or evidence of impaction is present in a fracture at the neck, the arm can be supported by a collar and cuff. Aspiration of the elbow joint is effective in relieving the patient's discomfort. If a fractured radial neck is evident and the articular surface tilts to the extent of 25 degrees or more, it is unlikely that this can be a satisfactory result. Plans for early operation should be made. Aspirating this elbow will lessen the patient's discomfort in the interim. Aspiration of the elbow posteriorly between the neck of the radius and the ulna has been most effective. This aspiration is done under local anesthetic following surgical preparation. A compression dressing is applied and a sling or a collar and cuff is then used.

Also, if a significant portion of the radial head is fractured off, then it is wise to recommend excision of the radial head within the next several days. The arm can be treated in the interim by aspiration. A word of caution regarding excision of the radial head must be given at this point. In one instance of fracture of the radial neck with significant angulation, two months after excision of the radial head the wrist was being forced into ulnar deviation

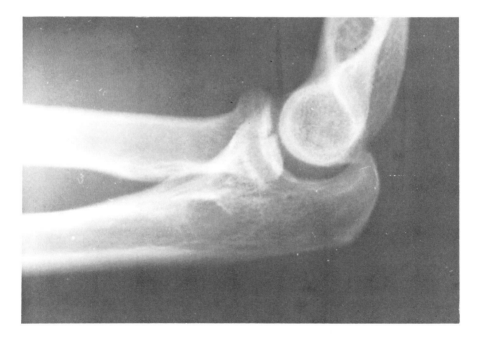

Fig. 8–8. Lateral roentgenogram of fracture through articular surface of radial head. Joint incongruity may require resection of this radial head, although one could justify six weeks immobilization of this elbow in a cast followed by trial of use.

because of proximal settling of the radius. A separation of the distal radioulnar ligaments had occurred at the time of the original injury—obviously unrecognized at the time of radial head excision. Subsequent attention to this detail during the examination has on occasion yielded evidence of injury to these ligaments; acute local tenderness on palpation and occasional roentgenographic evidence of distal radioulnar separation are evidences of this injury. When injury is identified, these distal radioulnar ligaments must be repaired at the time of the radial head excision. Temporary distal radioulnar fixation may be furnished by two transverse Kirschner wires.

Fracture of Olecranon Process

Fractures of the olecranon process of the ulna occur most commonly by direct blow but may be associated with an attempted anterior dislocation of the forearm in relationship to the humerus. The fractures occur from the level of the coronoid process proximally to the tip.

Examination. On examination, there will be definite tenderness over the fracture line of the olecranon process. A gap can be palpated between two bone ends when displacement is present.

Roentgenograms. Anteroposterior and lateral roentgenograms will confirm the diagnosis of fractured olecranon (Fig. 8–9) and indicate the extent of separation of the fragment(s) as well as the level of the fracture.

Treatment. Should no separation of fragments be present, the treatment is simple. A long arm cast is applied with the elbow extended 30 degrees short of full extension. This relieves the pull of the triceps from its insertion onto the olecranon process. In the elderly patient with a displaced or comminuted olecranon fracture, fragment approximation and union can sometimes be

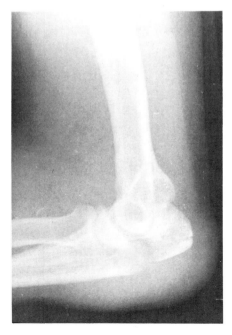

Fig. 8–9. Lateral roentgenogram showing fracture of olecranon process.

achieved by a long arm cast with the elbow extended. This position must be changed after three to four weeks by application of a new cast with the elbow flexed 40 degrees from full extension. However, should significant separation of fragments be present, operative approximation of the fragments must be accomplished in order to provide strong extension of the elbow. Fractures including up to 30% of the proximal olecranon process may be treated by excision of the proximal fragment and reattachment of the tendon of the triceps to the olecranon distal to the fracture; fractures involving more than 30% of the olecranon process warrant reapproximation and internal fixation.

The method of internal fixation varies from surgeon to surgeon. The wood screw has effectively held the fragments together, but in my own experience has rotated the proximal fragment sufficiently to cause modest joint incon-

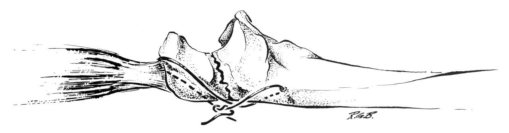

Fig. 8–10. Illustration of figure-of-8 wire used in treating uncomminuted displaced fracture of olecranon.

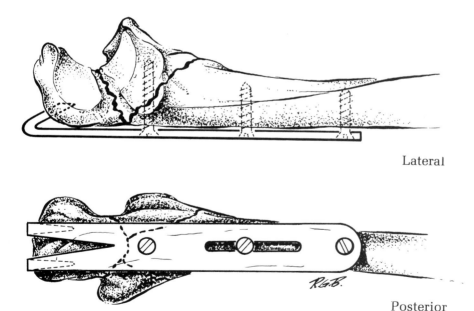

Lateral

Posterior

Fig. 8–11. Illustration of Zuelzer plate in use for fixation of comminuted fracture of olecranon process. Note that the screw spears fracture of coronoid process for antecubital fixation. (After Karl Alfred.)

gruity. More effective in reducing the olecranon fracture and in maintaining its reduction accurately has been a figure-of-8 wire passed under the tendon of the triceps and crossed at the site of the fracture on the dorsal side of the olecranon process. The wire is then passed through a hole drilled transversely in the dorsal ulna distal to the fracture (Fig. 8–10). Tightening the wire reduces and fixes the fracture fragments. The comminuted fracture of the olecranon process, which includes the coronoid process fracture, has been treated successfully by Alfred, who uses the Zuelzer plate along the dorsal olecranon surface. The tips of the hooks are bent into an acute angle and caught into the tip of the olecranon process. The central screw through the Zuelzer plate is so placed as to transfix the coronoid process into its normal position (Fig. 8–11).

After open reduction of an olecranon fracture it is good practice to immobilize the elbow for approximately two months. The arm is then placed in a collar and cuff or a sling, and a program of gentle range of motion exercises is initiated.

Fracture of Coronoid Process

An isolated fracture of the coronoid process occurs occasionally in the adult. It appears to be a product of hyperextension in which the capsule avulses a small segment of the coronoid process.

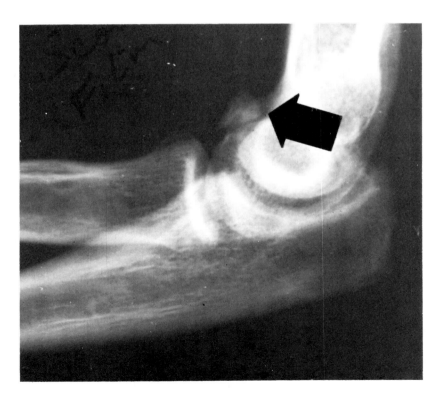

Fig. 8–12. Lateral roentgenogram of elbow in which coronoid process of the ulna has been fractured and displaced (arrow). Simple excision of this fragment is often the best treatment.

Examination. Palpation does not confirm a diagnosis except to pinpoint an area of tenderness at the anterior joint line of the elbow.

Roentgenograms. The lateral roentgenogram confirms the separation of a fragment from the coronoid process (Fig. 8–12). The anteroposterior roentgenogram is not particularly revealing.

Treatment. The treatment is immobilization in a long arm plaster of Paris cast with the elbow at 90 degrees flexion and the forearm in 45 degrees supination for approximately four weeks. A sling is used after this for comfort while range of motion exercises are gradually begun. Occasionally, surgical excision is necessary before symptoms subside.

INJURIES TO THE ELBOW IN CHILDREN

Injuries to the elbow occur frequently in children. Dislocations and supracondylar fractures are perhaps the most common, but fractures of the lateral condyle, the medial epicondyle, and the radial neck are also seen. In assessing and treating them, consideration must be given to the ossification centers, which appear at different stages in development. An ossification center appears in the capitulum about the second year of growth, in the epicondyle and the head of the radius about the fifth year, in the trochlea and the olecranon about the tenth year, and in the lateral epicondyle about the twelfth year.

Supracondylar Fractures—Posteriorly Displaced

Two types of supracondylar fracture tend to occur in the child. The more common supracondylar injury is the hyperextension injury with posterior displacement of the distal fragment and the elbow joint. This injury is fraught with potential vascular as well as median and ulnar nerve deficits.

Examination. A definite shift can be observed in the elbow. Palpation produces pain and reveals the olecranon prominence posterior to its usual position. The examination must include testing sensory and motor capability distal to the fracture. Palpation of the radial pulse and visualization of the nail beds are also an essential part of the examination.

Roentgenograms. The anteroposterior and lateral roentgenograms will show the fracture across the supracondylar segment of the humerus with the condyle and elbow joint posterior to the humeral shaft (Fig. 8–13). Adequate evaluation can be accomplished only by visualizing similar roentgenographic views of the opposite elbow.

Treatment. The undisplaced supracondylar fracture may be treated by flexing the elbow slightly greater than 90 degrees and maintaining this position either with a splint, a plaster of Paris cast, or a collar and cuff. If there is no evidence of neurologic or vascular deficit and the surgeon has adequate experience in dealing with this injury, the fracture may be reduced under general anesthesia by gentle hyperextension followed by manipulation of the distal humeral fragment anteriorly into its normal relationship with the proximal humerus. The manipulation is aided by the thumb. If accurate reduction is accomplished, the elbow will flex beyond 90 degrees without force. Maintenance of the radial pulse is monitored throughout the manipulation procedure. The arm is then maintained in slightly greater than 90 degrees flexion by the use of a posterior plaster of Paris mold and a collar and cuff. The

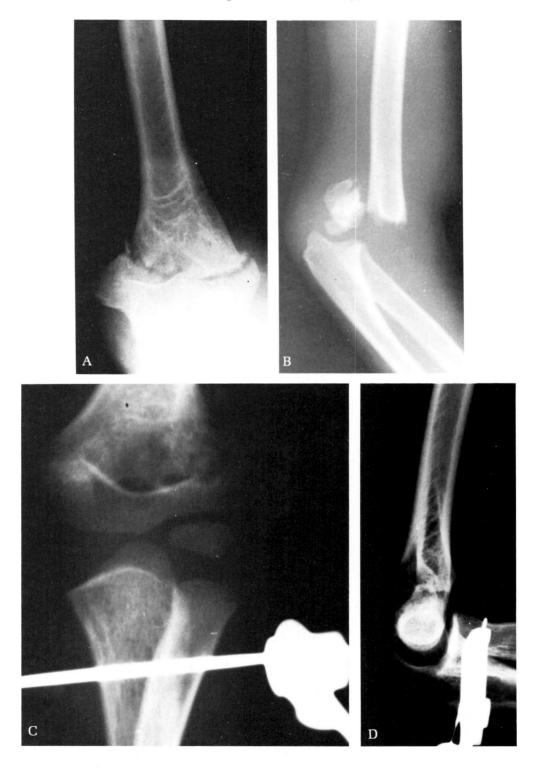

patient is watched closely for any evidence of undue pain or loss of normal pink color in the skin and the nail beds. Evidence of inability to flex the distal phalanges of the thumb, index, and middle fingers is checked. Any adverse change suggests a careful watch for other signs of a Volkmann's ischemic contracture (discussed later).

Should the physician treating a child with a displaced supracondylar fracture be inexperienced or should he have significant hesitancy regarding manipulation of the elbow under anesthetic, the safe approach is certainly to insert a Kirschner wire in the olecranon under general anesthetic and place this limb either in Dunlop's sidearm traction as used by Blount (Fig. 8–14) or in the overface type of traction as recommended by Smith (Fig. 8–4). I have treated a sizable group by each method and prefer the overface traction because it utilizes the effect of gravity to eliminate most of the swelling that occurs distal to the fracture. The three-point method of reduction as described by Smith uses the olecranon process and the medial and the lateral epipcondyles to monitor reduction and its maintenance. The traction methods of treatment allow constant monitoring of the radial pulse, as well as evaluation of the neurologic status from a sensory and motor standpoint. After approximately two weeks in traction, stability is generally present, and a long arm plaster of Paris cast or a collar and cuff can be applied with the arm flexed slightly greater than 90 degrees.

One of the most feared complications of the supracondylar fracture is Volkmann's ischemic contracture of the forearm. Bleb formation of the skin at

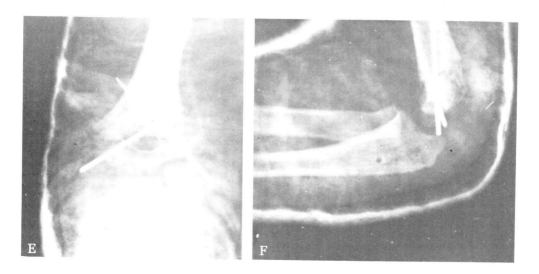

Fig. 8–13. Roentgenograms showing supracondylar fracture of the humerus in a six-year-old child. A, Anteroposterior view. B, lateral view. Note significant posterior displacement and swelling of soft tissue. C, Anteroposterior and D, lateral roentgenograms showing progress in reduction after two days of traction. Symptoms and signs of Volkmann's ischemic contracture ensued at this point, however, and operative fasciotomy of the forearm was combined with reduction and fixation of the fracture. E, Postoperative anteroposterior and F, lateral roentgenograms showing fracture anatomically reduced and fixed with crossed Kirschner wires.

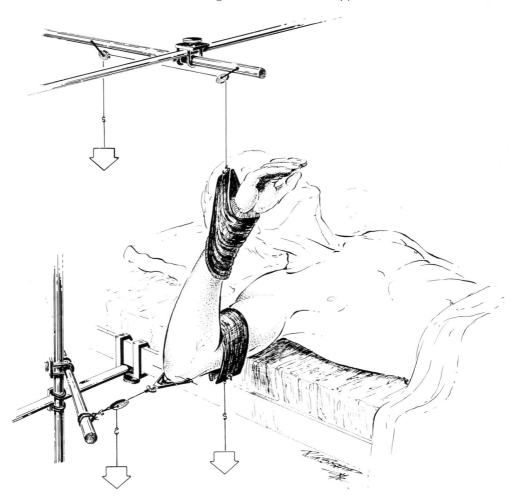

Fig. 8–14. Sidearm traction as used by Blount.

an early phase in the treatment of this injury has appeared to be a harbinger of impending Volkmann's ischemic contracture. Loss of pulse, progressive decrease in sensation, and weakness or loss of flexion capability of the thumb and the index and middle fingers at the interphalangeal joints are considered signs sufficiently diagnostic of Volkmann's contracture to warrant release of the fascia of the forearm. Once release of the fascia of the forearm is accomplished surgically, an adequate reduction of the fracture under direct visualization followed by internal fixation should be performed (Fig. 8–13E, F). In addition to exploring the brachial artery, elevation of the artery from its bed and injecting 1% local anesthetic about the artery and into its lumen have been helpful in reversing the process of Volkmann's ischemic contracture (Fig. 1–30). Too much emphasis cannot be placed on the need for early and adequate treatment of this complication.

Supracondylar Fractures—Anteriorly Displaced

The other type of supracondylar fracture is caused by a posterior to anterior force against the olecranon process. This is the rarer of the supracondylar injuries.

Examination. On examination, there will be an anterior shift of the distal humerus, radius and ulna. This causes a loss of the posterior definition of the elbow to palpation.

Roentgenograms. The anteroposterior and lateral roentgenograms confirm a fracture through the supracondylar portion of the humerus with an anterior shift of the condyles and the radius and ulna.

Treatment. Inasmuch as this type of supracondylar fracture has occurred by a force from posterior to anterior, some stability can be anticipated along the periosteum anteriorly. Accordingly, application of the cast while the arm is in a partially extended position would be indicated. A general anesthetic is necessary for reduction of this fracture. A long arm cast is applied with the elbow flexed 35 degrees short of full extension, and the cast is molded to provide three-point fixation, the proximal and distal points of force going posteriorly and the central point at the fracture site going anteriorly.

Fracture of Lateral Condyle of Humerus

Fracture of the lateral condyle of the humerus occurs when a hyperextension force is added to an adduction force to the elbow. The fracture line extends from the trochlea in the center of the humeral articular process up to the superior margin of the lateral epicondyle.

Examination. Examination of the elbow with a fracture of the lateral condyle may be unrevealing. The only sign may be an irritable child who has pain in the area of the elbow. Generally, in order to identify this injury by physical examination, there must be some displacement.

Roentgenograms. In order to evaluate injury to the lateral condyle, roentgenograms of both elbows must be taken with the anteroposterior and lateral views mirroring each other as much as possible. The fracture line should be evident from the midtrochlea proximal through the cortex of the lateral epicondyle on the anteroposterior view (Fig. 8–15). In the younger child, one must rely on the comparison views of the opposite elbow. The ossification centers can be misleading and confusing, even when utilizing the comparison views.

Treatment. If there is no or only slight displacement of the lateral condyle, the position may be maintained by placing the arm in a cast with the elbow flexed slightly greater than 90 degrees and the wrist extended. However, roentgenograms should be taken after two days and again after a week to be certain that displacement has not occurred. Since the extensor muscles of the wrist and fingers originate from this condyle, there is a tendency for the reduction position to be lost. In general, open reduction and internal fixation with two crossed Kirschner wires is the most effective treatment program for the displaced lateral condylar fracture because the extensor muscle origins will create a constant displacing force on this fragment. Following operation, a long arm cast is applied with the elbow flexed slightly above 90 degrees and with the wrist extended to the position of function. The pins can be removed at four

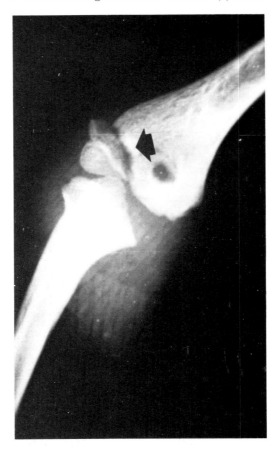

Fig. 8–15. Anteroposterior roentgenogram showing fractured lateral condyle (arrow) in a child. Internal fixation with threaded Kirschner wire is treatment of choice because extensor muscle origins will create constant displacing force on fragment.

weeks, and formal immobilization can cease at six weeks. An active program to increase range of motion should be started once the immobilization is no longer necessary.

Fracture of Medial Epicondyle

Medial epicondyle avulsion can occur from a valgus stress at the elbow from any cause. The epicondyle is an apophysis from which originates a portion of the flexor muscles to the wrist and the hand.

Examination. On examination, there may be observable swelling and ecchymosis over the medial epicondylar area. There will be distinct tenderness to palpation. There may be some crepitus palpable if the fragment is free. Active flexion of the wrist and fingers causes pain along the medial elbow, particularly if such flexion is only slightly resisted.

Roentgenograms and Treatment. The anteroposterior roentgenogram is most telling in showing the relationship of the ossific center of the medial epicon-

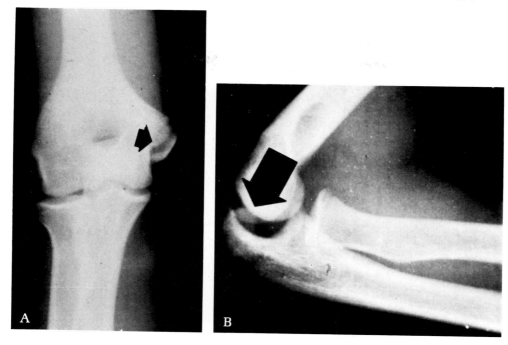

Fig. 8–16. A, Anteroposterior roentgenogram showing minimal slip of medial humeral epicondyle accompanied by widened epiphyseal plate (arrow points to widened area of lucency). B, Lateral roentgenogram of elbow in which medial humeral epicondyle has been avulsed and lies in elbow joint (arrow). This type of fracture requires operative removal and reattachment by Kirschner wire(s).

dyle (Fig. 8–16A). If the clear space between the ossific center and the lateral margin of the humerus is no more than 3 to 4 millimeters, the avulsion is incomplete and brief immobilization of ten days to two weeks should be sufficient. However, if the ossific center of the apophysis seems to be significantly displaced (more than 4 millimeters) and a comparison view of the opposite elbow confirms this, then open reduction and internal fixation is the treatment choice. Occasionally the epicondyle will be completely avulsed and dropped into the medial humeroulnar joint (Fig. 8–16B). A careful look at the roentgenogram and comparison with the opposite side will confirm this circumstance. The operative removal of the fragment from the joint and fixation to its bed of origin are essential.

Following either operative procedure, immobilization should be accomplished for three to four weeks with the long arm cast and the elbow flexed to 90 degrees. The pin(s) may be removed at four weeks and the arm then placed in a collar and cuff. A program of exercises to increase range of motion should be started.

Dislocations of Elbow

Dislocation of the elbow in the child is usually the posterior dislocation caused by a longitudinal force from distal to proximal along the ulna of a 45-degree flexed elbow.

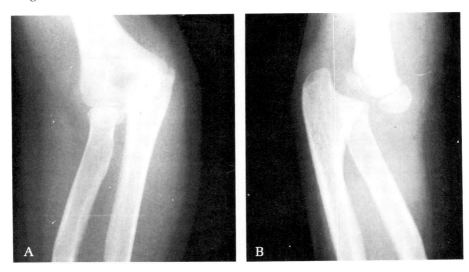

Fig. 8–17. Roentgenograms of posterior dislocation in elbow of five-year-old child. A, Anteroposterior view. The proximal radius and ulna overlie the distal humerus. B, Lateral view showing proximal radius and ulna lying posterior to distal humerus.

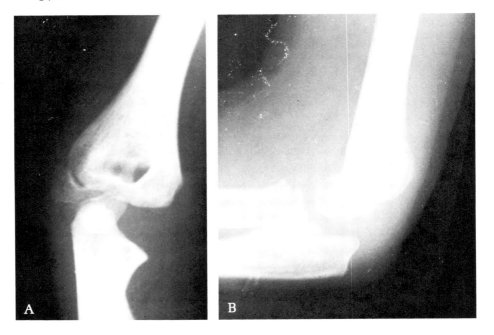

Fig. 8–18. Roentgenograms of distal humerus in eight-year-old child, showing pronation type of dislocation. A, Anteroposterior view. B, True lateral view of proximal radius and ulna. Note they lie toward an anteroposterior plane.

Examination. Examination of the arm with a dislocated elbow reveals the prominence of the olecranon process to be posterior to its usual position. The arm should be examined peripheral to the elbow for evidence of neurologic or vascular deficit; however, this is rare following dislocation of the elbow in the child.

Roentgenograms. The anteroposterior roentgenogram (Figs. 8–17, 8–18) shows the proximal radius and ulna superimposed on the distal humerus. The lateral roentgenogram will show the proximal radius and ulna resting posterior to the distal articular surface of the humerus. Comparison views of the opposite elbow are helpful to be certain no ossific center is in an abnormal position. However, fracture with a dislocation in the child is unusual.

Treatment. The dislocation, if seen early, can usually be reduced without a general anesthetic. It is well to give an analgesic agent such as meperidine prior to the reduction. The reduction is accomplished by longitudinal traction with the elbow flexed approximately 45 degrees and with minimal flexion-extension movements occurring while traction is applied. Countertraction is applied to the lower end of the humerus by an assistant. Once reduction is accomplished, the arm should be immobilized for four weeks with the elbow flexed to 90 degrees and the forearm in midrotation.

Fracture of Radial Neck

The line of force that creates a radial neck fracture is usually the longitudinal force transmitted up the shaft of the radius. This forces the head of the radius against the capitulum.

Examination. The child with a fracture of the radial neck will be irritable, and the elbow will be extremely tender to palpation. Any efforts at passive or active supination and pronation are painful, as are any efforts at flexion and extension.

Roentgenograms. The anteroposterior and lateral roentgenograms show typically a separation at the epiphyseal plate of the proximal radius with a small flake of the metaphysis of the radius attached to it (Fig. 8–19). The fracture is more than likely incomplete with minimal angulation, but any degree of angulation may be noted, however, up to total displacement of the radial head from the neck.

Treatment. The minimally angulated radial neck fracture is treated by applying a cast with the elbow flexed 90 degrees and the forearm in a neutral supination-pronation position. If the angulation is more than 20 degrees but less than 45 degrees, an effort should be made to gently "nudge" the head back into position while the forearm is supinated and pronated. This maneuver is best done under a general anesthetic. Improvement of position or maintenance of the angulation at less than 45 degrees, is acceptable as long as displacement is not present. However, if partial or total displacement is present or if the angulation is greater than 45 degrees and cannot be diminished by manipulation, then the operative approach is indicated. Since the potential growth of the proximal radius lies within the displaced fragment, it must be handled with extreme care. Under direct vision, this fragment should be placed onto the radial neck. An adsorbable suture may be placed from the periosteum of the radial neck into the radial head if such is deemed helpful. Only in the event of instability, with supination and pronation while flexed at 90 degrees, should a

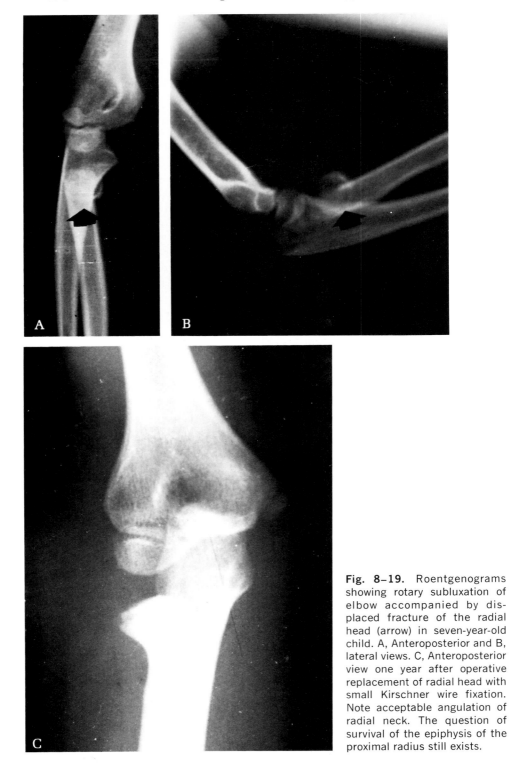

Fig. 8–19. Roentgenograms showing rotary subluxation of elbow accompanied by displaced fracture of the radial head (arrow) in seven-year-old child. A, Anteroposterior and B, lateral views. C, Anteroposterior view one year after operative replacement of radial head with small Kirschner wire fixation. Note acceptable angulation of radial neck. The question of survival of the epiphysis of the proximal radius still exists.

small threaded Kirschner wire be passed through the capitulum across the centrum of the head and down into the shaft of the radius. Such wire should be removed at three to four weeks. The head of the radius must never be excised in a growing child.

Dislocation of Radial Head

Isolated dislocation of the proximal radius will not occur without a concomitant fracture of the shaft of the ulna (Monteggia fracture-dislocation) and/or a tear of the annular ligament that holds the radius in its relationship with the ulna. The mechanism of injury is either a force from the dorsal side of the forearm fracturing the ulna and driving the radius anteriorly or a force to the volar surface of the forearm which will fracture the ulna, angulate it posteriorly, and dislocate the radial head posteriorly.

Examination. Either the Monteggia fracture-dislocation or a tear of the annular ligament is recognized by the angulation of the ulna and prominence of the radial head in the direction of the angulation.

Roentgenograms. Roentgenographic examination will confirm the fracture of the ulna with angulation toward the direction in which the radial head dislocates (Fig. 8–20).

Treatment. The treatment for the fracture-dislocation or the ligamentous tear is to attempt closed reduction of the ulna with return of the radial head to its relationships with the ulna and the capitulum of the humerus. Failure of reduction requires opening directly down to the neck of the radius and reestablishing the annular ligament. Once this is done it should not be

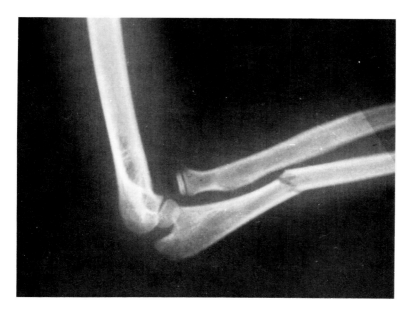

Fig. 8–20. Lateral roentgenogram of elbow of nine-year-old child in which dislocation of anterior radial head has accompanied angulated fracture of ulna. This is the Monteggia fracture dislocation. The both bone principle forces dislocation of the radial head.

necessary to consider any type of internal fixation in the ulna. Surgical or nonsurgical treatment requires approximately two months in a plaster of Paris cast for union of the ulnar fracture. Once the ulnar fracture is united in a reduced position, the radial head will remain reduced. An active range of motion exercise program should be started as soon as the cast is removed.

Nursemaid's Elbow

Nursemaid's elbow is most commonly caused by the nursemaid or parent lifting a child by one arm.

Examination. The examination reveals pain at the elbow and inability to actively or passively fully supinate and pronate because of pain. The arm is held in a guarded position with the elbow flexed.

Roentgenograms. The anteroposterior and lateral roentgenograms are invariably normal. It is thought that the pathology is a mobilization of the annular ligament up to the margin of the head of the radius where it becomes temporarily trapped.

Treatment. The treatment is most effectively accomplished by adduction of the elbow accompanied with a quick supination-pronation movement. The patient is immediately relieved, and although a sling or a collar and cuff may be used for several days, it is usually not necessary.

REFERENCES

1. Adams, J. C.: Outline of Fractures, Including Joint Injuries, 6th ed. Baltimore, Williams & Wilkins Co., 1972.
2. Alfred, K.: Personal Communication.
3. Blount, W. P.: Fractures in Children. Baltimore, Williams & Wilkins Co., 1954.
4. Charnley, J.: Closed Treatment of Common Fractures, 3rd ed., 1961, (Fourth Reprint) 1972. Edinburgh & London, Churchill Livingstone, 1972.
5. Ralston, E. L.: Handbook of Fractures. St. Louis, C. V. Mosby Co., 1967.
6. Rang, M. C.: Children's Fractures. Philadelphia, J. B. Lippincott Co., 1974.
7. Rockwood, C. A., and Green, D. P.: Fractures. Philadelphia, J. B. Lippincott Co., 1975.
8. Smith, L.: Deformity following supracondylar fractures of the humerus. J. Bone Joint Surg. 42-A:235, 1960.
9. Smith, L.: Deformity following supracondylar fractures of the humerus. J. Bone Joint Surg. 47-A:1668, 1965.
10. Smith, L.: Supracondylar fractures of the humerus treated by direct observation. Clin. Orthop. 50:37, 1967.
11. Watson-Jones, R.: Fractures and Joint Injuries, 4th ed., 2V. Baltimore, Williams & Wilkins Co., 1952-1955.

9

THE FOREARM

The unique requirements of the forearm for flexion and extension, as well as for supination and pronation, require some unusual anatomic features to make this accommodation. The joint at the elbow is a ginglymus or moving hinge type of joint. This accomplishes the movement of bringing the hand from a distal position up to a proximal position toward the body. When the forearm is at full supination, the radius and the ulna are relatively parallel to each other, the radius having a modest lateral bow to it. As the forearm is brought from this position into a full pronation position, the radius remains anchored to its proximal relationship with the ulna while the distal radius rotates about the fixed shaft of the ulna a full 180 degrees. This allows the hand to be moved from a fully supinated or palm-up position into one of full pronation (palm down).

The distal radius is anchored to the distal ulna by a series of small ligaments that maintain stability but allow the mobility necessary for rotation to occur. Deep to the ligaments, between the radius and the ulna, lies a triangular cartilage which appears to serve as something of a buffer (Fig. 9–6). An interosseous membrane is attached from the radius to the ulna throughout the entire length of the forearm. It divides the anterior compartment from the posterior compartment of the forearm. The fibers of this interosseus membrane run obliquely from the ulna distally to the radius proximally and provide a certain stability for the forearm against a longitudinal force. They also provide stability for the forearm should resection of the radial head be necessary.

All of the muscles that provide external control for flexion or extension of the wrist and hand arise from the forearm. Control of supination of the forearm is provided through the supinator muscle running from the medial surface of the ulna to the lateral surface of the radius on the dorsal side. In addition, the tendon of the biceps by inserting into the radius at the bicipital tuberosity provides a certain amount of supinator force. Pronation of the forearm is primarily controlled by the pronator teres muscle which originates in the superficial flexor wad at the medial anterior elbow and inserts onto the radius at approximately its midshaft. The pronator quadratus lies on the volar aspect of the distal forearm and assists the pronator teres by adding to the strength of pronation.

Isolated Fracture of Ulnar Shaft

The isolated fracture of the ulnar shaft most likely occurs from a direct blow to the ulna but may be the product of an excessive supination or pronation force that allows the ligamentous structures to remain intact and rotate the ulna beyond its elastic capability. In keeping with the both bone principle, when one bone of a two-bone system is fractured *and* displaced, there is obligatory fracture of the other bone of the system or a separation of the ligamentous structures connecting these two bones. The isolated ulnar fracture does not tend to displace.

Examination. Examination of the forearm in which an isolated ulnar fracture exists is usually not very revealing. There may be minimal evident deformity, ecchymosis, or swelling at the area of the fracture; no gross deformity occurs in the single bone fracture as indicated in the both bone principle. Longitudinal compression between the wrist and the olecranon process will create pain sufficiently localized for the patient to point accurately to the fracture site.

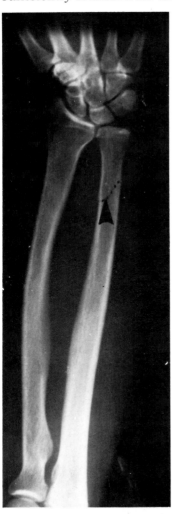

Fig. 9–1. Anteroposterior roentgenogram showing isolated fracture of ulna (arrow). This fracture heals well if appropriately immobilized for eight to ten weeks.

Roentgenograms. The anteroposterior (Fig. 9–1) and lateral roentgenograms will reveal the evidence of an isolated fracture in the shaft of the ulna. This fracture may occur at any point within the shaft.

Treatment. Treatment of the isolated ulnar shaft fracture should be immobilization in a long arm cast for between eight and twelve weeks, depending upon roentgenographic evidence of union. In a review of patients with isolated ulnar shaft fractures treated at the Cook County Hospital, Altner and I found that union almost invariably ensued with little problem unless an operative approach has been made to this fracture. It had been my impression that the isolated fracture would be prone to nonunion unless some type of internal fixation was accomplished because the ulna served as the post around which the radius rotated. The study effectively changed that opinion and subsequent experience has borne out the value of simple immobilization.

Isolated Fracture of Radial Shaft

The isolated fracture of the radial shaft is most commonly the product of a direct injury to the radius. A fracture in the more distal radius at a point 2 to 3 inches proximal to the wrist joint has a very distinct tendency toward redisplacement, even should adequate reduction be accomplished. This has been referred to, because of a study by the Piedmont Orthopaedic Society pointing up the redislocating hazard of this fracture, as the Piedmont fracture. This entity may also be referred to as a Galeazzi fracture.

Examination. The examination of the injury to the radial shaft is not particularly revealing. Minimal angulation may be observed. The proximal one half of the radius is covered by muscles; hence, a fracture in this area is seldom evident on observation. However, longitudinal pressure along the shaft of the radius from the wrist to the elbow will create pain at the fracture site.

Roentgenograms. The roentgenograms will confirm the fracture (Fig. 9–2A, B). The major concern is the level of the fracture.

Treatment. Fractures in the proximal two thirds of the shaft of the radius may be treated by application of a cast if bony contact is present. If bony contact is not present, closed reduction is difficult, and an open reduction followed by internal fixation may be the best approach. In the so-called Piedmont fracture, it will be most unlikely that reduction can be maintained without internally fixing the fracture (Fig. 9–2C, D); because of this, internal fixation with a Rush pin or a four-hole plate where possible is the treatment of choice. In either instance, immobilization for approximately ten to twelve weeks following reduction is essential before roentgenographic evidence of union will be seen.

Fractures of Both Bones of Forearm

Fractures of both bones of the forearm are usually a product of direct injury, with fractures occurring commonly at the point of impact. As mentioned in Chapter 1, the both bone principle dictates that when one bone of a two-bone system is fractured *and* displaced, there is obligatory fracture of the other bone or a tear of the ligamentous attachments at either end. Nowhere is this better shown than when both bones of the forearm are fractured. Fractures of both bones of the forearm in the adult are usually difficult ones in which to maintain reduction by closed means.

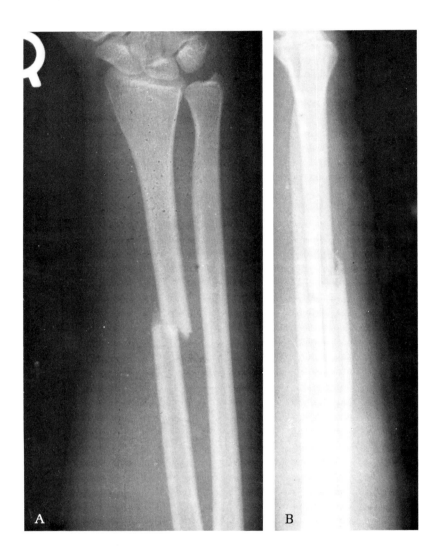

Fig. 9–2. Isolated fracture of radius. A, Anteroposterior roentgenogram. B, Lateral roentgenogram.

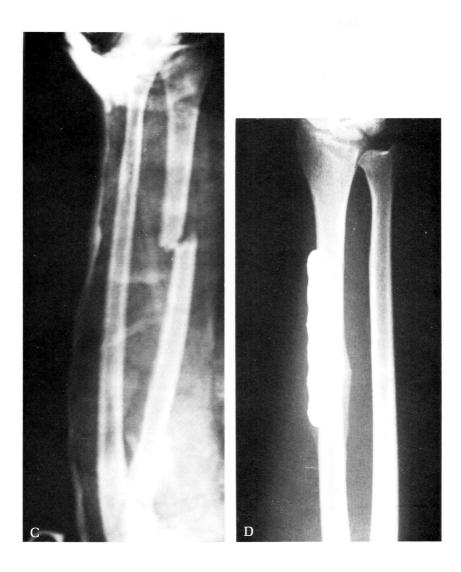

Fig. 9–2. (Cont'd)   C, Roentgenogram showing that fracture does not retain reduction in cast. Accordingly, internal fixation was accomplished with a compression plate after open reduction. D, Anteroposterior view six months after reduction and internal fixation.

Examination. If both bones of the forearm are fractured, the examination will reveal an angulation deformity. Because of potential vascular or neurologic deficit peripheral to the injury, a careful examination for defects in circulation, sensation, and motor control must be performed before any treatment program is started.

Roentgenograms. Anteroposterior and lateral roentgenograms (Fig. 9–3) confirm the fractures and indicate the exact location as well as obliquity and comminution.

Treatment. One group of orthopaedic surgeons treats fractures of both bones in the forearm of the adult by closed reduction under general anesthetic followed by immobilization in a cast. Their results are very satisfactory. Only in rare instances, however, has this method been satisfactory in my practice. The

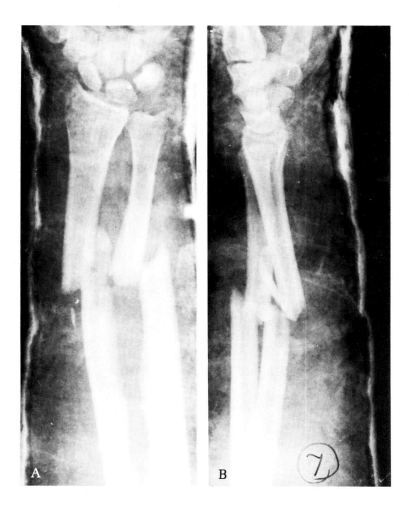

Fig. 9–3. Roentgenograms showing fractures of both bones of forearm. A, Anteroposterior view. B, Lateral view. Open reduction and internal fixation were necessary to treat this injury in an adult.

open treatment has provided better results. If open reduction and internal fixation of fractures of both bones is planned, it is well to attempt to maintain length of the forearm by getting some end-to-end apposition of at least one of the fractured bones. The arm can then be maintained in a long arm cast until such time as an operative approach is feasible.

As for internal fixation devices—plates, intermedullary devices, and a combination of the two—all have their proponents who seem to get good results with the system they use. In the radial shaft fracture from midshaft proximally, it is more difficult to obtain fixation with an intramedullary device other than a plate. However, in the more distal radial shaft fracture, the intramedullary fixation may be utilized. Good fixation can be obtained in the ulna with intramedullary fixation in any shaft fracture as low as the junction of the middle and distal thirds. Below this, the intramedullary rod may need to be inserted from distal to proximal or some type of plate fixation may be used. Following surgical fixation, a safe practice is to utilize the long arm cast for ten to twelve weeks, depending upon evidence by roentgenogram of union of the fractures. Nonunions of radial and ulnar fractures have occurred, but if so, there are generally extenuating circumstances such as inadequate immobilization or massive initial injury.

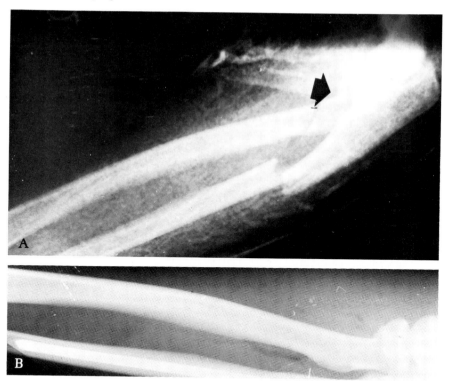

Fig. 9–4. A, Lateral roentgenogram showing displaced fracture of proximal ulna accompanying fracture of radial head (arrow). These meet criteria of the both bone principle. B, Roentgenogram after reduction and Rush rod fixation of ulna were accompanied by reduction of radius and union of both bones.

Monteggia Fracture-Dislocation

The Monteggia fracture-dislocation is the product of a force striking the forearm generally at the junction of the proximal and middle one thirds from either the volar or the dorsal surface. Often a pronation force is added to the direct dorsal midshaft blow when the anterior (extension) type of fracture-dislocation occurs. A supination force may be added when the dorsal (flexion) type of injury occurs. The forces cause a fracture of the shaft of the ulna and a dislocation of the radial head. The annular ligament must be torn from its position encircling the radial neck in order for the radial head to dislocate. The both bone principle is graphically demonstrated with this injury (Fig. 9–4). In addition, because of severity of the trauma, this injury is not uncommonly an open injury with the radial head as well as the ulnar fracture communicating to the exterior.

Examination. Examination of an arm in which a Monteggia fracture-dislocation has occurred, shows an angulation of the forearm with a usually palpable dislocated radial head in a position opposite to the direction of angulation of the distal forearm. Thus, in the anterior type, the radial head dislocates into the antecubital fossa and the distal forearm angulates dorsally. In the dorsal type of Monteggia fracture-dislocation the radial head is dislocated dorsally while the distal forearm angulates in a volar direction.

Roentgenograms. The anteroposterior and lateral roentgenograms (Fig. 9–5) are helpful in assessing the exact mechanism of injury. The anteroposterior view will show the fracture of the ulna and usually a superimposition of the

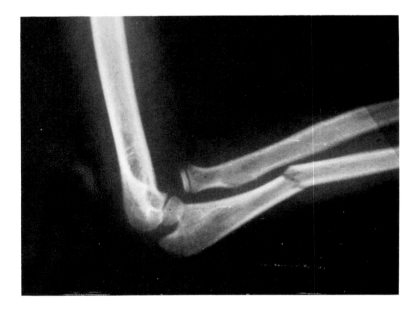

Fig. 9–5. Lateral roentgenogram of forearm in nine-year-old child, showing volar dislocation of radial head accompanying volar displacement of ulnar fracture. This is a Monteggia fracture dislocation. Operative reduction and fixation of ulna are usually necessary in the adult and occasionally may be necessary in the child. Open reduction of radial head may be necessary.

radius over the distal humerus. The lateral view, however, will show the anterior or posterior positioning of the radial head, as well as the angulation of the ulnar fracture. The pathology in this instance has been a tearing of the annular ligament from its position about the neck of the radius and thus a loss of structure providing major stability for the relationship between the radius, the ulna, and the capitulum.

Treatment. If the fracture is closed, an effort should be made to reduce this fracture-dislocation, by closed means. Usually a general anesthetic is required. After relaxation, the radial head is directed toward its normal position at the elbow. In the anterior type of fracture-dislocation, this maneuver is done by digital pressure against the radial head and a simultaneous supination force to the forearm (opposite to dislocating force) associated with correction of the ulnar angulation. The posterior fracture-dislocation is reduced in the opposite direction. Once the fracture has been reduced, if stability seems present, a long arm cast may be applied with particular effort to accommodate the molding of the cast to oppose the direction of the original deformity. However, most commonly the ulna is not stable and the fracture must be openly reduced and internally fixed. Usually internal fixation of the ulna provides a stability to the relationship of the radial head with the ulna and capitulum.

If the fracture is open, the wound must be excised and then a decision must be made regarding internal fixation. On occasion it has been necessary to retract the annular ligament from obstructing reduction of the radial head. In this instance, reconstruction of the annular ligament is necessary after reduc-

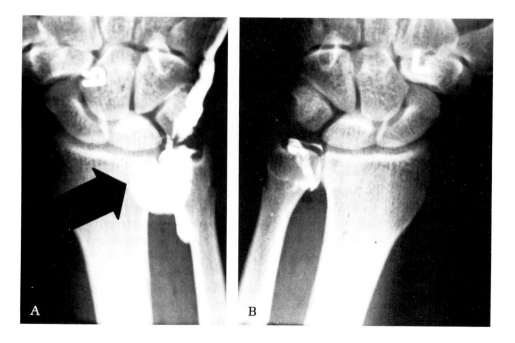

Fig. 9–6. A, Arthrogram of radioulnar joint following tear of dorsal ligament. Compare escape of radiopaque material (arrow) with the normal side, B.

tion of the head. Immobilization in a long arm cast must follow the operative procedure for ten to twelve weeks until there is roentgenographic evidence of adequate union occurring at the ulnar fracture. Removal of the plaster of Paris cast must be followed with intensive active range of motion exercises in order to obtain the fullest motions possible at the elbow and through the forearm.

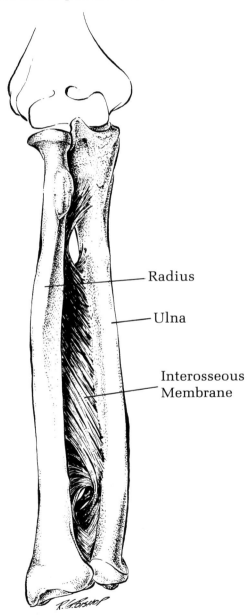

Radius

Ulna

Interosseous
Membrane

Fig. 9–7. Illustration of interosseous membrane between radius and ulna. These fibers explain at least in part how stability can follow radial head resection.

Radioulnar Injury with Radial Neck Fracture

The radioulnar injury combined with fracture of the radial neck occurs by a longitudinal force along the axis of the radius, causing fracture of the neck or head of the radius and separation of the ligamentous fibers that maintain stability between the distal radius and the ulna (Fig. 9–6). As discussed in Chapter 8 under Fracture of the Radial Head and Neck, resection of the radial head without recognition of the distal radioulnar injury may lead to subsequent radial settling and enforced radial deviation of the wrist (Fig. 9–7).

FRACTURES OF THE FOREARM IN CHILDREN

Fractures of both bones in the forearm of the child usually are the product of a fall onto an outstretched hand. The mechanism is generally produced with a dorsal and supination directed force.

Examination. Examination of the fractured forearm shows dorsal angulation of the more distal forearm. Because of pain, the child will allow no palpation. A brief sensory examination is necessary, however, before treatment is begun.

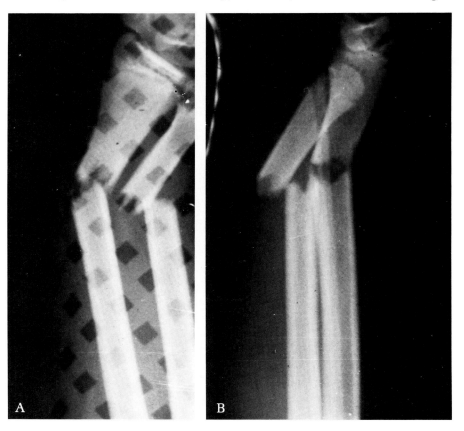

Fig. 9–8. Roentgenograms showing fracture of both bones of forearm. A, Anteroposterior view. To effect reduction, the distal fragments must be brought into relationship with supinated proximal fragments. B, Lateral view. Dorsal angulation of distal fragments will also need to be corrected at time of reduction under general anesthetic.

Roentgenograms. The anteroposterior and lateral roentgenograms (Fig. 9–8) will identify the level of the injury as well as the obliquity and comminution. If any periosteum is intact in the forearm with fractures of both bones, it will be on the concave side of the fracture. In addition, the level of the fracture allows the treating physician to anticipate the type of muscle pull that will be occurring on each fragment. For example, in the fracture occurring at the junction of the middle and proximal thirds of the forearm, the supinator muscle will tend to have supinated the proximal fragment while the pronator teres and the pronator quadratus will have combined to pronate the distal fragment. Any reduction method must aim to bring the distal fragment into a position to meet the proximal fragment because the distal fragment is the only fragment over which the physician has any control.

Treatment. Reduction of fractures of both bones under general anesthetic is the treatment of choice. This should only be done after a careful study of the roentgenograms and a determination of useful information to be used in the reduction of this fracture as well as in the maintenance of that reduction.

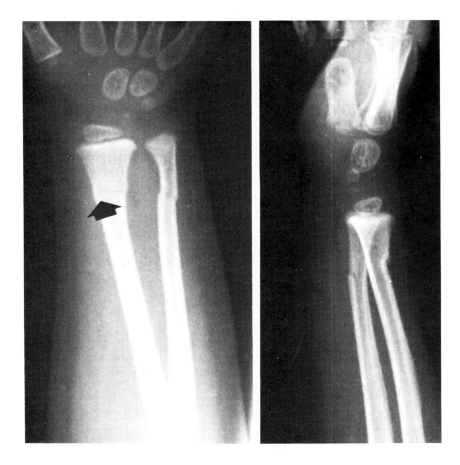

Fig. 9–9. Torus fracture is seen just above arrow on radius. This fracture is caused by a longitudinal compressive force buckling the cortex.

Reduction is generally accomplished by increasing the deformity and, with the surgeon's thumb, pressing the distal fragments on the concave side of the injury. Once the distal fragments have been aligned to the proximal fragments, the hand and wrist are brought out of the increased deformity position back to the reduction position. Not only has it been necessary to use angulation forces, but pronation or supination directed forces have also been used in the reduction of this fracture.

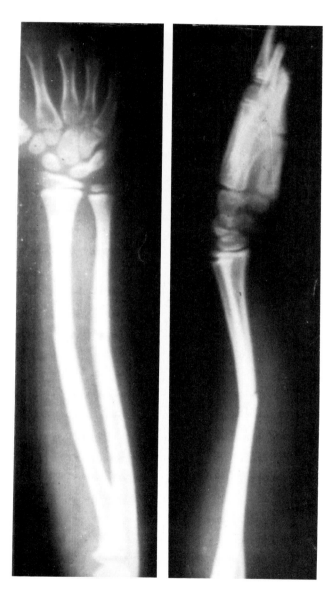

Fig. 9–10. Greenstick fractures of radius and ulna. If angulation is too great, these fractures must be completed and then reduced.

At this point the reduction may be maintained by three-point fixation with a long arm plaster of Paris cast. In the three-point fixation, the aim is to keep the intact periosteum taut by force applied by the cast. Tautness is accomplished, in essence, by a force toward the intact periosteum at the fracture site combined with forces away from the intact periosteum at the most distal and proximal points of this portion of the forearm.

In fractures of both bones with greenstick angulation, angulation up to about 15 degrees of the midportion of the shafts is acceptable. It must be recognized, however, that sufficient clearance needs to be maintained for the radius to rotate about the ulna in supination and pronation. The angulation of the midshaft will only slowly and minimally correct itself, hence the small degree of allowable angulation. Any amount of rotation of one fragment in relationship to its opposing fragment is not acceptable because the growth of the child cannot accommodate to rotation deformities. Angulation or an offset near the epiphyseal plate is acceptable, particularly if it is in the line of motion of the adjacent joint. The torus fracture (Fig. 9–9), which is a buckling of the cortex caused by a longitudinal compressive force, can generally be treated by simple immobilization for four to six weeks. Greenstick fractures of the mid forearm in which angulation (Fig. 9–10) has occurred but the fractures are incomplete through the radius and ulna are usually best treated by completing the fractures and then placing the limb in a long arm cast. This procedure can be done without a general anesthetic but is most easily accomplished with the patient anesthetized. Once the fractures are completed, the fragments tend to maintain good position if the arm is simply held by the fingers and a plaster of Paris cast is applied with the elbow flexed to 90 degrees and the forearm held in midrotation.

REFERENCES

1. Adams, J. C.: Outline of Fractures, Including Joint Injuries. 6th ed. Baltimore, Williams & Wilkins Co., 1972.
2. Altner, P. C. and Hartman, J. T.: Isolated fractures of the ulnar shaft in the adult. Surg. Clin. North Am. 52:1, 1972.
3. Blount, W. P.: Fractures in Children. Baltimore, Williams & Wilkins Co., 1954.
4. Charnley, J.: Closed Treatment of Common Fractures, 3rd ed., 1961, (Fourth Reprint). Edinburgh & London, Churchill Livingstone, 1972.
5. Hughston, J. C.: Fractures of the distal radial shaft. J. Bone Joint Surg. 39-A:249, 1957.
6. Ralston, E. L.: Handbook of Fractures. St. Louis, C. V. Mosby Co., 1967.
7. Rang, M. C.: Children's Fractures. Philadelphia, J. B. Lippincott Co., 1974.
8. Rockwood, C. A., and Green, D. P.: Fractures. Philadelphia, J. B. Lippincott Co., 1975.
9. Watson-Jones, R.: Fractures and Joint Injuries, 4th ed., 2V. Baltimore, Williams & Wilkins Co., 1952-1955.

10

THE WRIST

The articulation of the carpal bones with the radius and the intercarpal articulations provide for dorsiflexion and palmar flexion of the wrist, as well as for its ulnar and radial deviation. For the hand to be placed in a rotated position requires the supination or pronation efforts of the forearm. Each of the carpal bones has its soft tissue attachments which provide the blood supply for that specific bone. The one bone that has a particularly precarious circulation arrangement is the navicular. The nutrient artery to the navicular enters the bone about the junction of its distal and middle thirds (Fig. 10–1). The artery then arborizes to supply those portions of the navicular bone distal and proximal to this point of entrance. The distal articular surface of the radius has a volar tilt of 30 degrees and an ulnar opening tilt of 35 degrees (Fig. 10–2).

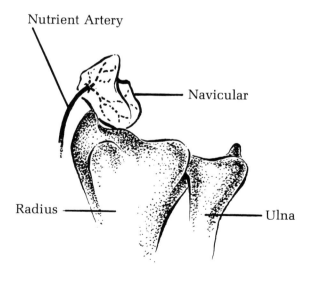

Fig. 10–1. Illustration of wrist joint with particular emphasis on blood supply to navicular. Blood enters the navicular bone through ligaments attaching at its waist and turns to supply the proximal and distal portions. Any fracture (with displacement)) proximal to the entrance of the artery is likely to leave the proximal part of the bone without blood supply.

These must be considered in the treatment of any fracture that enters into the joint. The distal and lateral projection of the radial styloid process is thought to play a role in fracturing the navicular bone when a strong radial deviation force occurs at the wrist.

Colles' Fracture

Colles' fracture, by far the commonest fracture at the wrist and perhaps the most commonly occurring of any single fracture, was described by Abraham Colles in 1814. This is a dorsiflexion and supination injury with the force creating a fracture across the distal radius at a point within one inch of the wrist joint; a small chip fracture of the ulnar styloid process accompanies this injury.

Examination. The examination of a patient with the Colles' fracture shows a deformity resembling a silver fork. The wrist is noticeably dorsiflexed and radially deviated.

Roentgenograms. The anteroposterior (Fig. 10–3A) and lateral roentgenograms confirm the fractures across the radius as well as of the ulnar styloid

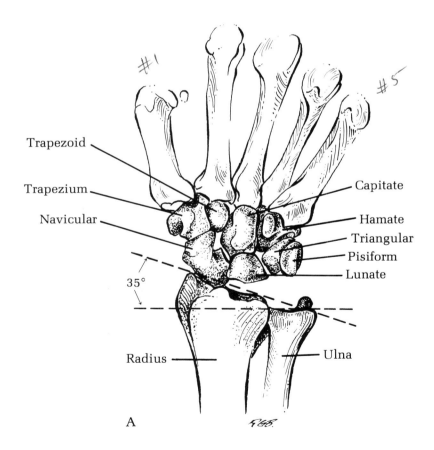

Fig. 10–2. A, Anterior view of distal radius and ulna. Note normal 35-degree angle of radial articulation from styloid process to its medial joint surface.

process. Often there is some comminution of the distal radial fragment. On the anteroposterior roentgenogram, there is loss of the usual 35-degree ulnar angulation of the joint surface (assessed by drawing a line from the tip of the lateral radius to its medial joint surface). On the lateral roentgenogram, as well, there is loss of the volar opening of the radial joint surface (Fig. 10–3B). The Colles' fracture may occur with no displacement, but this is the exception rather than the rule. Occasionally the bony prominence produced by the sharp

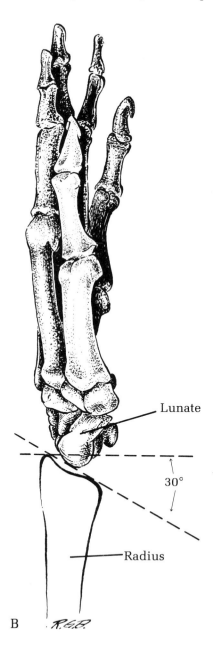

Lunate

30°

Radius

Fig. 10–2. (Cont'd) B, Lateral view of distal radius demonstrating normal angle opening to volar surface at 30 degrees off of perpendicular.

B

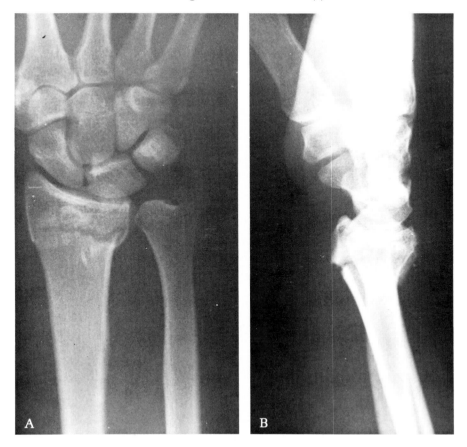

Fig. 10–3. Roentgenograms of Colles' fracture of distal radius and the ulnar styloid process. A, Anteroposterior view. Loss of normal angle of distal radius is evident. B, Lateral view. The distal radius is fractured and displaced dorsally, causing loss of normal angle of distal radial joint surface.

dorsiflexion deformity at the radiocarpal level causes a median nerve injury; this will usually resolve following reduction of the proximal fragment out of the carpal tunnel.

Treatment. Treatment of the Colles' fracture may vary in the undisplaced or in the slightly displaced and impacted fractures. In the latter, application of an immobilizing device is indicated for approximately six weeks. When the fragments are significantly displaced, the full relaxation of a general anesthetic may be required for reduction. The patient may be given an injection of Demerol for analgesia and 1% local anesthetic may be injected into the fracture hematoma of the radius following surgical preparation of the wrist. Reduction of this fracture is accomplished by increasing the deformity in the direction of the concavity and using the thumb to position the distal fragment(s) so that the cortices of the concave side are matching (Fig. 10–4A, B). Following this maneuver, the wrist and hand are brought toward a volar reduced position

Anteroposterior   Lateral View

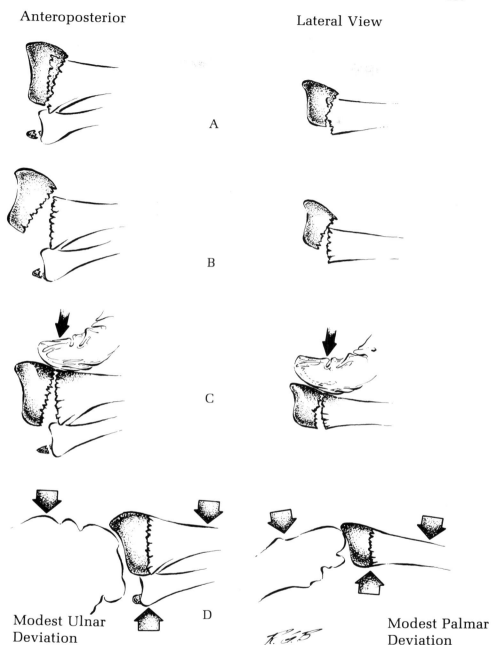

Modest Ulnar
Deviation

Modest Palmar
Deviation

Fig. 10–4. Reduction of Colles' fracture. A, Position of displaced fragments. B, The deformity is first increased with the angle of concavity dorsal and lateral being increased. C, The cortex of the distal fragment(s) is brought into alignment with that of the proximal fragment. The wrist along with the distal radial fragments is moved into a volar and ulnar position to tauten the periosteum on the dorsal and radial sides at the fracture. D, The arm is then immobilized in this position to maintain reduction by three-point fixation.

(Figs. 10–4C, D). Maintenance of the reduction can be accomplished with a modest volar and ulnar deviation. A long arm cast is then applied, utilizing three points of fixation. The force at the fracture site is from the volar and ulnar sides across the fracture and toward the intact dorsal periosteum; the proximal and distal forces oppose the central one. The most effective factor in maintenance of reduction of the distal fragment is the gentle molding of the distal radial fragment toward the ulnar and volar sides rather than sharp volar and ulnar angulation at the wrist (Fig. 10–5). The Colles' fracture, complex or otherwise, when treated by the cast method alone requires a long arm cast for six weeks (Fig. 10–6) followed by a less inclusive form of immobilization such as a short arm cast or splint for an additional four to six weeks.

The comminution present in the Colles' fracture may preclude an adequate reduction, and in this instance a traction method may be used with a Kirschner wire. In Colles' fractures that are difficult to hold reduced, Green uses a Kirschner wire through the second and third metacarpal necks along with a Kirschner wire through the proximal ulna. Both wires are then incorporated into a short arm plaster of Paris cast. He leaves the palmar aspect of the fingers

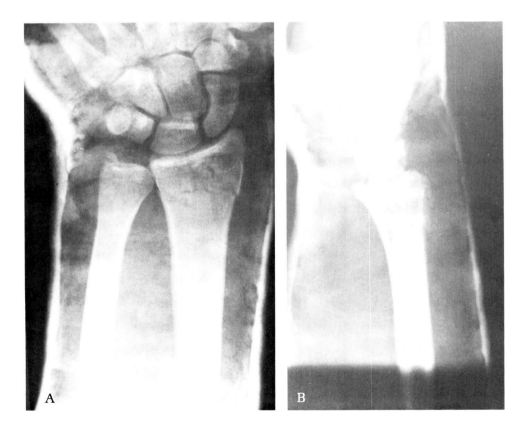

Fig. 10–5. Roentgenograms of reduced Colles' fracture (Fig. 10–3A) that is being held in plaster of Paris cast by three-point fixation. A, Anteroposterior view. B, Lateral view. Note restoration of angle of distal radius.

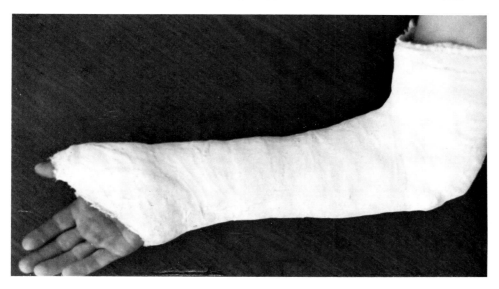

Fig. 10-6. Classic long arm cast to maintain reduction of fragments and prevent supination or pronation of forearm.

open for mobility from the metacarpophalangeal distally as early as the patient can tolerate this action.

In the comminuted Colles' fracture, I prefer application of traction to Kirschner wires in the distal metacarpal of the thumb and in the proximal dorsal ulna. Following reduction, the wires are incorporated into a long arm cast. The wires can be removed at a cast change in six weeks. The long arm cast will still be needed for an additional four to six weeks, depending on roentgenographic evidence of union.

The most frequent complication of the Colles' fracture is the settling that occurs because of the comminution of the fragments. Roentgenograms taken through the plaster cast at three days, one week, and often two weeks are essential in order to be certain that the reduction of the fracture is being maintained. An intermediate to late complication that occurs with some patients following Colles' fracture is the reflex sympathetic dystrophy of Sudeck (see section on complications in Chapter 1). This is a difficult complication to manage, and treatment is a long tedious process. Sympathetic nerve blocks are often helpful. An intensive but active physical therapy program including the use of paraffin is beneficial. In many instances the monamine oxidase inhibitors have aided the reversal of this osteoporotic process. The use of a monamine oxidase inhibitor, however, must be undertaken with full knowledge of the drug and its potential complications. An often accompanying complication in any injury to the forearm, wrist, and hand is periarthritis or pericapsulitis at the shoulder, which may well be caused by an unrecognized injury to the shoulder at the time of the original wrist injury. This complication can often be prevented by repeated emphasis to the patient of the need for his performing range of motion exercises of the shoulder.

A late complication that may be seen with the Colles' fracture is the carpal tunnel syndrome. This is caused by loss of a portion of the carpal tunnel space due to the bony deformity. Compression of the median nerve thus occurs because of decrease in the space through which it must traverse. If a perineural injection of methylprednisolone acetate (Depo-Medrol) does not relieve the signs and symptoms, surgical release of the volar carpal ligament usually solves this problem. Lastly, degenerative changes may occur in the joint in which there is significant incongruity. Symptoms of pain at the wrist following the Colles' fracture may be helped by resection of the distal ulna.

Smith's Fracture

Smith's fracture is a reverse of the Colles' fracture (Fig. 10–7). The mechanism of injury is one of extreme pronation accompanied by a force causing an abnormal amount of volar flexion.

Examination. A deformity will be observed toward the radial and volar side of the wrist with a pronation position of the hand.

Roentgenograms. The anteroposterior and lateral roentgenograms confirm the abnormal positions with the distal radius lying anterior and slightly lateral to its usual position with the more proximal radius. The dorsal or volar displacement of the fracture fragments cannot be determined without seeing a lateral view.

Treatment. Smith's fracture is reduced in the opposite fashion to the Colles' fracture—that is, by volar flexion first, gentle positioning of the distal fragment(s), and then a dorsiflexion of the wrist with supination to bring it into its reduced position (Fig. 10–7C, D). This fracture would be treated in a long arm cast with supination of about 45 degrees and wrist dorsiflexion of approximately 30 degrees. After six weeks, if sufficient evidence of early union is seen on roentgenograms, the long cast may be replaced by a less extensive mobilizing device such as a well-molded short arm cast for an additional four to six weeks.

Carpal Bones

Fractures of the carpal bones present special problems, depending on the specific bone involved. For this reason they will be discussed individually.

Fracture of the Navicular

The navicular is the most common bone in the carpal group to fracture and can be fractured at any point throughout its body. The most typical point for a

Fig. 10–7. Roentgenograms of Smith type of fracture of distal radius and ulna. A, Anteroposterior view. The dorsal or volar displacement of fracture fragments cannot be determined without seeing a lateral view. B, Lateral view showing clearly a volar displacement of the radial fragments. The mechanism of fracture is one of extreme pronation of the forearm accompanied by a force causing an abnormal amount of volar flexion. C, Anteroposterior view of reduced Smith fracture with reduction being maintained by full supination in a long arm cast. (Note bowing of radius and ulna without a crossed position.) D, Lateral view, showing dorsiflexion of wrist maintained by long arm cast.   →

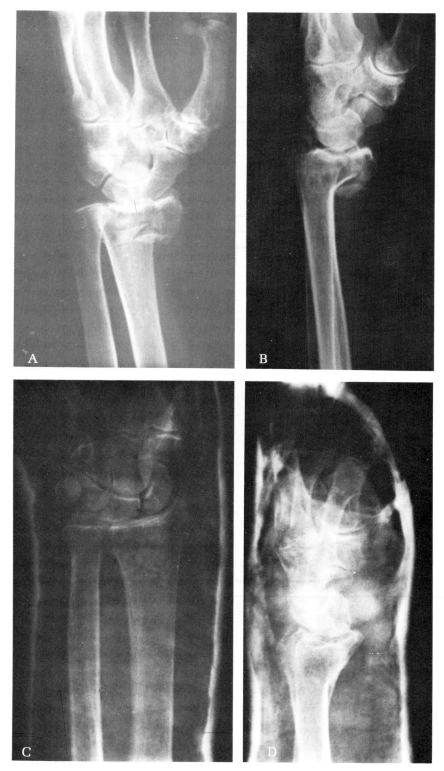

fracture appears to be at the waist where the styloid process of the radius would impinge against the navicular during a radial deviation maneuver. It is thought by some that a rotary mechanism of the wrist plays some role also in the fracture of the navicular.

Examination. The navicular fracture is not always easy to identify. On examination there is pain at the anatomic snuff box on the dorsum of the wrist between the long extensor and the long abductor tendons of the thumb. A longitudinal compressive force from the thumb to the wrist usually causes pain at this point also. Radial deviation of the wrist is particularly painful to the patient with a navicular fracture.

Roentgenograms. A series of roentgenograms specifically designed to show various points of rotation of the carpal bones is essential in order to see the fracture of the navicular. The necessary views include the anteroposterior (Fig. 10–8), the true lateral, and an oblique view in which the hand is placed on the cassette with the thumb opposing the index finger. This will most commonly show the navicular fracture. On the roentgenograms some variation in width of the two fragments indicates that some rotation is present.

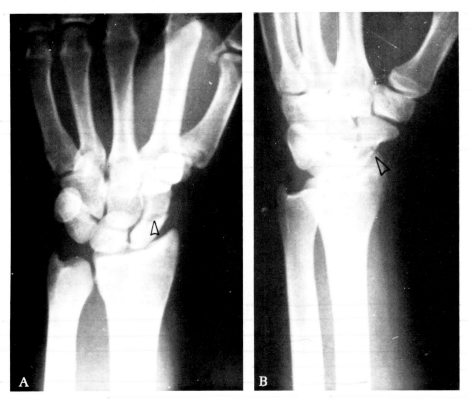

Fig. 10–8. A, Anteroposterior and B, oblique roentgenograms showing fracture at waist of carpal navicular bone (arrows). The appropriate position for immobilization is the functional position with the wrist slightly dorsiflexed and in ulnar deviation. A short arm cast is then applied to the second through fifth metacarpal heads and the thumb enclosed to the interphalangeal joint.

Treatment. Should a strong suspicion be present but no x-ray evidence be seen, immobilization in a short arm cast extending to the knuckles of the second through the fifth fingers and to the tip of the thumb with the thumb in an opposing position to the index finger is in order for two weeks. Roentgenograms at this time will often show slight bone resorption at the fracture site as the early stage of healing begins to be manifest.

The usual treatment of a fractured navicular is accomplished by application of a short arm cast which extends to the metacarpophalangeal joints of the second through the fifth fingers and to the tip of the thumb. The thumb is placed in a position of opposition. A cast change at six weeks is often helpful in maintaining a well-fitting cast. Generally three months are required for evidence of union of the navicular. Watson-Jones has stated that all fractures of the navicular will unite if immobilized for sufficient time. Nonunion of the navicular fracture does occur, particularly when the blood supply into the more proximal part of the navicular has been interrupted. An avascular necrosis of the proximal navicular can also occur as a result of inadequate blood supply. Should evidence of adequate healing of the navicular not be seen at three months, serious consideration must be given to bone grafting across the fracture site.

Fracture of Lunate

The lunate bone is not commonly fractured. Physical examination is rarely helpful in the diagnosis, and roentgenograms are necessary before a diagnosis can be made. Once a diagnosis is established, this fracture can usually be managed by using a short arm cast which is extended to the metacarpophalangeal joints of the second through fifth fingers and on to the proximal phalanx of the thumb. Roentgenograms seldom show evidence for union of the lunate short of ten to twelve weeks of immobilization.

Carpal Fractures

Fractures have been reported in all of the carpal bones, most of those not detailed here being the avulsion type of fractures. Examination seldom provides information of help in the diagnosis. The roentgenogram usually confirms the diagnosis. Treatment of these fractures is the same as for the lunate.

Perilunate Fracture-Dislocation

A sudden, sharp dorsiflexion supination force, particularly in young adults, may cause a fracture across the waist of the navicular and leave its proximal portion attached to the lunate and the radius. The remaining proximal and distal carpal rows dislocate as a unit from their relationship to the proximal navicular, the lunate, and the radius.

Examination. A prominence will be seen on the dorsum of the wrist with distinct pain to palpation. Any motion of the wrist is painful.

Roentgenograms. The roentgenogram must include the anteroposterior and lateral views and often an oblique carpal view in order to be able to assess fully what has happened. The roentgenograms must be studied carefully to identify the full extent of this injury (Fig. 10–9). Occasionally, comparison views of the opposite wrist are helpful in assessing the injured wrist.

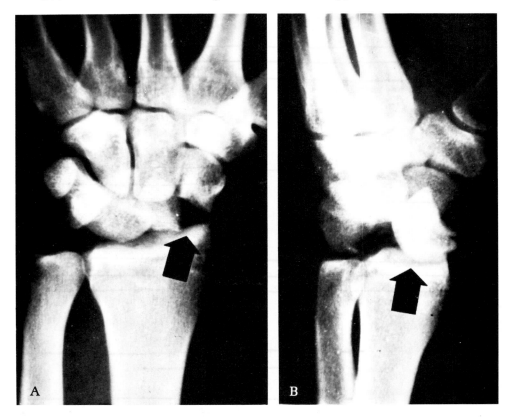

Fig. 10–9. Perilunate fracture-dislocation of wrist. A, Anteroposterior roentgenogram. Arrow points to abnormal relationship of lunate bone and proximal navicular fragment to distal radial articulation. Distal carpal row remains attached to triangularis and pisiform bones as well as to distal navicular fragment. This entire complex is dislocated on the proximal navicular fragment and the lunate. B, Lateral roentgenogram. Arrow points to carpal lunate bone which is tipped into volar flexed position with its navicular fragment. The remainder of the carpi are dislocated dorsally about this unit.

Treatment. When the perilunate fracture-dislocation is seen early, closed reduction is possible but not necessarily probable. The effort to reduce this fracture-dislocation should be made in the operating room so that one can proceed if necessary with open reduction of the carpal bones and the navicular fragment. Once the fracture-dislocation has been reduced, transfixation of the reduced navicular fracture with Kirschner wire is recommended. The results of treatment of this severe injury have been rather poor even in the best of circumstances. Late complications include nonunion of the fractured navicular, avascular necrosis of the navicular, and considerable stiffness of the wrist with pain. Occasionally the wrist in which this injury has occurred requires an arthrodesis before adequate comfort is obtained.

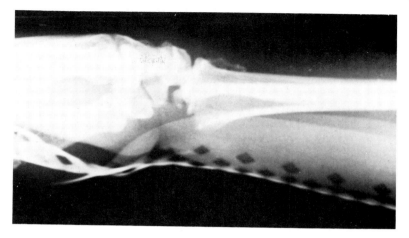

Fig. 10–10. Lateral roentgenogram showing fracture dislocation of wrist (radiocarpal fracture-dislocation). The dorsal distal one third of articular surface of radius has been fractured and lies in normal relationship to proximal carpal row.

Radiocarpal Dislocation

Most commonly a dorsiflexion force is necessary to dislocate the wrist. In this injury, the entire proximal carpal row is shifted dorsally in relationship to the radius. The remainder of the carpal bones and other bony structures of the hand retain their relationship to the proximal carpal row. This injury causes greater soft tissue damage to the volar aspect of the wrist than to the dorsal.

Examination. The carpal prominence of the wrist is seen on the dorsal side while a prominence of the radius is seen on the volar side of the wrist. The median nerve may become entrapped in this particular injury.

Roentgenograms. The anteroposterior roentgenograms reveal a superimposition of the dorsal carpal row over the distal radius. On the lateral view, loss of the contact relationship between the distal radius and the proximal carpal row is noted (Fig. 10–10).

Treatment. Reduction of the radiocarpal dislocation is occasionally possible by using a combination of meperidine and diazepam for analgesia and relaxation. More commonly, a general anesthetic is required to secure sufficient relaxation for reduction. Once reduced, a long arm cast is applied with the wrist held in approximately 20 degrees of palmar flexion and 45 degrees of pronation. Immobilization for four to six weeks should be sufficient for this dislocation to achieve stability.

Dislocation of Lunate

The most common single dislocation in the carpal bones is dislocation of the lunate. The more typical lunate dislocation occurs from a fall on the dorsiflexed wrist in which the lunate loses its stabilizing effect between the proximal capitate and distal radial articulations. The lunate bone is forced in a volar direction into the carpal tunnel.

Examination. Some fullness of the volar aspect of the wrist can be observed if

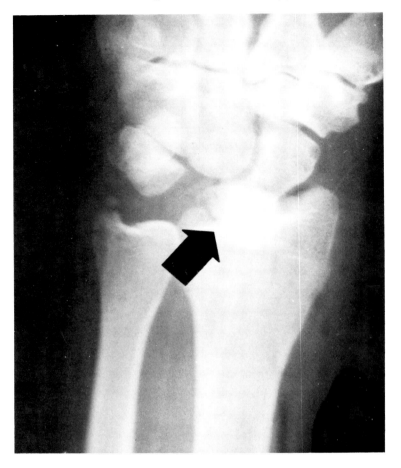

Fig. 10–11. Anteroposterior roentgenogram showing dislocated carpal lunate (arrow). To its left is the space from which this lunate has been dislocated. This is the most common dislocation of a carpal bone.

the lunate is dislocated. Wrist movement is restricted. There may also be evidence of compression of the median nerve and of the long flexor tendons.

Roentgenograms. The anteroposterior roentgenograms will show loss of position of the lunate from its usual relationship between the radius and the capitate (Fig. 10–11). On the lateral roentgenogram the usual quarter-moon shaped lunate resting against the distal radial joint surface will be absent and lying free in the volar space. The pathology in this circumstance is that the lunate has been torn from its dorsal ligamentous attachments but most likely will still have some volar ligament attachments which maintain its vascularity.

Treatment. Treatment of this dislocation, if seen early, can often be accomplished by using meperidine and diazepam for analgesia and relaxation. With the wrist then dorsiflexed and a modest traction applied longitudinally, dorsally directed digital pressure applied against the volar aspect of the dislocated lunate will often bring it back into position. Should the relocation not be possible or should this injury be seen late, open reduction should be accomplished. Great care should be given to maintaining the soft tissue attachments, for these provide the blood supply to the bone. In the circumstance in which the lunate has beeen completely severed from all soft tissue attachments, better results have occurred following excision of the lunate. When free of ligamentous attachments, the lunate that is reduced by the closed method will undergo aseptic necrosis. Following reduction, a short arm cast is applied and maintained for approximately four weeks.

WRIST INJURIES IN CHILDREN

In children injuries to the epiphyseal plate of the distal radius and ulna are more common than other injuries to the wrist. Wrist injuries seen occasionally are dislocation of the lunate, fracture of the navicular, and soft tissue injuries.

Epiphyseal Injury to Distal Radius and Ulna

A not uncommon occurrence in the child between the ages of six and ten is a separation through the epiphyseal plate of the distal radius or of the distal radius and ulna. This is generally caused by a dorsiflexion force with some supination element added. The epiphyseal injury is usually of the Type II separation, as described by Salter, in which there is a portion of the metaphysis of the radius on the dorsal and radial side.

Examination. The deformity in epiphyseal separation is obvious and has much the same appearance as does the deformity of the Colles' fracture in the adult. It is impossible to determine the detail of bony injury from physical examination alone.

Roentgenograms. The anteroposterior and lateral roentgenograms should serve to point out that there has been the epiphyseal separation (Fig. 10–12A, B). Most often it will be associated with a triangle of metaphysis attached along the dorsal and radial side. Because this separation through the epiphyseal plate occurs in the zone of hypertrophic cells, one would anticipate little tendency toward growth abnormality. Careful study of the roentgenograms is essential to be certain of the type of epiphyseal injury. As pointed out in the section on epiphyseal injuries (Chapter 2), certain epiphyseal injuries require perfect reduction, even though this can be accomplished only by operation.

Treatment. If seen promptly, the epiphyseal separation may often be reduced under local anesthetic by increasing the deformity gently and then bringing the hand and wrist into a reduced position. General anesthesia may be required to secure sufficient relaxation to proceed with reduction. Maintenance in a long arm cast for six weeks is usually sufficient. Because of increased vascularity following injury some increased growth may occur in this limb. This is usually inconsequential.

Injuries to the Carpus

Occasionally a dislocation of the lunate occurs in the child. It is recognized and treated in the same fashion as the dislocated lunate in the adult.

Fractures of the navicular also occur in the child and are usually undisplaced. The roentgenograms should be taken in the same fashion as described

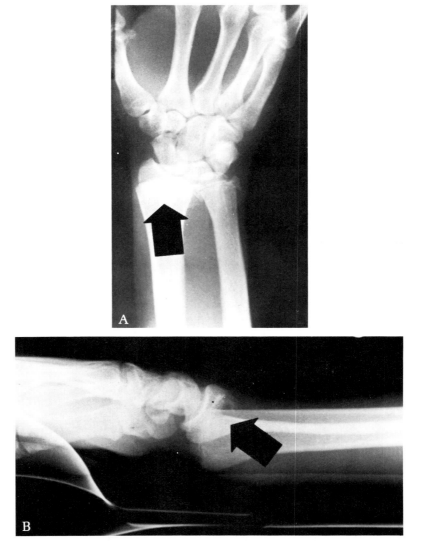

Fig. 10–12.   Roentgenograms of distal radial epiphyseal slip. A, Anterior view. The epiphysis overlies the distal metaphysis. Note triangular segment of radial metaphysis attached to epiphysis (arrow). B, Lateral view. A small triangular fragment of metaphysis is attached to dorsally dislocated distal radial epiphysis (arrow).

for adults. Comparison views of the opposite wrist are essential for adequate evaluation. Should a fractured navicular be strongly suspected but not confirmed by roentgenograms, it is well to apply a short arm cast extending to the thumb tip and to the metacarpophalangeal joints of the second through the fifth fingers. At the end of two weeks, roentgenograms are obtained again. If a fracture indeed exists, it should show at this point by resorption of a segment of the bone at the fracture site. Fractures of the navicular generally require three months of immobilization for union to occur.

Soft Tissue Injuries

The ligamentous injuries of the wrist in the child generally require two to three weeks of immobilization to achieve stability.

REFERENCES

1. Adams, J. C.: Outline of Fractures, Including Joint Injuries, 6th ed. Baltimore, Williams & Wilkins Co., 1972.
2. Blount, W. P.: Fractures in Children. Baltimore, Williams & Wilkins Co., 1954.
3. Charnley, J.: Closed Treatment of Common Fractures, 3rd ed. (Fourth Reprint). Edinburgh & London, Churchill Livingstone, 1972.
4. Colles, A.: On the fracture of the carpal extremity of the radius. Edinburgh Med. Surg. J. 10:182, 1814.
5. Green, D.: Pins and plaster treatment of comminuted fractures of the distal end of the radius. J. Bone Joint Surg. 57-A:304, 1975.
6. Ralston, E. L.: Handbook of Fractures. St. Louis, C. V. Mosby Co., 1967.
7. Rang, M. C.: Children's Fractures. Philadelphia, J. B. Lippincott Co., 1974.
8. Rockwood, C. A., and Green, D. P.: Fractures. Philadelphia, J. B. Lippincott Co., 1975.
9. Salter, R. B., and Harris, R. W.: Injuries involving the epiphyseal plate. J. Bone Joint Surg. 45-A:587, 1963.
10. Watson-Jones, R.: Fractures and Joint Injuries, 4th ed., 2V. Baltimore, Williams & Wilkins Co., 1952-1955.

11

THE HAND

The anatomic structure of the hand is such as to make man one of the few animals capable of prehension. The bases of the metacarpals are placed in a neat relationship to the distal carpal row in such fashion as to allow cupping of the hand to occur in a medial to lateral and a proximal to distal direction. The carpometacarpal joints flex to an average of 110 degrees from the fully extended position. In the process of flexing metacarpophalangeal joints two through five individually, the flexion is accomplished in such a manner as to allow each fingertip to point to the navicular bone in the proximal carpal row. The condylar flares of the metacarpal heads opposing the plateau bases of the proximal phalanges provide the side-to-side stability for the metacarpophalangeal joints. The interphalangeal joints also are provided some measure of side-to-side stability by the condylar shapes of the phalangeal heads and the plateau shapes of the opposing bases. Flexion of metacarpophalangeal joints two through five is accomplished by the intrinsic musculature of the hand, specifically the lumbrical and interosseus muscles. The proximal interphalangeal joints of the second through the fifth fingers are flexed by the superficial flexor muscles from the forearm; the distal second through fifth finger interphalangeal joints are flexed by the deep flexor muscles from the forearm. The flexor pollicis longus from the forearm flexes the interphalangeal joint of the thumb.

On the dorsum of the wrist the long extensors attach into the base of the proximal phalanges of fingers two through five to extend the metacarpophalangeal joints; the lumbricales and interossei by a system of tendinous slips passing from a palmar to a dorsal position at the sides of the proximal phalanges insert into the extensor hood and extend the interphalangeal joints. Extension of the thumb is accomplished by the extensor pollicis brevis which inserts at the base of the proximal phalanx and the extensor pollicis longus which inserts into the base of the distal phalanx. Both of these extensor tendons originate from muscles in the dorsum of the forearm. A long abductor of the thumb allows abduction strength by its insertion into the radial side of the base of the first metacarpal bone. It is aided by the abductor pollicis brevis which is inserted into the proximal phalanx. The action to bring the thumb into opposition to the other fingers is accomplished by the opponens pollicis, a small muscle in the palmar thenar mass; adduction of the thumb is provided by the adductor pollicis, also an intrinsic muscle in the thenar muscle group.

Carpometacarpal Dislocation

Dislocation of the base of the metacarpal of the second, third, fourth, or fifth fingers from its relationship to the distal carpal row often occurs by direct force creating a dorsiflexion-like maneuver of the midhand. However, a forced flexion as created in fisticuffs can dislocate the base of the metacarpals dorsally.

Examination. The examination will reveal a prominence either volar or dorsal of the base of the involved metacarpal with distinct tenderness at this area.

Roentgenograms. Anteroposterior, lateral (Fig. 11–1A), and often oblique roentgenograms (Fig. 11–1B) are necessary in an effort to identify the injury in question. In fact, often comparison views of the opposite hand are necessary before making a final decision regarding carpometacarpal dislocation.

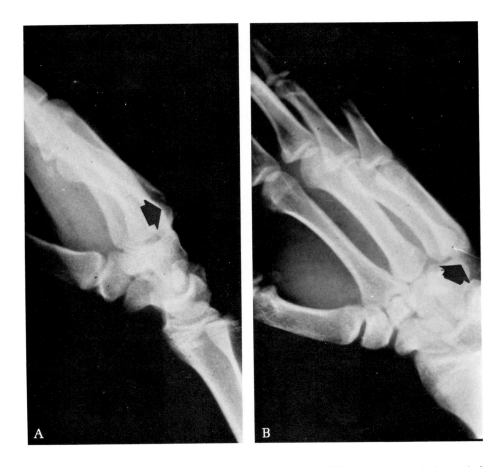

Fig. 11–1. Roentgenograms showing dislocation of base of fifth metacarpal. A, Lateral view showing base elevated away from its contact with hamate bone (arrow). B, Oblique view. Arrow points to dislocation of base of fifth metacarpal in relation to distal carpal row. Reduction of this fracture can sometimes be held by gauntlet cast and finger splint. Usually, however, this dislocation requires fixation with Kirschner wires for several weeks to achieve stabilization.

Treatment. If this dislocation is seen early, it probably can be reduced by direct manipulation under either an analgesic agent or 1% local anesthetic injected into the dislocated joint capsule. Following reduction of this dislocation, immobilization in a gauntlet cast with a splint supporting the involved finger is usually sufficient. The metacarpal is held in an extended position while the phalanges are slightly flexed. Immobilization is maintained for about four weeks. Once relocation is accomplished, one has to beware of the tendency for redislocation. Occasionally, it may be necessary to transfix this metacarpal base with two crossed Kirschner wires in order to maintain reduction.

Bennett's Fracture of the Thumb Metacarpal

The mechanism of injury for Bennett's fracture of the medial base of the thumb metacarpal is adduction and longitudinal compression against the greater trapezium bone of the distal carpal row. This injury may partially tear the capsule of the carpometacarpal joint on its radial side.

Examination. On the examination there is a very marked tenderness along the medial base of the thumb. There may be a palpable prominence on the radial aspect at the carpometacarpal articulation.

Roentgenograms. Roentgenograms will show an oblique fracture through the medial cortex of the first metacarpal extending down into the carpometacarpal joint (Fig. 11–2).

Treatment. Because Bennett's fracture is an adduction type of injury, theoretically an adduction and traction force followed by abduction of the

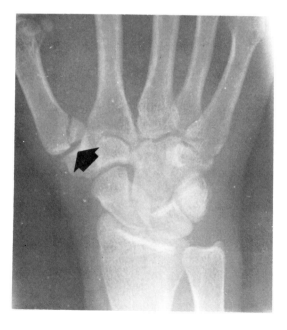

Fig. 11–2. Anteroposterior roentgenogram showing Bennett's fracture of thumb metacarpal base. The ulnar half of joint surface is displaced slightly distally (arrow). These usually require reduction followed by Kirschner wire fixation.

thumb should obtain and maintain reduction. This is possible occasionally, but more likely than not, the reduction cannot be maintained without internal fixation. A percutaneous Kirschner wire can be placed across the base of the metacarpal and into the greater trapezium to maintain reduction. This hand can then be immobilized in a gauntlet cast. The pin should be removed at three to four weeks, but immobilization should be continued to an approximate total of six weeks. Another method for treating this fracture is by placing a wire through the distal phalanx of the thumb. Traction is then applied to this wire from an outrigger on a gauntlet cast to reduce and maintain the reduction of this fracture-dislocation.

Metacarpal Fracture

Direct or indirect forces usually are present to create the metacarpal fracture. These fractures are often oblique, may be transverse, or may be spiral.

Examination. In a metacarpal fracture examination reveals swelling in the area of the metacarpal bone involved. Rotational deformity of the finger distal to the fracture often occurs. The tip of the flexed finger should point to the navicular bone in the normal hand.

Roentgenograms. A study of roentgenograms will identify the type of fracture present (Fig. 11–3). The treatment that will be necessary can be determined after study of the hand and the roentgenogram.

Treatment. Transverse fractures of the metacarpal may be reduced following an appropriate nerve block accomplished with 1% local anesthetic. Immobilization of this injury is accomplished by incorporating a splint in a gauntlet cast and extending it under the involved finger to the fingertip (Fig. 11–3C). Special attention must be given to prevent rotational deformity inasmuch as this can be a most disabling complication of the metacarpal fracture.

The oblique or spiral fracture may be treated by a traction pin through the distal phalanx attached to an outrigger device on a gauntlet cast. Again, attention must be directed to the position necessary for accurate reduction *without* rotary malunion. It may be optimum treatment to surgically reduce and transfix the metacarpal fracture with Kirschner wires.

Immobilization by any one of these methods is required for eight to ten weeks or until adequate evidence of union is seen on roentgenograms. Usually traction can be discontinued after four to six weeks, and immobilization can be continued in a gauntlet cast for four to six weeks more. Intensive efforts at regaining a full range of motion must be undertaken as soon as the immobilization is stopped.

Boxer's Fracture

The mechanism of injury of the boxer's fracture is a dorsal force driving the fifth (or fourth and fifth) metacarpal head into the palm of the hand. A protected blow with the fist can cause this injury.

Examination. On examination of the hand with boxer's fracture, the injury is evident with loss of the fifth metatarsal head dorsally (the knuckle). The metacarpal head is palpated in the palm of the hand.

Roentgenograms. Anteroposterior, lateral, and oblique roentgenograms will determine the extent of the flexion deformity of the metacarpal head(s) (Fig. 11–4). They will also indicate whether impaction is present.

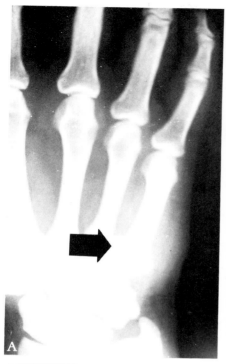

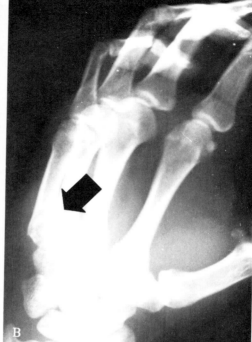

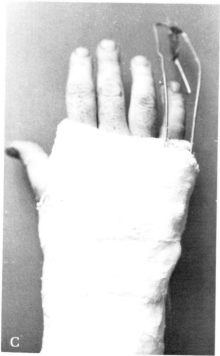

Fig. 11–3. Roentgenograms showing metacarpal fracture of hand. A, Anteroposterior view. Arrow points to a fracture at base of fifth metacarpal. This fracture occurred while patient was engaged in fisticuffs. B, Oblique view. Dorsal displacement of distal fragment is noted at arrow. C, Immobilized hand. Traction was applied to fifth finger by Kirschner wire through distal phalanx to achieve and maintain reduction. An outrigger on dorsum of gauntlet cast was used to furnish traction post for rubber band from Kirschner wire. Four to six weeks of such traction are sufficient to achieve early union. Continued immobilization in a gauntlet cast for the total immobilization period of eight to ten weeks is sufficient.

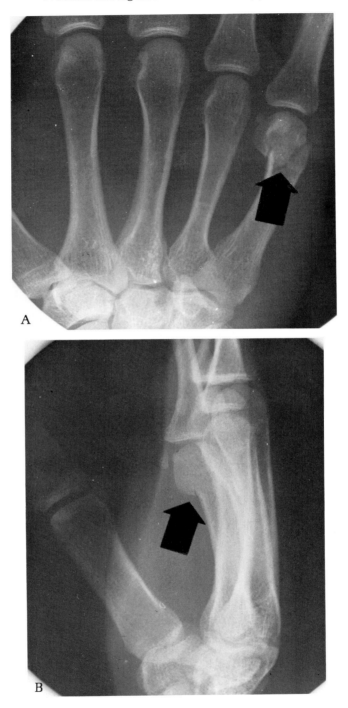

Fig. 11–4. Boxer's fracture. A, Fracture of fifth metatarsal neck is seen just distal to the arrow. B, Arrow points to palmar displacement of fifth metacarpal head. Some palmar displacement can be accepted, but too much will leave an unhandy mass in the palm.

Treatment. If the fracture is impacted and in an acceptable position, it need only be supported by a palmar splint until comfortable. If the fracture is not impacted, however, one may be able to bring the metacarpal head into adequate position and utilize the gauntlet cast with a splint elevating the metacarpal head. According to Phalen, as much as 35 degrees of angulation is acceptable without significant disability. When the fracture is comminuted sufficiently to preclude stability on a splint, the head must be reduced into an adequate position and internally fixed. Usually this can be accomplished under an ulnar nerve block. After surgical preparation the Riordan wire on the hub of a syringe may be utilized to drill percutaneously through the head of the fifth metacarpal and down on the shaft. The wire can then be cut off just beneath the skin and immobilized for three to four weeks. At this point the pin is removed and further immobilization on a splint for a total of six weeks is usually sufficient. If the Riordan pin is not available, a No. 18 needle can be used and the local anesthetic can be injected through it as it is guided into position for fixation of the distal fragment onto the shaft of the fifth metacarpal. Should this fracture require open reduction, another method of fixation is to transfix the fifth metatarsal head by two Kirschner wires to the fourth metatarsal neck. This avoids entering the joint and the subsequent restriction of its motion. Rotation of any metacarpal fracture on its longitudinal axis should be avoided.

Metacarpophalangeal Dislocation

The metacarpophalangeal dislocation occurs most commonly from a force striking the palmar surface of the hand and driving the base of the proximal phalanx dorsally over the head of the metacarpal from the second through the fifth fingers.

Examination. On inspection, the deformity of the metacarpophalangeal dislocation is evident as a dorsal prominence of the phalanx at the metacarpophalangeal joint.

Roentgenograms. The roentgenograms will confirm the metacarpophalangeal dislocation. On the lateral roentgenogram, the base of the phalanx lies dorsal to the metacarpal head. On the anteroposterior view, the base of the phalanx overlies the metacarpal head (Fig. 11–5).

Treatment. The metacarpophalangeal dislocation can usually be simply reduced by closed methods under an appropriate nerve block. The capsule occasionally entraps the dislocated metacarpal head, however, and prevents its being reduced other than operatively under direct vision. Entrapment is particularly prone to occur in the metacarpophalangeal dislocation of the index finger or the thumb. In this event, operative reduction is necessary. Immobilization for three to four weeks following the dislocation appears sufficient for stability.

Phalangeal Fracture

Fractures may occur at any point along the phalanges from the base distally. These are often caused by hyperextension forces that create dorsal displacement but may occur from any mechanism.

Examination. The examination shows the displacement (often dorsal) of the phalanx distal to the fracture. Rotation may be present and can be judged by the

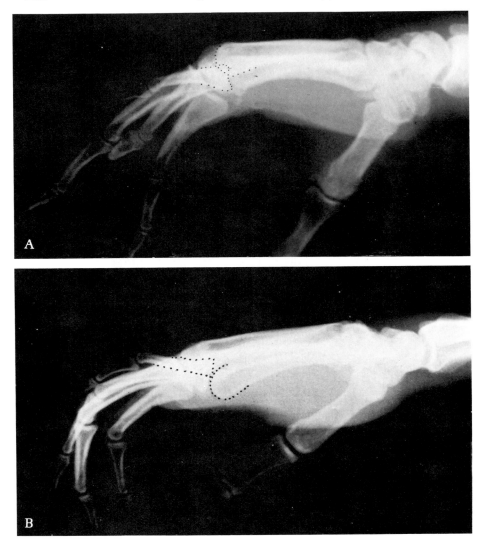

Fig. 11–5.   A, Lateral roentgenogram showing volar dislocation of base of proximal phalanx in relation to fifth metacarpal head (outlined by dotted line). B, Dorsal dislocation of base of proximal phalanx on fifth metacarpal head (outlined by dotted line). The metacarpal head may become entrapped by a tear in the volar plate, requiring operative relief.

position of the nail bed of the involved finger as compared to that of the other fingers.

Roentgenograms. Roentgenograms confirm the fracture deformity and its displacement (Fig. 11-6). The roentgenogram can indicate the likelihood of stability once the fracture is reduced. The transverse fracture should be stable while the oblique and the spiral fractures may tend to redislocate. Roentgenograms can indicate a rotational deformity of the phalanx. When the rotational deformity is present, the lateral view roentgenogram of the head proximal to

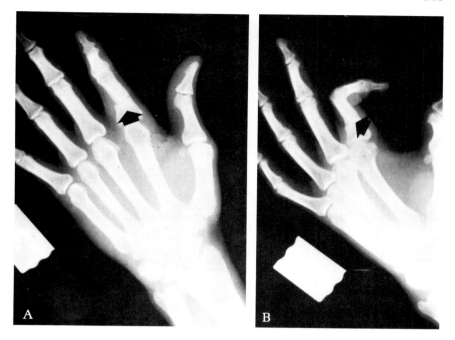

Fig. 11–6. Transverse fracture of proximal phalanx of index finger (arrows). A, Anteroposterior roentgenogram. B, Oblique roentgenogram. A flexed splint will likely maintain reduction of fracture, which is relatively stable. Of primary importance in treating this fracture is prevention of any rotary deformity.

the fracture will show an anteroposterior or oblique condylar view of the distal portion of that phalanx. Similarly, an anteroposterior view of the head proximal to the fracture will include lateral or lateral oblique views of that portion of the phalanx distal to the fracture.

Treatment. An appropriate nerve block or digital block can be accomplished for reduction of the transverse fracture. Generally, immobilization of this fracture on a volar metal splint is sufficient to maintain reduction. Of primary importance in treating this fracture is the prevention of any rotary deformity.

Of special concern is the displaced fracture of the proximal phalanx. It must be accurately reduced and held especially as regards rotation along its longitudinal axis. Open reduction and Kirschner wire fixation may be necessary to obtain a good functional result.

Interphalangeal Joint Dislocation

Interphalangeal joint dislocation usually occurs by a volar force driving the base of the proximal or middle phalanx dorsally.

Examination. A dorsal prominence representing the base of the phalanx is noted on examination.

Roentgenograms. An anteroposterior roentgenogram confirms the dorsal displacement of the proximal part of the phalanx with superimposition of the

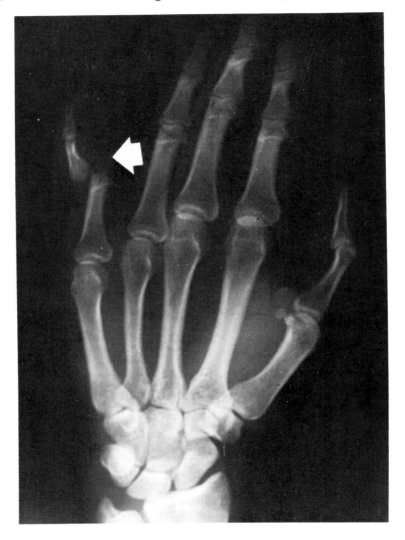

Fig. 11–7. Anteroposterior roentgenogram showing dorsal dislocation at proximal interphalangeal joint of fifth finger (arrow).

dislocated base on the adjacent phalangeal head. A lateral roentgenogram will show the base of the phalanx dorsal to its adjacent phalangeal head (Fig. 11–7).

Treatment. If seen early, the interphalangeal joint dislocation can often be reduced simply with the use of a digital nerve block. After reduction, immobilization on a flexed splint is necessary for three weeks. Should a fracture of a portion of the base of the phalanx occur with the dislocation, and be small in size, the injury may be treated as a dislocation. Once reduced, if this fragment is sufficiently large, internal fixation may be necessary in order to obtain the best result.

Base Fracture of the Distal Phalanx

Avulsion fracture of the dorsum of the distal phalanx is associated with drop of the distal phalanx. The avulsed fragment is attached to the extensor tendon. This is the so-called baseball finger often occurring because of a blow to the tip of a slightly flexed finger.

Examination. On examination the patient is unable to actively extend the distal phalanx completely while extending the remainder of the finger competently.

Roentgenograms. Roentgenograms will confirm a dorsal proximal fragment avulsed from the distal phalanx (Fig. 11–8). Occasionally a tendon rupture at this point gives the same clinical picture without avulsing the fragment of bone.

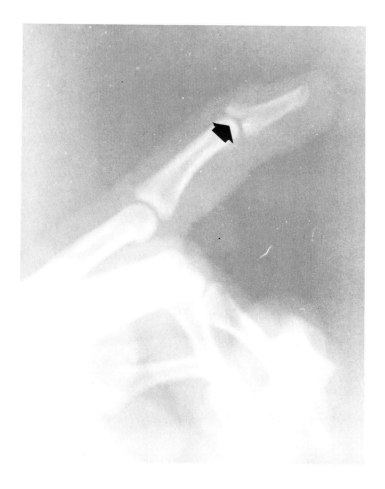

Fig. 11–8. Lateral roentgenogram showing avulsion fracture at dorsal base of distal phalanx. Reduction and its maintenance by hyperextending the distal phalanx is the best treatment. The metacarpophalangeal and proximal interphalangeal joints may need to be flexed to reduce the pull of the extensor hood into its insertion at this dorsal fragment.

Treatment. Treatment of the base fracture should be aimed at relaxing the extensor pull onto the distal phalanx. Relaxation can be accomplished by flexing the proximal interphalangeal joint and extending the distal interphalangeal joint. A number of methods for accomplishing this have been devised. Probably as effective as any method is molding of this position by a well-fitting plaster of Paris cast. A splint may be bent to provide the flexion at the proximal interphalangeal joint with extension at the distal interphalangeal joint; the finger, however, must then be taped into this position with the splint, a process sometimes creating circumferential constriction. The distal phalanx may also be fixed in the hyperextended position by passing a Kirschner wire up the longitudinal axis of the distal phalanx and across the extended distal interphalangeal joint. Immobilization can be discontinued at three to four weeks but it will likely take several months before full active extension is available to the joint. The tuft or distal phalangeal fracture needs to be splinted only for the patient's comfort. Splinting of most phalangeal fractures can be discontinued at two to three weeks.

INJURIES TO THE HAND IN CHILDREN

NOTE: The inability to adequately reduce any of the fractures or fracture-dislocations in the child can be a relative indication for open reduction. This is done to prevent a deformity that is not correctable with the growth of the child.

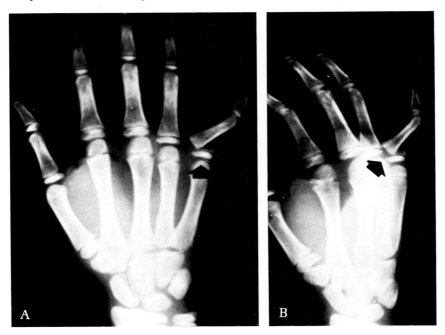

Fig. 11–9. A, Anteroposterior roentgenogram showing Type II slip at epiphysis of proximal phalanx of fifth finger (arrow). The ulnar deviation of the finger distal to this slip must be corrected. A digital or an ulnar block should relieve symptoms and allow reduction. B, Oblique roentgenogram showing dorsal deviation of fifth finger distal to slip at epiphysis (arrow) of fifth finger. Once reduced, immobilization for three to four weeks should be sufficient.

Metacarpal fractures are usually the product of a dorsal force and create a dorsal angulation. They are treated much as are the metacarpal fractures in the adult so long as the epiphyseal plate is not involved.

Metacarpophalangeal dislocation and *interphalangeal dislocation* are also essentially the identical injury of the adult and are treated in like manner.

Epiphyseal Fracture of the Phalanx

Especially is the epiphysis of the proximal phalanx in the child prone to a separation injury. This occurs most commonly at the fifth finger and is usually a dorsally directed abduction force.

Examination. Inspection of the finger with an epiphyseal separation will reveal dorsal angulation, or in the fifth finger, a dorsomedial angulation.

Roentgenograms. Anteroposterior and lateral roentgenograms show a separation of the metaphysis from the epiphysis in the involved finger (Fig. 11–9). The roentgenograms are essential for the accurate assessment of the extent of the injury and in the decision regarding the method of treatment.

Treatment. Reduction of the epiphyseal fracture of the phalanx is done after appropriate nerve block and is usually accomplished by increasing the deformity slightly and then reducing the distal finger back into its neutral relationship. It is often necessary to use the thumb of the surgeon as the fulcrum for reduction. Any angulation of the adjacent joint will disappear quite effectively within several months. Reduction can generally be maintained over a flexed splint that is attached to a gauntlet cast. This immobilization need only be provided for three to four weeks.

REFERENCES

1. Adams, J. C.: Outline of Fractures, Including Joint Injuries, 6th ed. Baltimore, Williams & Wilkins Co., 1972.
2. Blount, W. P.: Fractures in Children. Baltimore, Williams & Wilkins Co., 1954.
3. Boyes, J. H.: Bunnell's Surgery of The Hand, 5th ed. Philadelphia, J. B. Lippincott Co., 1970.
4. Charnley, J.: Closed Treatment of Common Fractures, 3rd ed., 1961, (Fourth Reprint). Edinburgh & London, Churchill Livingstone, 1972.
5. Phalen, G. S.: Personal Communication.
6. Ralston, E. L.: Handbook of Fractures. St. Louis, C. V. Mosby Co., 1967.
7. Rang, M. C.: Children's Fractures. Philadelphia, J. B. Lippincott Co., 1974.
8. Rockwood, C. A., and Green, D. P.: Fractures. Philadelphia, J. B. Lippincott Co., 1975.
9. Watson-Jones, R.: Fractures and Joint Injuries, 4th ed., 2V. Baltimore, Williams & Wilkins Co., 1952-1955.

12

THE PELVIS

Three distinct entities comprise the bony pelvis, namely, the innominate bones, the sacrum, and the coccyx. The innominate bone is the product of coalesence of the growth centers of the ilium superiorly, the pubis bones anteroinferiorly, and the ischium posteroinferiorly. These three bones meet at the triradiate cartilage to form the acetabulum about the femoral head. Inferiorly, the anterior pubis and the posterior ischium send projections to meet each other, thus forming the obturator foramen.

The iliac bone from each side of the pelvis articulates with the sacrum in an amphiarthrodial joint—a slightly mobile joint united by strong interosseous fibers. These interosseous fibers comprise the complex known as the sacroiliac ligament. Many anatomists believe the sacroiliac ligament to be the strongest ligament in the human body. Each pubic bone sends a projection anteromedially to meet the like projection from its fellow of the opposite side. Each ischium sends a like projection anteromedially to join the pubis. They meet to form the symphysis pubis, an amphiarthrodial joint stabilized by a complex of pubic ligaments. The obturator foramen is surrounded by walls of bone forming a rigid circle. The larger ring formed by the bony structures of the pelvis in their articulations is semirigid (Fig. 12–1). Because of the rigidity of these pelvic circles, any *displaced* fracture or dislocation occurring through the pelvis must be associated with another fracture or a ligamentous separation within that ring. This is one of the few "always" rules in medicine.

Avulsion Fractures

The avulsion of the bony origin of any of the muscles arising from the pelvis is possible as a result of an acute forceful contraction of that muscle. This type of avulsion fracture tends to occur in the adolescent when the bony origin is ossified but not strongly united to the pelvis. The more common sites for this to occur are both anterior iliac spines and the ischial prominences.

Roentgenograms. Generally the avulsed bony fragment is seen to best advantage on the anteroposterior roentgenogram. Should the injury be greater than two weeks old, new bone formation may be seen between the avulsed fragment and pelvis (Fig. 12–2).

Treatment. The injured part should be protected by bed rest or no weight bearing initially until the patient becomes asymptomatic. Gentle active range of

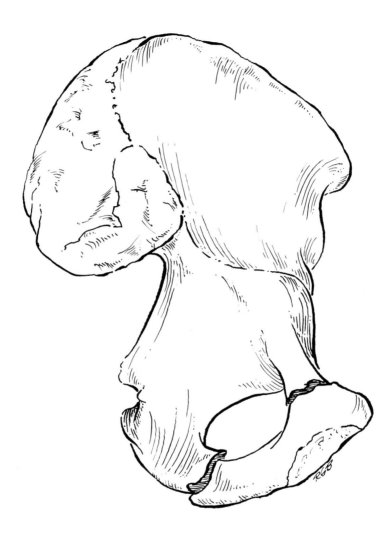

Fig. 12–1. Illustration of pelvis. For a fracture with displacement to occur in the major ring or in the obturator rings, there must be a compensatory break or joint separation elsewhere in that ring.

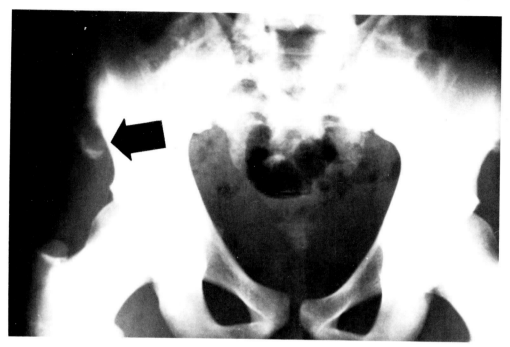

Fig. 12–2. Avulsion fracture of bony prominence (arrow) which occurs most often in the adolescent and following strong contraction of the muscle originating from that prominence.

motion exercises can be begun as soon as the pain subsides. These should be progressively performed until the full ranges of motion of the hips are obtained. In the more severe avulsion fracture, achieving the full range of motion can require up to two months. Following this time, progressive resistance exercises should be performed until full strength is reattained. These injuries do not require operative reattachment of the avulsed fragment. Rarely will one find a long-term disability from this type of fracture.

Isolated Fractures to the Pelvis and Sacrum

An isolated fracture of the pelvis is one in which the energy of the injuring force is absorbed by creating a loss in continuity in the bony pelvis or sacrum without significant displacement of the fragments.

Examination. The major complaint in the isolated fracture of the pelvis or sacrum is one of pain in the pelvis and posterior sacral areas, following known trauma of significant extent. Ecchymosis is often present over the area of injury. Compression of the iliac crest will usually cause pain at the area of fracture in the patient with pelvic or sacral fracture, even though undisplaced. These injuries are rarely unstable.

Roentgenograms. The anteroposterior roentgenogram of the pelvis may or may not show a fracture. Oblique views (Fig. 12–3) of the pelvis can be extremely helpful in visualizing the "hidden" pelvic or sacral fracture when the anteroposterior view has failed to demonstrate evidence of fracture.

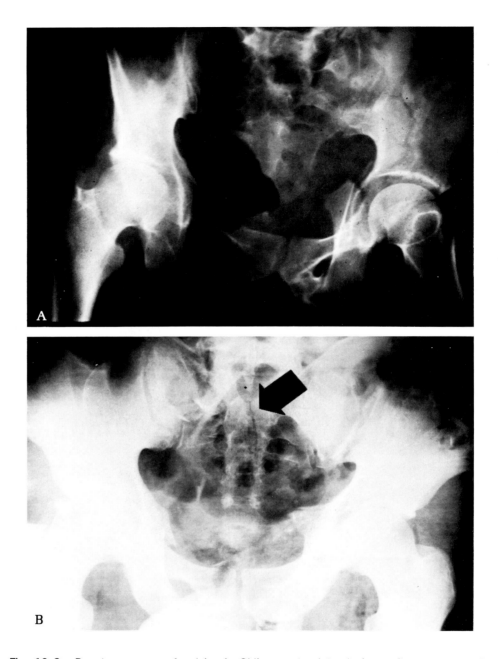

Fig. 12–3. Roentgenograms of pelvis. A, Oblique anterolateral view—often necessary to demonstrate specific pelvic injury such as fractures at midacetabulum and into its superior weight bearing dome. Note multiple fractures of wing, isthmus, and acetabulum of left pelvis. B, Frontal oblique view which may demonstrate sacral injuries not otherwise seen. Arrow points to vertical fracture of sacrum.

Treatment. Bed rest is recommended to relieve symptoms of the isolated fracture and is followed by ambulation with or without crutch support as necessary. This is an individual matter for each patient. Disability for longer than three months following this type of fracture would be unlikely.

Displaced Fractures and/or Dislocations

Any force sufficiently great to cause a fracture of the pelvis and to displace the fragments causes a second fracture or joint separation within the ring involved. A direct blow to the symphysis area may fracture the pubis and the ischium across the obturator foramen. Displacement of this bony segment is at times combined with the similar injury to the pubis and ischium of the opposite side. However, the single fractures of the pubis and ischium may be associated with the separation of the symphysis pubis. In this injury, if the sacroiliac joints and the remainder of the pelvis are intact, this should be a stable injury allowing early weight bearing without complication.

Should the fracture of the pubis and ischium be associated with a vertical fracture of the ipsilateral ilium lateral to the sacroiliac joint, associated with a dislocation of the sacroiliac joint following separation of the sacroiliac ligaments, or associated with a vertical fracture of the sacrum just medial to the sacroiliac joint on the same side, an instability results. This is the so-called Malgaigne fracture (Fig. 12–4). Similar circumstances that create an immediately unstable injury are those in which the symphysis pubis is separated in association with a vertical fracture of the ilium lateral to the sacroiliac joints, in association with a dislocation of the sacroiliac joint following disruption of

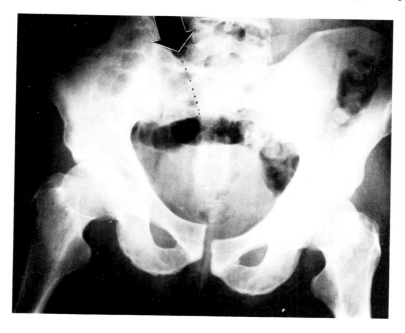

Fig. 12–4. Anteroposterior roentgenogram of pelvis showing separation of symphysis pubis associated with longitudinal sacral fracture (arrow). Note superior shift of right hemipelvis.

the sacroiliac ligaments, or in association with a vertical fracture of the sacrum just medial to the sacroiliac joint. In the aforementioned injuries of the symphysis or the pubis and the ischium associated with a fracture of the ilium or of the sacrum adjacent to the sacroiliac joint, stability of the fractured pelvis will be seen as soon as union of the fracture adjacent to the sacroiliac joint occurs. However, in symphysis or pubic and ischial injuries associated with separation of the sacroiliac joint, regardless of other pelvic injuries, there will tend to be a pelvic instability even after "healing" (see treatment). Ligamentous healing alone seldom provides sufficient strength for needed weight bearing to occur without sacroiliac displacement or discomfort.

Because of its cancellous bone, the pelvis has an abundant blood supply and thus provides an excellent source of blood for hematoma, subsequent clot formation, and rapid fracture healing. Accurate radioactive tracer studies on blood volume have shown that the average pelvic fracture causes a blood loss of about 1500 cc into the surrounding tissues.

Examination. When trauma of sufficient magnitude to cause any displaced fracture or joint separation has occurred, the patient's primary complaint is pain in the pelvic area involved. Separation of the symphysis pubis is often palpable when present. Fracture in this area is indicated by palpation of crepitus. When the Malgaigne type of injury is present, a proximal shift of one entire side of the pelvis may be present. This is best illustrated by an *apparent* leg length shortening on the involved side. This is the measurement of the leg length from the umbilicus to the tip of the medial malleolus. The true leg length as measured from the anterior superior iliac spine to the tip of the medial malleolus will be unchanged from the preinjury length, and will under ordinary circumstances be equal to the true length of the uninjured side (Fig. 12–5).

The patient with a pelvic injury of this significance, because of the usual heavy loss of blood into the extravascular space, may well be in shock on arrival at an emergency unit (Fig. 12–6). An immediate typing and cross matching of blood should be accomplished at the same time that a central venous catheter is introduced into the vein, inasmuch as the patient may go into shock during the triage. Major arterial or venous bleeding can occur in association with pelvic fractures because of vascular injury to the common iliac or branch vessels. The best means of gauging this injury and indeed the patient's general condition is the central venous pressure. Arteriograms have been utilized in an effort at more complete assessment of injury but are difficult to interpret because of the multiplicity of vessels within the pelvis.

Another complication occurring not uncommonly in the displaced pelvic fracture is injury to the genitourinary system. A ruptured bladder or severed urethra should be recognized immediately. All males should be asked to void, and the specimen should be examined microscopically. Should red cells be abundant in the urine or should the patient be unable to void spontaneously, an indwelling catheter should be inserted into the bladder. In the female, a catheterized specimen is examined, and the catheter is left in the bladder if red cells are present to any degree. Urologic consultation should be obtained to assess the need for cystograms or other diagnostic measures. Treatment of any disruption of the urinary tract assumes precedence over the orthopaedic injuries.

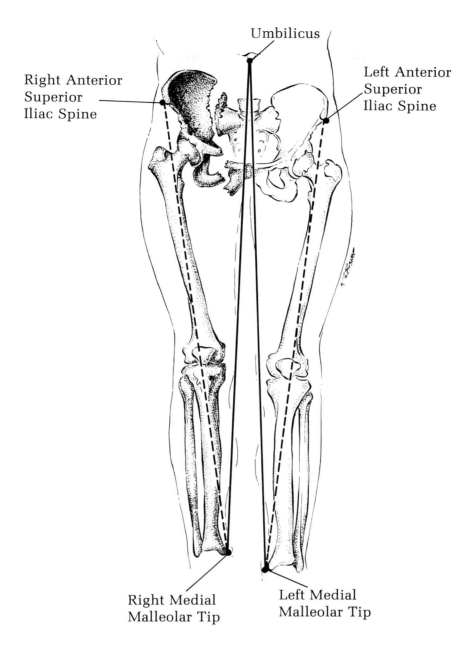

Umbilicus

Right Anterior
Superior
Iliac Spine

Left Anterior
Superior
Iliac Spine

Right Medial
Malleolar Tip

Left Medial
Malleolar Tip

Fig. 12–5.   Illustration showing apparent shortening of leg length associated with superior shift following Malgaigne fracture (Fig. 12–4). True leg length from anterior superior iliac spine to medial malleolus has not changed, but effective leg length from umbilicus to medial malleolus (apparent leg length) is decreased on affected side.

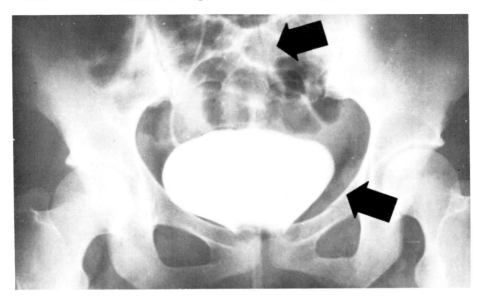

Fig. 12–6. Intravenous urogram showing displacement of bladder (lower arrow) by hematoma associated with pelvis injury on same side. Upper arrow points to fracture line in sacrum. Just inferior to lower arrow is a fracture of pubis and ischium.

Less common, but a complication that may be associated with the fractured pelvic ring near the sacroiliac joint is injury to the fourth lumbar nerve and/or the lumbosacral plexus. This is identified by sensory decrease or loss at the base of the great toe and/or weakness in the anterior compartment muscles. A residual weakness in the anterior compartment of the lower leg and thus weak ankle or toe dorsiflexion can result.

Roentgenograms. The most helpful roentgenographic view for routine evaluation of any pelvic injury is the anteroposterior one. Any break in the cortical continuity of the pubis or the ischium should be noted. Separation of the symphysis also may be seen on this view. Extension of a fracture line adjacent to the sacroiliac joint on the iliac or sacral side is often difficult to visualize. Should this injury be suspected, the anteroposterior rotational views may help clarify the full extent of bony injury. When complete disruption of the pelvic ring exists, the wing of the ilium on the injured side appears wider than that of the uninjured side because of an external rotation of the pelvis that occurs on the injured side when bony continuity of the entire hemipelvis is lost.

Treatment. Fractures of both pubic and ischial bones usually require only bed rest initially. Once the acute symptoms begin to subside, the patient may begin ambulation with the use of crutches and a four-point gait. In this instance, the sacroiliac joints have not been disrupted, and the pelvis should be stable.

Fractures of the pubis and ischium or the separation of the symphysis associated with a fracture adjacent to the sacroiliac joint or dislocation of that joint requires skeletal traction on the involved side. An effective method for

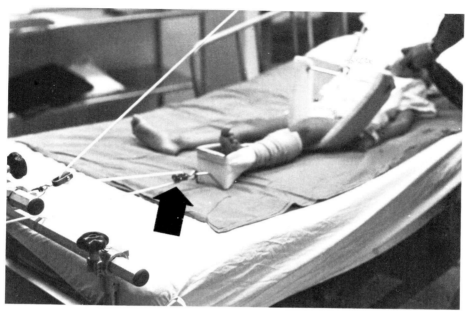

Fig. 12–7. Management of fractured pelvis of youthful patient by Russell's traction, an effective method of traction for treatment of pelvic and hip injuries. Arrow points to pulley which reverses line of pull of rope and doubles effect of weight.

pelvic and hip injuries is Russell's traction, combining a sling under the knee with a pin through the distal tibia and fibula (Fig. 12–7). Ten to 15 pounds of weight is usually sufficient for this type of traction. The fractured side is then reduced to its normal position as judged by a roentgenogram and/or by measuring apparent leg lengths from the umbilicus to the tip of the medial malleoli. On occasion, a pelvic sling (Fig. 12–8) may be used in addition to the longitudinal traction, particularly when both sides of the pelvis are fractured. When the pelvic sling is used, a compressive force not otherwise available may be added by crossing the ropes from the sling to the weights on the opposite sides. The amount of weight used should be just sufficient to lift the buttocks from the bed. Such traction may need to be maintained for ten to twelve weeks because of the soft cancellous callus which occurs. However, six to eight weeks in traction may be sufficient to allow guarded weight bearing. Should the proximal injury be a sacroiliac disruption, a trial of protective weight bearing is indicated following traction; however, the surgeon must be alert to a settling that can occur across this joint following injury. If such settling does occur, or if the joint is painful, a sacroiliac fusion is the only means of offering painless stability. When bony healing is achieved in pelvic fractures without the sacroiliac disruption, then the pelvis should have achieved sufficient stability for weight bearing. A method of progressive weight bearing is useful in rehabilitating the patient.

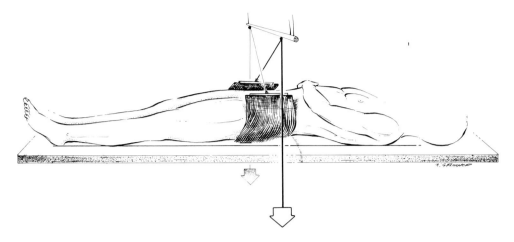

Fig. 12–8.   Illustration of patient being treated in pelvic sling. Crossed ropes to weights off side of bed create medial compressive forces, most beneficial in treatment of fractures of both sides of pelvis. Weights should be sufficient to allow passage of flat of hand under buttocks.

Fractures of the Acetabulum

Acetabular fractures will be most commonly found at one of three points, depending upon the direction of the force creating the fracture. One type of acetabular fracture occurs when the femur is extended and a force along the shaft drives the femoral head into the acetabulum superiorly (Fig. 12–2A).

Another type of acetabular fracture often seen is in the medial acetabular wall. An external force on the greater trochanter drives the femoral head medially into the acetabular wall (Fig. 12–9).

When the hip is at the 90-degree flexion position, a force along the shaft of the femur, if of sufficient magnitude, will drive the femoral head out of the acetabulum posteriorly. Either the posterior capsule must tear, or the posterior acetabular wall will fracture. Combination fractures of the foregoing three types can occur.

Examination. In any fracture of the acetabulum, there will be pain on movement of the hip. A compression force across the trochanters is painful at the fracture site. In the fracture of the superior acetabulum, the true leg length may be shortened, particularly if any significant superior shift of the acetabular roof has occurred.

A fracture of the medial wall of the acetabulum may not cause other signs to allow identification of the specific injury on examination. Evidence of ecchymosis may be seen overlying the greater trochanter on the symptomatic side in this injury. Movement of the involved hip is painful and limited. Pain on motion associated with loss of normal active hip motion is present in any patient with an acetabular fracture even though no dislocation of the hip is present.

When a posterior dislocation of the hip occurs along with a fractured acetabulum, it is usually recognized clinically by the characteristic position of the hip in flexion, internal rotation, and adduction. There is apparent shorten-

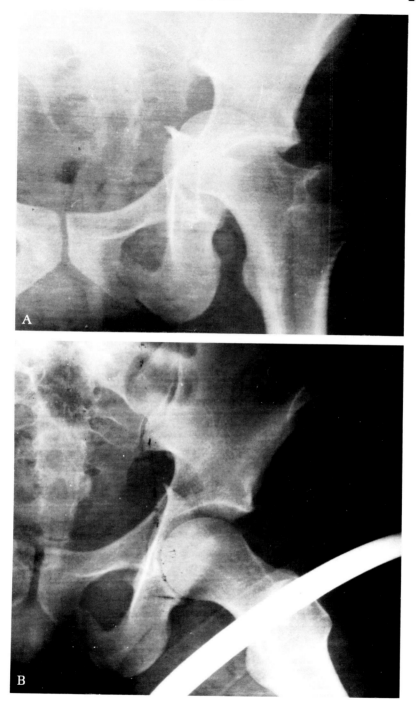

Fig. 12–9. A, Anteroposterior roentgenogram showing medial displacement of femoral head associated with acetabular fracture. B, Balanced skeletal traction applied to reduce femoral head and acetabulum into reasonably good relationship as shown in this roentgenogram.

ing of this extremity. The sciatic nerve emerges from the pelvis at the sciatic notch and courses immediately posterior to the acetabulum. A posterior dislocation or fracture dislocation of the hip may have the complication of a partial or complete sciatic palsy.

Roentgenograms. The anteroposterior roentgenogram should reveal the fracture of the superior weight bearing surface. In addition, a fracture of the medial wall of the acetabulum should be visualized on the anteroposterior roentgenogram. The full extent of these injuries may be better clarified by oblique (anteroposterior) roentgenographic views. The posterior fracture dislocation may not be readily apparent on the anteroposterior roentgenogram (Fig. 12–10, 12–11). However, a true lateral roentgenogram of the pelvis should demonstrate the loss of continuity of the acetabulum as well as the posterior dislocation of the femoral head (Fig. 13–1B). This type of roentgenogram is secured with the injured side lying against the film cassette. The x-ray technique is identical to that for taking the lateral view of the lumbosacral spine, except that the roentgenographic tube is centered over the greater trochanter. In this technique for the true lateral view of the pelvis the dislocated femoral head and the involved acetabulum will be smaller than that of the normal side. This is because the involved femoral head and acetabulum are closest to the film and subject to less magnification by the roentgen rays. A careful study in this situation reveals the femoral head resting posterior to the acetabulum with an irregularly shaped ossicle lying near it. The cross table lateral roentgenogram of the involved hip may help in a more complete assessment.

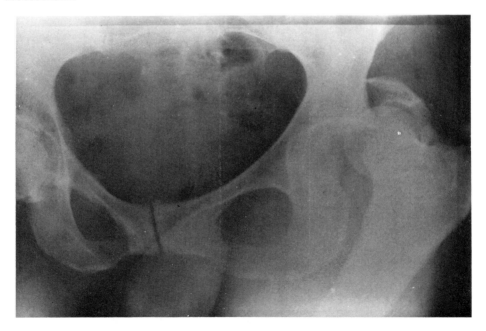

Fig. 12–10. Anteroposterior roentgenogram showing fracture of lateral superior acetabular lip. This is a problem only if sufficient weight bearing surface is lost to allow dislocation of hip. In that instance, surgical fixation may be in order.

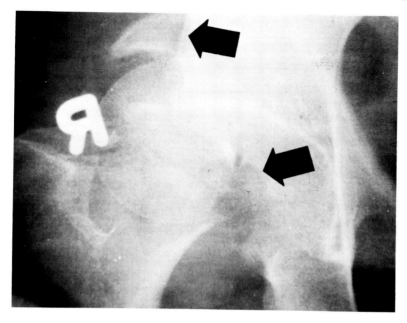

Fig. 12–11. Anteroposterior roentgenogram demonstrating fracture of posterior acetabulum in addition to femoral neck fracture and head dislocation. Upper arrow points to fragment and lower arrow indicates acetabular defect. If size of fragment is significant, surgical fixation may be required for stability of femoral head in acetabulum.

Treatment. In order to avoid the possible long-term complication of avascular necrosis of the femoral head, the posterior fracture-dislocation of the hip should be reduced as soon as possible. Reduction is usually accomplished under heavy analgesia or general anesthesia as necessary. The injured hip is flexed to 90 degrees and adducted, and longitudinal traction is applied to the femoral shaft. While the traction is on, countertraction is placed against the iliac crest by an assistant. Small internal and external rotation jogs are often helpful in bringing the head into the acetabulum. Once the fracture-dislocation has been reduced, the stability of the reduction should be tested by flexing the hip to 30 or 35 degrees and pressing the femoral head into the acetabulum (from neutral rotation and adduction-abduction position). Should the hip injury be innately unstable, it will redislocate at this point. This instability provides an indication for open reduction and internal fixation of the posterior fragment, particularly with little comminution of the posterior fragment(s).

When operative means are not necessary, then Russell's traction should be applied for six weeks to allow the posterior fragments to adhere to their point of origin and/or for the capsule to heal. Then the patient may begin ambulation by crutch walking, with no weight bearing on the affected side, and over the next six weeks may progress to full weight bearing which in the uncomplicated injury should be achieved three months following injury. Because of the potential of avascular necrosis, roentgenograms must be taken every four to six months for several years (at least three years).

Depending upon the size of the superior fragments and whether they can be held in a position congruous to the head, the fracture of the weight bearing dome of the acetabulum may be treated by open or closed methods. If the fragment is large and noncomminuted and does not reduce with traction, then open reduction and fixation with screw(s) or Kirschner wire(s) is indicated to stabilize the femoral head in the acetabulum. If the fragments are comminuted, then skeletal traction of the Russell's type is usually preferred. Traction for eight weeks when indicated is followed by ambulation with no weight bearing for an additional eight weeks. Because of the soft callus formed by the cancellous bone, there can be settling and development of joint incongruity should weight bearing be permitted too early.

A combination of fractures of the medial wall and the superior rim occurs which may tend to collapse the acetabular fragments about the femoral head. In this instance, modest Russell's traction for comfort until the acetabular fragments have been stabilized is the recommended treatment. Stabilization usually requires eight weeks in traction followed by an additional eight-week period of no weight bearing.

Any fracture of the acetabulum that creates a joint incongruity must dictate only a fair long-termed prognosis for that hip joint. Degenerative arthritis often ensues, and arthoplasty may be necessary.

Fractures of the medial wall of the acetabulum may be treated in Russell's traction with a sling under the knee and the Kirschner wire through the distal tibia and fibula for the traction. They may also be treated in balanced skeletal traction with the ring of the Thomas splint against the ischium and the pin in the proximal tibia (just posterior to the tibial tubercle). Progress roentgenograms will be necessary during traction. Should the medial fragment(s) and the femoral head not be moved back into an acceptable position under the weight bearing dome of the acetabulum with this traction, then a lateral eye hook (Scuderi bolt or Miller pin) or a Kirschner wire may be placed into the greater trochanter to provide for direct lateral pull in addition to that of the longitudinal traction. Following reduction, this traction should be maintained for two months before ambulation with crutches is allowed. The ambulation with crutches should be nonweight bearing for an additional six weeks, and then progressive weight bearing can be initiated as tolerated and indicated by examination and roentgenogram following this.

PELVIC FRACTURES IN CHILDREN

Pelvic fractures do occur in the child and are more often the result of significant trauma. Diagnostic and treatment consideration are similar to those for the adult.

REFERENCES

1. Adams, J. C.: Outline of Fractures, Including Joint Injuries, 6th ed. Baltimore, Williams & Wilkins Co., 1972.
2. Blount, W. P.: Fractures in Children. Baltimore, Williams & Wilkins Co., 1954.
3. Clarke, R., Topley, E., and Flear, C.T.G.: Assessment of the blood-loss in civilian trauma. Lancet 1:629, 1955.
4. Larson, C. B., and Linning, J. E., Jr.: Indications for closed and open treatment of fracture dislocations of the hip. J. Bone Joint Surg. 46A:1366, 1964.
5. Ralston, E. L.: Handbook of Fractures. St. Louis, C. V. Mosby Co., 1967.

6. Rang, M. C.: Children's Fractures. Philadelphia, L. B. Lippincott Co., 1974.

7. Rockwood, C. A., and Green, D. P.: Fractures. Philadelphia, J. B. Lippincott Co., 1975.

8. Rowe, C. R., and Lowell, J. D.: Prognosis of fractures of the acetabulum. J. Bone Joint Surg. *43A*:30, 1961.

9. Stewart, M. J., and Milford L. W.: Fracture-dislocation of the hip, an end-result study. J. Bone Joint Surg. *36A*:315, 1954.

10. Watson-Jones, R.: Fractures and Joint Injuries, 4th ed., 2V. Baltimore, Williams & Wilkins Co., 1952-1955.

13

THE HIP

The ball and socket joint of the hip is a remarkable arrangement allowing motion in all spheres, but especially useful are flexion and extension, abduction and adduction, and internal and external rotation. The capsule of the hip joint attaches along the base of the femoral neck laterally and along the periphery of the entire acetabulum medially. This attachment makes the femoral head and neck predominately intra-articular. The fibers of the capsule as viewed anteriorly run in an inferolateral direction. Thus they will tend to be taut with extension and internal rotation and to relax with flexion and external rotation. The primary blood supply for the femoral head arises from a terminal branch of the medial femoral circumflex artery which has passed posterior to the hip joint capsule (Fig. 13–1). This vessel follows the capsule laterally to its insertion along the base of the neck whence it penetrates the capsule and turns proximally along the posterior-superior margin of the femoral neck. There may be a number of these vessels at this point, but all lie within the visceral periosteum of the femoral neck. This positioning of vessels is hence fraught with a certain vulnerability. After passing superomedially along the neck, the vessels divide at the neck-head junction so that one branch of the vessel will serve the metaphyseal area of the femoral neck and another branch will serve the femoral head. This is at the point where the epiphyseal plate existed in the immature hip. Little, if any, direct anastomosis or circulation of vessels occurs across the epiphyseal plate in the child or across the area in which this epiphyseal plate existed in the adult. After any dislocation of the femoral head from its relationship to the acetabulum in the child or the adult there is a distinct risk of loss of blood supply to the femoral head. Furthermore, because these vessels lie in the visceral periosteum of the femoral neck, any fracture of the femoral neck with displacement may well cause a loss of blood supply to the femoral head. These factors demand special consideration in the treatment of injuries about the hip joint.

Hip Dislocations

Posterior dislocation of the hip is typically a product of trauma. The dislocating force runs along the longitudinal axis of the femur when it is flexed to about 90 degrees and slightly adducted. This dislocation of the hip most commonly occurs to the rider in the right front seat of an automobile. On impact his knee(s) strikes the dashboard to provide longitudinal force.

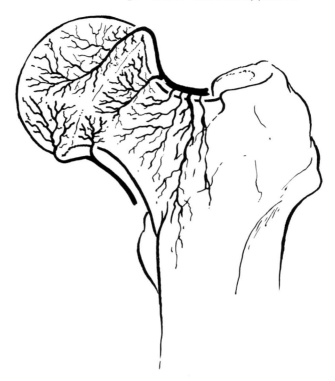

Fig. 13–1. Composite concept of blood supply of proximal femur after Trueta and Crock. Since femoral head and neck are entirely intracapsular and arterial flow is primarily from distal neck proximally, the precarious nature of hip dislocations and displaced femoral neck fractures is evident.

Examination. Examination of the patient with the posterior dislocation of the hip will reveal classic pathognomonic signs. The thigh of the involved side is held in a partially flexed, internally rotated and adducted position. This is an obligatory position because the femoral head is locked posterior to the acetabulum. As part of the examination, the sensory and motor competence of the lower extremities distal to the hip on the involved side must be tested, as a sciatic nerve deficit is not an uncommon complication associated with posterior dislocation of the hip.

Roentgenograms. Adequate roentgenograms to determine the posterior dislocation of the hip include the anteroposterior view as well as a true lateral view of the pelvis (Fig. 13–2). In the true lateral view the same technique is used as in taking the lateral views of the lumbosacral spine, except that the tube is focused over the greater trochanter. The hip suspected of dislocation is placed against the cassette so that it will be the "small" femoral head and acetabulum (being farthest from the tube and thus having less magnification) when studying the roentgenogram. On the anteroposterior view, one *may* see that the femoral head is obviously not in relationship to the acetabulum. However, just often enough the femoral head lies posterior to the acetabulum in

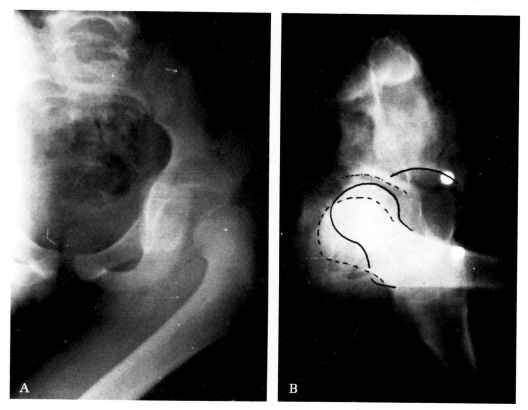

Fig. 13–2. Roentgenograms demonstrating dislocation of femoral head from acetabulum. A, Anteroposterior view. Adduction of femur accompanied by internal rotation is classic for posterior dislocation of hip. Inability to visualize lesser trochanter indicates internal rotation is present. B, True lateral roentgenogram, often helpful in more fully assessing extent of injury to hip. Dotted lines outline normal femoral head and acetabulum superior to it. Intact lines show dislocated femoral head and acetabular roof under which it should rest.

such a position as to appear to be "in place" on the anteroposterior view. Dislocated hips have been missed owing to this *apparent* position of the femoral head. Because the head is posterior to the acetabulum in a forced internal rotation position, the lesser trochanter will be less visible than in the normal position. On the true lateral roentgenogram of the pelvis, the femoral head will be seen posterior to the acetabulum on the involved side. One can compare the dislocated (smaller) head and acetabulum to the normal (larger) ones. The cross table lateral view of the involved hip is also often confirmatory of the loss of the relationship of the head to the acetabulum.

Treatment. Because of potential loss of blood supply to the femoral head in the dislocated hip, reduction at the earliest possible time is recommended. An effort may be made to reduce the hip, utilizing the analgesia and relaxation provided by a combination of meperidine and diazepam. To accomplish the reduction of the hip the surgeon must stand astride the involved joint (Fig.

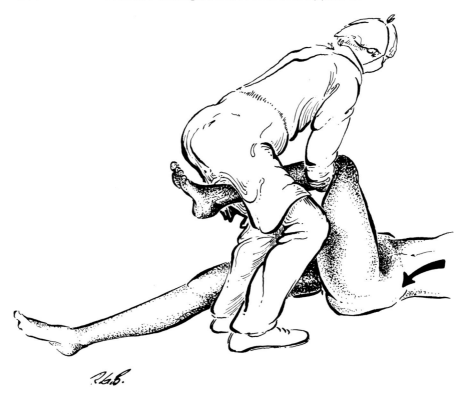

Fig. 13-3. Method of reducing posterior dislocation of hip. Hip must be held at 90-degree angle to trunk and adducted before traction is applied. Then steady longitudinal traction is applied along axis of femur while countertraction is placed against wing of ilium. Short internal and external rotary jogs often help final reduction to occur.

13-3). The hip is flexed to 90 degrees and adducted approximately 15 degrees. Traction is then applied distally along the axis of the femur while countertraction is applied against the iliac crest by an assistant. With steady traction followed by several small rotational movements, the hip should move back into position. If relaxation is not possible under analgesia, then a general anesthetic must be used to secure sufficient relaxation for reduction of the dislocated hip. Once the patient is relaxed, the same method is used to reduce the dislocated hip. It is extremely rare for the hip not to come into socket at one of these two attempts. However, if it does not reduce by manipulation, the leg should be placed in Russell's skeletal traction (Fig. 12-6) with a 15-pound weight and with the foot of the bed elevated. This system slowly but progressively tires the muscle spasm to the extent that the hip can often drop into location spontaneously. The weights may be increased to as much as 30 pounds in 5-pound increments if necessary. Only after these efforts to reduce the hip have failed should operative reduction be considered. Since the incidence of avascular necrosis of the femoral head rises geometrically after the hip has remained dislocated for eight or more hours, a certain deliberate haste must be made in the nonoperative treatment before making a decision to operate.

After reduction, the hip should be maintained in traction for approximately three weeks to allow for some capsular healing. The patient can then begin ambulation with no weight bearing on the involved side for an additional period of two months. Exercises to improve range of motion and strengthen the muscles must then be pursued to obtain the best result. Roentgenograms should be taken of this hip at three-month intervals for the first year and at six-month intervals after that for a total of three years. In some instances, evidence of avascular necrosis of the femoral head has been noted several years after dislocation. Should any symptoms arise in the hip in subsequent years, attention should be directed to the possibility of an avascular necrosis.

Anterior Dislocation of the Hip

Anterior dislocation of the hip can only occur from an adducted position with the hip slightly flexed. A strong external rotation force must be then added to dislocate the hip.

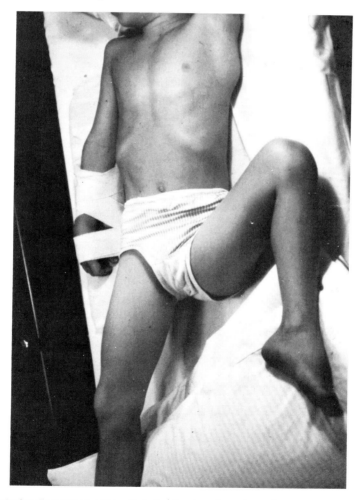

Fig. 13–4. Anterior dislocation of hip. Note leg lies in external rotation. Adduction, traction, and internal rotation should complete reduction of this dislocation. Abduction and internal rotation will maintain reduction.

Examination. On examination of the anteriorly dislocated hip, the leg lies externally rotated and often slightly flexed (Fig. 13–4). It may lie in adduction, but this position is not obligatory. The patient cannot actively flex the hip when it is dislocated in this position. The femoral head is palpable anterior to the femoral triangle.

Roentgenograms. The anteroposterior and cross table lateral roentgenograms of the involved hip should indicate the dislocation of the femoral head from its relationship to the acetabulum. In addition, with the external rotation present in the anterior dislocation, on the anteroposterior roentgenogram the femoral neck will appear shorter, the lesser trochanter will appear to be larger, and a portion of the greater trochanter will recede into a superimposition over the femoral neck.

Treatment. After administering a combination of meperidine and diazepam for analgesia and relaxation, this anterior dislocation of the hip can often be reduced. Reduction requires longitudinal traction with the hip in adduction. This is followed by internally rotating the hip. Once the head is in the acetabulum, abduction and internal rotation will be the position of stability. Should the hip not reduce by this method, then a general anesthetic must be administered. Once the patient is relaxed, the previously described maneuver is performed. The limb should then be positioned in abduction and kept in Russell's type of traction for three weeks (Fig. 12–6). This period is followed by crutch walking with no weight bearing for a total of eight weeks. Repeated roentgenographic examination of the hip over the first year at three-month intervals and for the subsequent two years at six-month intervals is necessary to make certain that no evidence of avascular necrosis is encountered.

Obturator Dislocation of the Hip

The uncommon obturator dislocation of the hip is caused by a forced hyperabduction of the neutral hip which uses the greater trochanter against the pelvis to lever the femoral head out of the acetabulum. This forces the head inferiorly into the obturator foramen.

Examination. On inspection, the hip will be clearly fixed in the abducted position and cannot be brought to neutral without pelvic accommodation to the fixed femoral head. Neurologic deficit is seldom seen in this injury.

Roentgenograms. The anteroposterior roentgenogram is pathognomonic of the obturator dislocation, as the femoral head rests in the obturator foramen (Fig. 13–5). The cross table lateral view of the involved hip will provide assurance that the femoral head is not resting anterior or posterior to the obturator foramen.

Treatment. The reduction of the obturator dislocation, which has occurred by tearing the inferior capsule, has been said to be most easily possible by converting it to an anterior or a posterior dislocation, and then reducing either of these in the appropriate manner. My experience, however, suggests that an abduction traction on the femur with countertraction against the pelvis is essential. A firm lateral pressure is then placed against the medial side of the femoral head as slight internal and external rotation movements of the femur are performed. Adduction to neutral then completes this reduction. This has proved an effective means of reducing this particular dislocation. Since this

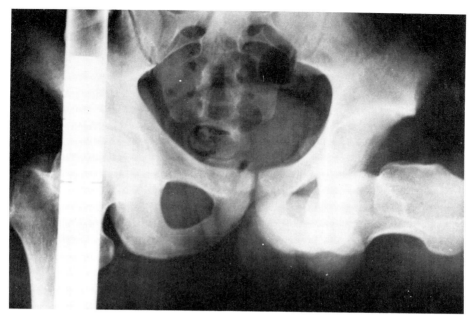

Fig. 13–5. Anteroposterior view of obturator dislocation of hip with femoral head lying in obturator foramen. Since this dislocated head has moved toward its blood supply, the likelihood of ensuing avascular necrosis is diminished.

dislocated head has not moved in a direction to damage its blood supply, the patient can begin crutch walking with no weight bearing after becoming asymptomatic from several days of bed rest. The patient should continue nonweight bearing for six weeks and have roentgenographic examinations at two- to three-month intervals for the first year and at six-month intervals for the following two years. The likelihood of avascular necrosis is slight because of the direction of dislocation.

Subcapital Hip Fractures

The subcapital fracture of the hip may occur by a variety of mechanisms of injury. It is not clear in many instances whether a patient falls and fractures the hip or whether he fractures the hip and falls. At any rate, if abduction forces are associated with the fall, the fracture line runs more toward the horizontal across the neck of the femur. The adduction force creates a fracture line that tends to be more vertical through the neck of the femur. A fall on the lateral aspect of the hip may cause an impacted fracture.

Examination. On examination, the hip in which there is an impacted fracture tends to be fixed in a slight external rotation position. Definite stability is present. In the other fractures of the femoral neck, there is definite loss of continuity of the femoral neck; hence, the entire lower extremity lies in 90 degrees of external rotation. If the fracture is not impacted, crepitus can be palpated with any attempted passive movement of the hip.

Roentgenograms. The anteroposterior and lateral roentgenograms allow a more effective assessment of the type of subcapital fracture (Fig. 13–6). Purely from the standpoint of prognosis, the more horizontal the line of fracture, the more likely will adequate union occur without avascular necrosis ensuing. As the fracture line moves toward the vertical, the shearing force becomes greater, and the chances of union of the fracture are less. Associated with the increasingly vertical fracture line is an increased potential for an aseptic

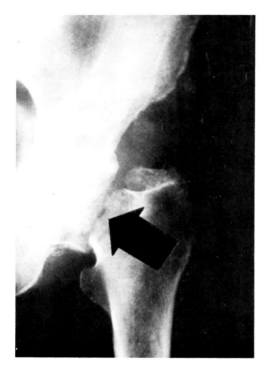

Fig. 13–6. Arrow points to subcapital fracture of femoral neck. Fracture line is vertical, increasing shear at fracture site and increasing likelihood fo nonunion.

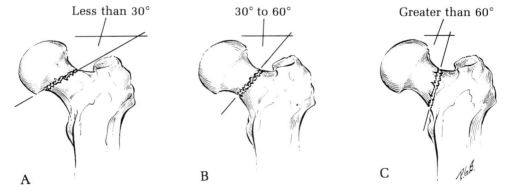

Less than 30°   30° to 60°   Greater than 60°

A   B   C

Fig. 13–7. Illustration of concept of Pauwels: the more horizontal the fracture line, the better the chances for union. A, Type I fracture line intercepts horizontal at less than 30 degrees. B, Type II fracture line intercepts horizontal plane at between 30 and 60 degrees. C, Type III fracture line intercepts horizontal at greater than 60 degrees.

necrosis of the femoral head. This has led a German orthopaedic surgeon, Pauwels, to classify femoral neck fractures as types I, II, or III (Fig. 13–7). The Pauwels I fracture is the fracture line that is less than 30 degrees from horizontal. The line of the Pauwels II fracture intercepts the horizontal plane at between 30 and 60 degrees, and the fracture line of the Pauwels III fracture intercepts the horizontal plane at greater than 60 degrees. The lower the Pauwels number, the greater are the chances of fracture union without avascular necrosis. From the discussion of the vascular anatomy of the hip, one recognizes that any significant displacement of the femoral neck fracture is associated with a significant increase in the chances of interruption of the blood supply to the femoral head.

Treatment. The treatment of choice in the impacted femoral neck fracture is three-pin fixation, provided the impaction does not force the weight bearing lines of the inferior femoral head into a greater valgus position than the inferior neck (Fig. 13–8). Fahey points out that the hyperabducted impacted fracture has a strong tendency toward an avascular necrosis. In this instance a primary prosthetic replacement would probably be in order. Some treating surgeons, however, place the patient with the impacted femoral neck fracture in bed for several days to determine stability of impaction and, if disimpaction does not occur, then permit mobilization on crutches with no weight bearing. The displaced subcapital fractures with a fracture line intercepting the horizontal plane at less than 60% should be reduced and internally fixed by the surgeon's method of choice. My preference is for a sliding type of nail that will allow the settling necessary following concomitant resorption of the fracture line. No weight bearing is allowed on the limb until evidence of some trabecular pattern coursing the fracture line is seen on a roentgenogram. The fracture lines that intercept the horizontal plane at greater than 60 degrees have less chance of union, and a primary prosthesis should be considered.

Intertrochanteric Fractures

The intertrochanteric fracture tends to occur more often in the older aged patient and is often comminuted. A common mechanism of injury is not clearly identified.

Examination. The examination reveals essentially the same findings as in the femoral neck fracture. The entire lower limb lies in external rotation.

Roentgenograms. The anteroposterior and cross table lateral roentgenograms are most valuable in determining the approach necessary for reduction of the intertrochanteric fracture. The fracture is clearly seen on the anteroposterior view. However, posterior comminution and loss of stability is not clear without a good cross table lateral roentgenogram (Fig. 13–9). This may not be obtained in some instances until the patient is in the operating room on the fracture table.

Treatment. The treatment of choice in the intertrochanteric fracture is open reduction and internal fixation. If a significant loss of the posterior portion of the lesser trochanter occurs by comminution, then stability cannot be expected without some medial displacement of the shaft. The method of open reduction described by Dimon and Hughston has been most effective. In this method a medial displacement of the femoral shaft is accomplished to provide bony

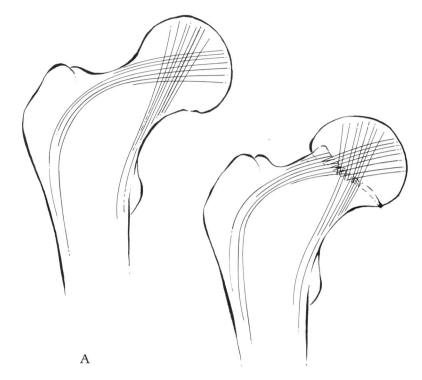

A

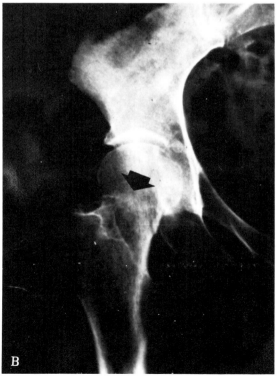

B

contact between the inferior femoral neck and the shaft. Internal fixation can be secured with Jewett and Holt nails or the lag screw combined with the compression plate. Following nailing, the patient with the intertrochanteric fracture should not be allowed to bear weight on this extremity until evidence of early union is present. This will most likely require three months.

Should it be necessary for various medical reasons, the intertrochanteric fracture may be treated in skeletal traction. The Russell's type of traction with a Kirschner wire through the distal tibia and fibula is used. Approximately 10 pounds of weight will maintain reduction of the intertrochanteric fracture while callous formation ensues (Fig. 12–6). About three months are required for the callus to be sufficiently firm to allow the patient out of traction. He should be kept nonweight bearing until the callus is seen on roentgenogram to have matured.

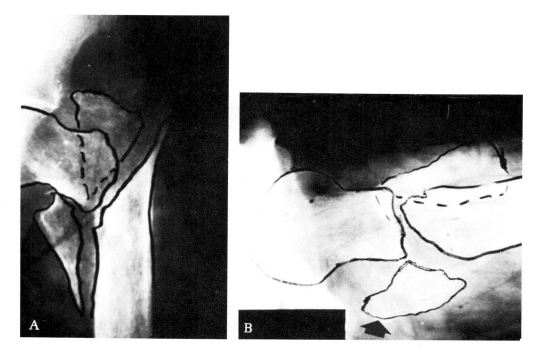

Fig. 13–9. Roentgenograms with fragments of comminuted intertrochanteric fracture outlined. A, Anteroposterior view. B, Lateral view. Arrow points to fragment that drops posteriorly and allows instability of fracture. To achieve stability distal fragment must be shifted medially and fixed surgically to major neck and head fragments.

Fig. 13–8. A, Illustration of Fahey concept of impacted femoral neck fractures. If the head is forced into too severe a valgus position in relation to its neck, then avascular necrosis is prone to ensue. Note interruption of stress lines. B, Arrow points to line of increased density representing impacted fracture of the femoral neck.

Subtrochanteric Fracture

The subtrochanteric fracture is seen particularly in the elderly adult following a fall and appears to be a result of a transmitted rotational force. Often the subtrochanteric fracture has a spiral configuration.

Examination. The involved limb of the patient with the subtrochanteric fracture will tend to lie in external rotation. This is not obligatory, however, since the iliopsoas tendon is attached proximal to the fracture. However, there will be shortening of the involved extremity.

Roentgenograms. The anteroposterior and lateral roentgenograms are essential for the evaluation of the subtrochanteric fracture (Fig. 13–10). There is a tendency for the proximal fragment of the subtrochanteric fracture to flex and externally rotate because the iliopsoas tendon is attached to the lesser trochanter. The head and neck appear to be short because of the flexed position of the proximal fragment.

Treatment. If the fracture is such that major fragments allow stability with fixation, then open reduction and internal fixation is the treatment of choice. The Jewett nail is an excellent fixation device for the subtrochanteric fracture. It is important, however, in using the Jewett nail not to place a screw superior to the fracture site. When a screw is so placed, it has a tendency to maintain

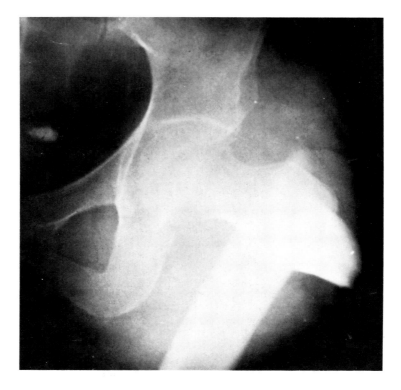

Fig. 13–10. Anteroposterior roentgenogram showing subtrochanteric fracture of femur. Note proximal fragment is abducted and externally rotated. For proper union distal fragment must be brought to meet proximal fragment surgically or by traction.

separation of fragments. Should the subtrochanteric fracture be so comminuted as to defy internal fixation surgically, then it can be treated by the Russell's type of skeletal traction. Ten pounds usually provides sufficient weight to maintain reduction of this fracture. The traction method must align the distal fragment to the proximal fragment(s). This alignment occasionally requires significant flexion and abduction of the thigh (Fig. 14–1). To accomplish this by traction may require ingenuity on the part of the treating physician (and *patience* on the part of the patient).

Weight bearing should not be allowed on an extremity in which this type of fracture has occurred until roentgenographic evidence of early union is seen. Certainly a minimum period of time is three months. The patient who is treated in traction will need to be in traction for those three months.

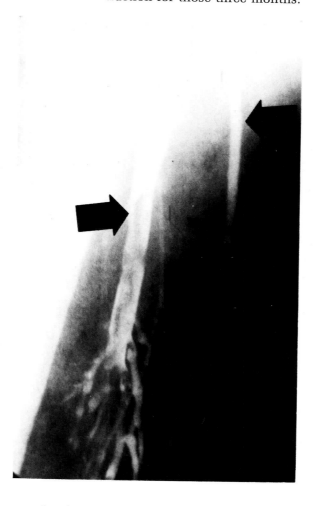

Fig. 13-11. Venogram of patient following use of Jewett nail for intertrochanteric fracture. Note dark tail of thrombus trailing up superficial femoral vein (left arrow) and increased filling of saphenous vein by contrast medium (right arrow)—often seen in partial or complete deep obstruction.

Complications

Silent venous thrombosis is a not uncommon complication of any hip injury. The incidence of this complication runs slightly in excess of 50% in those series in which no preventive measures are employed (Fig. 13–11). A statistically significant lowering of silent venous thrombosis has been achieved by elevation of the foot of the bed by 15 to 20 degrees. Other prophylactic measures or treatment such as anticoagulants and elastic stockings, may be employed, depending upon circumstances and the experiences of the surgeon.

Nonunion of the femoral neck fracture may occur because of the relationship of the fracture line to horizontal. As indicated previously, the more vertical the fracture line, the greater the shear and the more likely a nonunion will occur.

The adequacy of reduction will also play a role in nonunion. The perfectly reduced fracture in most instances will proceed to better union.

Adequacy of fixation is another determining factor in good union. The type of fixative device will play a role as will the stability provided by that device for that specific fracture. For example, the Jewett nail is an excellent fixation device for the intertrochanteric fracture. If posterior comminution exists, however, then a shift of the distal fragment toward the most proximal fragment is necessary in order to provide needed stability, even with the Jewett nail. The nail is only as good as the bone in which it is used.

HIP INJURIES IN CHILDREN

Any prognosis given regarding a hip injury in a child must be guarded so far as the future of the hip is concerned. Not only is it possible that the growth potential can be altered, but there also may be avascular necrosis because of interruption of the blood supply to the hip. In addition, nonunion of femoral neck fractures have been reported in children.

Dislocations of the Hip

Although rare, traumatic dislocation of the hip in the child does occur. This almost always is the posterior dislocation of the hip caused by a force along the longitudinal axis of the flexed femur.

Examination. In the posterior dislocated hip, an obligatory flexion, adduction, and internal rotation, each to a modest degree, are noted. However, none of these is correctable because of the fixed position of the femoral head posterior to the acetabulum.

Roentgenograms. Roentgenograms should include the anteroposterior view as well as the true lateral view of the pelvis (Fig. 13–2).

Treatment. The urgency of reduction of the dislocated hip in the child obtains because the circulation to the femoral head is even more precarious than that of·the adult (see anatomy of hip). The hip is reduced in a manner identical in that of the adult, and the limb is maintained in a Russell's type of traction with a traction boot for three weeks. Nonweight bearing is enforced for six weeks following this injury. The child must be followed for some five or more years after this to be certain of the status of the vascularity in the head.

Fractures of the Femoral Neck

Fractures of the femoral neck in the child are not common but do occur generally following significant trauma.

Examination. The injured limb will lie in external rotation whether or not the fracture is impacted. The hip is an irritable one in an irritable child. If the fracture is impacted, however, the hip can often be put through a gentle limited range of motion. Any effort to examine the leg of the hip fracture that is displaced is met with failure.

Roentgenograms. Anteroposterior and lateral (the cross table view may be the easiest to obtain) roentgenograms may show a line of increased density at the neck, indicating impaction. However, there may be a radiolucent line across the femoral neck without evident displacement, or there may be significant displacement of the femoral head from the femoral neck (Fig. 13–12).

Treatment. If the fracture of the femoral neck is undisplaced, a spica cast can be placed on for ten to twelve weeks, at which time roentgenograms should show reasonable evidence of beginning union. If there is any significant displacement of the fragments as viewed on the anteroposterior and lateral roentgenographic views, consideration must be given to internal fixation of this fracture following open reduction. Callahan believes that opening the capsule relieves the pressure within the capsule. This intracapsular pressure could well cause occlusion of the artery to the femoral head. He recommends that the capsule be left open following the internal fixation with three pins. This system was followed at the Cook County Hospital with good overall results. The operative approach to the femoral neck fracture appeared more effective than did attempting traction and/or casting of this extremity in a spica cast.

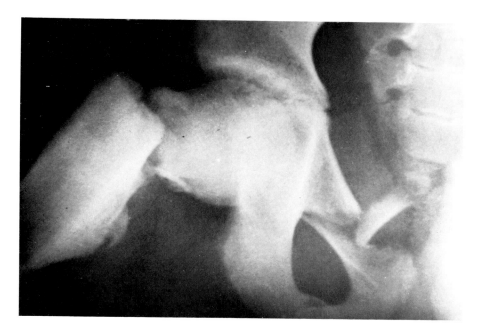

Fig. 13–12. Anteroposterior roentgenogram showing midfemoral neck fracture in fourteen-year-old boy. I prefer open reduction and internal fixation with pins associated with capsular decompression for treating this fracture.

Traumatic Epiphyseal Slip

The traumatic epiphyseal slip is the product of acute injury and should be treated much as one treats the femoral neck fracture. This is a true orthopaedic emergency demanding early definitive care.

Examination. On inspection, the involved lower limb is seen to lie in external rotation. The patient is anxious and resists any effort at examination of the involved extremity.

Roentgenograms. The anteroposterior and lateral roentgenographic views confirm a separation of the femoral head away from the femoral neck through the epiphyseal plate (Fig. 13–13). On occasion on one of the roentgenographic views, a segment of metaphysis of femoral neck will be seen to be still attached

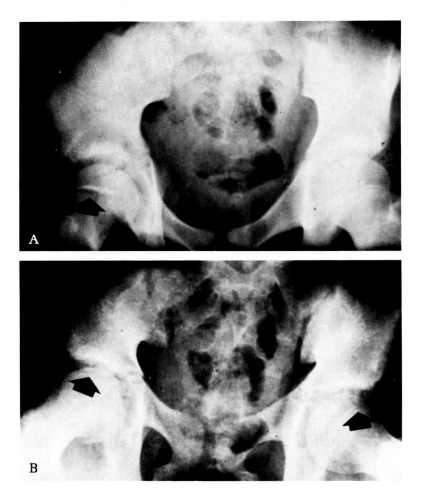

Fig. 13–13. Roentgenograms of hips of fourteen-year-old boy complaining of pain in hips and knees. A, Anteroposterior view showing perhaps some widening of epiphyseal plate on right (arrow). B, Lateral view showing slipping of capital femoral epiphyses (arrows), the right being more advanced than the left. This slipping is seldom related to trauma, although an acute slip can be superimposed upon a chronic condition.

to the epiphyseal plate. This would imply the type II separation as described by Salter and Harris. This is more common in the traumatic slip of the capital femoral epiphysis. The nontraumatic slip of this epiphysis occurs in the zone of cartilage proliferation and is a different pathologic entity, even though similar treatment methods are used. Following open reduction and internal fixation, the patient with this injury should not be allowed to bear weight on this extremity for eight to ten weeks. The evaluation of progress of this hip should be continued for every two to three months for the first year and every six months after that for several years—at least until one is confident of the outcome of treatment.

REFERENCES

1. Blount, W. P.: Fractures in Children. Baltimore, Williams & Wilkins Co., 1954.
2. Bunata, R. E., Fahey, J. J., and Drennan, D. B.: Factors influencing stability and necrosis of impacted femoral neck fractures. J.A.M.A. *223*:41, 1973.
3. Callahan, J. J.: Personal Communication.
4. Crock, H. V.: Blood Supply to the Lower Limb Bones in Man. Edinburgh, Churchill-Livingstone, 1967.
5. Donaldson, S. W., Badgley, C. E., and Hunsberger, W. G.: Lateral view of pelvis in examination for hip dislocation. J. Bone Joint Surg. *30A*:512, 1948.
6. Dimon, J. H., and Hughston, J. C.: Unstable intertrochanteric fractures of the hip. J. Bone Joint Surg. *49A*:440, 1967.
7. Pauwels, F.: Pauwels' classification of fractures of neck femur according to angle of inclination (Fig. 6–89), Vol. 1, p. 587. *In* Campbell's Operative Orthopaedics, 5th ed., edited by A. H. Crenshaw. St. Louis, C. V. Mosby Co., 1971.
8. Ralston, E. L.: Handbook of Fractures. St. Louis, C. V. Mosby Co., 1967.
9. Rockwood, C. A., and Green, D. P.: Fractures. Philadelphia, J. B. Lippincott Co., 1975.
10. Trueta, J.: Studies of the Development and Decay of the Human Frame. Philadelphia, W. B. Saunders Co., 1968.
11. Watson-Jones, R.: Fractures and Joint Injuries, 4th ed., 2V. Baltimore, Williams & Wilkins Co., 1952-1955.

14

THE FEMUR

The femoral shaft throughout its extent is covered by a thick envelope of muscle. Because of this covering and the absence of subcutaneous borders, the femur is not as prone to be involved in an open fracture as are bones with subcutaneous borders. In the high shaft fracture, there is a tendency for the proximal femoral fragment to move into a flexed and externally rotated position (Fig. 14–1). A similar occurrence has been mentioned in the discussion of subtrochanteric fractures (see Chapter 13). In the distal femoral shaft fracture or in the supracondylar femoral fracture, there is a definite tendency for the distal fragment to move into a position of hyperextension. This position is thought to be primarily due to the origin of the gastrocnemius muscle along the posterior margin of the lower femur.

Fracture of Femoral Shaft

Femoral shaft fractures are usually the product of rather severe trauma, the forces creating the individual fracture being extremely variable.

Examination. On examination of a lower limb in which a femoral shaft fracture has occurred, the limb distal to the fracture tends to lie in external rotation. The thigh is shortened and its muscle mass appears to be much increased.

Roentgenograms. The anteroposterior (Fig. 14–2) and lateral roentgenograms will confirm the specific type of fracture and whether it is oblique, spiral, transverse, or comminuted.

Treatment. The decision regarding treatment will depend to some extent upon the information obtained from the roentgenograms. To effect reduction, the distal fragment must be brought into a position to meet the proximal fragment. If the fracture can be adequately fixed by internal fixation with an intramedullary nail or a heavy plate such as the compression plate, then this is considered to be the treatment of choice for the uncomplicated femoral shaft fracture. The internally fixed femoral shaft fracture should be protected from full weight bearing for some six to eight weeks until there is roentgenographic evidence of early union across the fracture site. For this fracture, the proponents of the cast brace would use traction for two to four weeks. Once a certain stability is achieved, the cast brace would be utilized. This has the advantage of allowing the patient to be mobile without an operation. Weight bearing has a

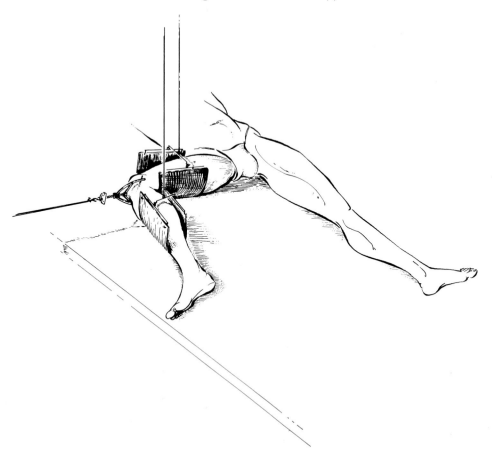

Fig. 14–1. Illustration of 90-90-90 method of traction, often necessary to reduce fracture of proximal femoral shaft. Abduction, flexion, and external rotation are unopposed on the proximal fragment. To effect reduction the distal fragment must be brought into position to meet the proximal fragment.

beneficial effect on fracture healing. Loss of some leg length is a common accompaniment to use of the cast brace.

Should the fracture be sufficiently comminuted that treatment by internal fixation or cast brace is not feasible, the balanced skeletal traction method works well. This traction is best applied to a Kirschner wire inserted into the tibia just posterior to the tibial tubercle. An alternative position for the Kirschner wire is through the distal femur. This type of treatment requires that the patient remain in traction for approximately twelve weeks; following roentgenographic evidence of union of the fracture fragments, the patient may begin ambulation in an ischial weight bearing caliper. This is used for an additional four months. One must not underestimate the magnitude of the effect of the femoral shaft fracture in the life of an individual and his(her) family.

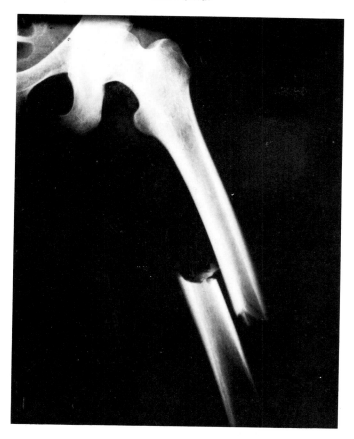

Fig. 14–2. Anteroposterior roentgenogram fracture of femoral shaft. This midshaft fracture with minimal comminution is ideal for internal fixation with an intramedullary nail.

Supracondylar and Intercondylar Fractures of Femur

The supracondylar fracture tends to occur most commonly by direct force onto the dorsum of the distal thigh just above to the knee. This fracture can occur, however, through forced hyperextension of the lower leg onto the knee. The distal fragment moves into a position of hyperextension because of the spasm of the gastrocnemius muscle. This muscle originates posteriorly at the condyles of the femur.

Examination. On the examination of the patient with a supracondylar injury the deformity is first seen just proximal to the knee. This may be an extension deformity and/or it may angulate toward the medial or lateral side. This latter angulation depends often upon the injuring force and the direction from which it came. There is, on occasion, interruption of the blood supply to the lower limb distal to the fracture site as well as possible injury to the sciatic nerve. The examination must indicate any findings in this regard.

Roentgenograms. The anteroposterior and lateral roentgenograms (Fig. 14–3) give detail of the fracture. A fracture line is seen proximal to the femoral condyles. In the intercondylar fracture, there is also seen a radiolucent line running between the condyles. Comminution of the fragments is not uncommon (Fig. 14–4).

   Treatment. The supracondylar fracture may be treated by a moderately flexed, gently molded long leg cast. Should this not maintain reduction, however, the fracture can be treated in balanced skeletal traction. If this is done, the knee needs to be flexed to 90 degrees in order to relax the gastrocnemius and allow reduction of the distal fragment(s) in relationship to the proximal fragment. The skeletal traction is derived through a Kirschner wire deep to the tibial tubercle. Maintenance of this position in traction for approximately six weeks is usually sufficient to then allow application of a cast or a cast brace (Fig. 14–9). An alternative to the traction treatment is to openly reduce the

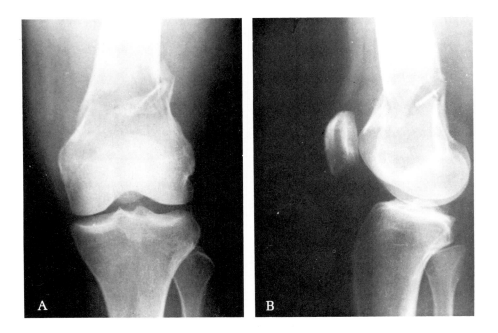

Fig. 14–3. Roentgenograms of supracondylar fracture in an adult. A, Anteroposterior view. B, Lateral view indicating that force caused hyperextension to occur at fracture site. This fracture may be treated by a moderately flexed, gently molded long leg cast. Should this not maintain reduction, however, skeletal traction through the proximal tibia may be necessary until the fracture shows "stickiness" at the fracture site. A moderately flexed long leg cast can then be used until roentgenographic evidence of union is seen.

Fig. 14–4. Roentgenograms of severely comminuted supracondylar and intercondylar fracture of femur. A, Anteroposterior view. B, Lateral view. Balanced skeletal traction was applied from pin in proximal tibia. To effect reasonable reduction of fragments, attachment to Thomas splint was flexed about 60 degrees. C, Anteroposterior view of healed fracture. D, Lateral view. Although some malunion is present, there is no significant ligamentous laxity at the knee, and patient can flex knee from 5 degrees to 90 degrees.

→

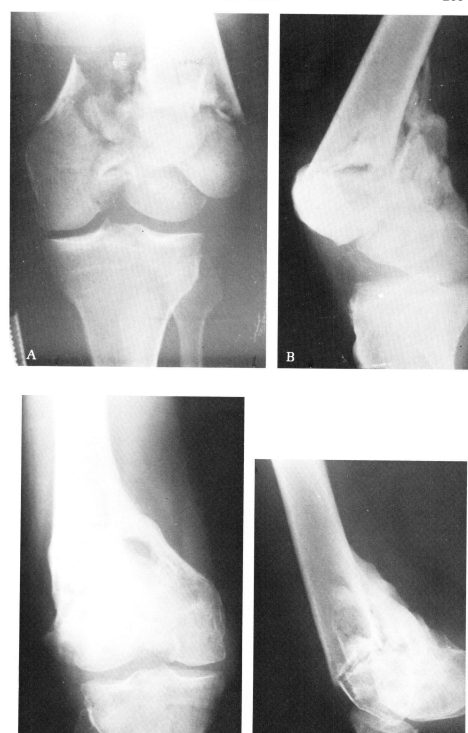

fracture(s) and internally fix it with a blade plate, crossed Rush pins or Kirschner wires. In order to be able to openly reduce and fix this fracture, there must be a fragment or fragments of sufficient size to retain the fixation. The cast brace can be used to treat this fracture once stabilization has been achieved from traction. This requires experience in the use of the cast brace, as this fracture can easily displace or settle if inadequately managed. Again, as in the femoral shaft fracture, the internal fixation allows early mobilization of the patient. No weight bearing can be allowed until evidence of union is seen on a roentgenogram (usually fourteen to sixteen weeks). The proponents of operative management point out that this method of treatment gives the most congruous surfaces for articulation with the tibial plateaus.

One of the potential complications of the supracondylar or intercondylar injury, particularly when treated in traction, is a silent venous thrombosis. The deep fascia leashes the popliteal vessels in place and will not allow them to shift away from their posterior femoral relationship. Pressure of a hematoma or of the displaced fracture in this space can thus create venous occlusion and distal hemostasis, resulting in venous thrombosis. Treatment of this complication is by the method(s) of preference of the surgeon.

Isolated Condylar Fractures of the Femur

The isolated fracture of a femoral condyle can involve the medial or the lateral condyle. The size of the condylar fragment most likely depends on whether the fracture is a product of a "push-off" or a "pull-off" force. The former fragments tend to be larger than do the latter. Either type of fragment can interrupt the articular surface of the involved condyle. A fragment that is entirely intra-articular likely has no blood supply and thus tends to undergo avascular necrosis.

Examination. The patient with an isolated condylar fracture of the femur will have a painful knee, with the pain being localized to the side of fracture. There will be a bloody effusion of the involved knee joint. This effusion is less massive in the knee with a displaced fracture (allowing extra-articular escape of the blood) than it is in the knee with an undisplaced fracture of the condyle.

Roentgenograms. An anteroposterior roentgenogram will usually show a radiolucent fracture line in the involved condyle whether or not the fragment is displaced (Fig. 14–5A). On the lateral roentgenogram, a fracture of the condyle is evident only if it is displaced (Fig. 14–5B). If neither of these views shows evidence of a fracture and one strongly suspects its existence (from the history of injury, localized pain, and presence of a significant knee effusion), anteroposterior rotational roentgenograms may help identify the presence of a fracture line.

Treatment. In the undisplaced or minimally displaced condylar fracture, a long leg plaster of Paris cast may be used for eight weeks. A walking heel may be applied for the last four weeks of this immobilization. Nonweight bearing should be continued until roentgenographic evidence of union can be seen.

When the condylar fragment is displaced significantly, it should be reduced to minimize joint incongruity and effect improved blood supply to the fragment. This most often means open reduction of the fragment followed by internal fixation with screw(s) or Kirschner wire(s). The postoperative management is the same as the treatment for the undisplaced fracture.

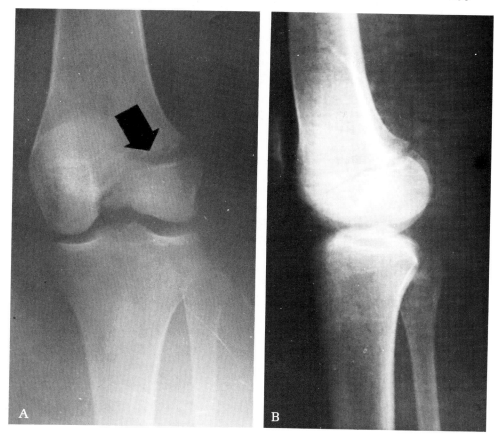

Fig. 14–5. Anteroposterior and lateral roentgenograms of knee showing fracture through lateral femoral condyle (arrow). Because this fragment is probably entirely intra-articular, it is most likely without vascular supply and thus tends to undergo avascular necrosis. For this reason, internal fixation is treatment of choice.

On occasion, circumstances preclude operation on the fractured femoral condyle. In this event the leg can be placed in a Thomas splint with a Pearson attachment, and balanced skeletal traction may be applied with a Kirschner wire through the distal tibia and fibula. The line of pull should be so placed as to correct any displacement if possible. The splint should be converted to an exerciser at two weeks so that the patient can flex and extend the knee joint. At six weeks the traction may be discontinued in favor of a long double upright brace. A dial pad should be placed appropriately at the knee to resist the anticipated deforming force. A cast brace can be used rather than the long double upright brace.

FRACTURES OF THE FEMUR IN CHILDREN

A prime consideration in the treatment of fractures of the femur in children is the growth potential of the fractured femur, regardless of the site of the fracture or the method of reduction chosen.

Fractures of the Femoral Shaft

Femoral shaft fractures in children are usually the product of severe trauma. The mechanism of injury can be variable. According to Blount, about 70% of all fractures of the femoral shaft in children occur in the middle third, 18% in the proximal third, and the remaining 12% at the distal end. The spiral fracture is a product of torsional forces, but the transverse fracture usually occurs from direct injury.

Examination. The examination of the child with a femoral shaft fracture reveals the affected limb to be externally rotated from the fracture site distally. The child is apprehensive and will not consent to any examination. However, the neurologic and vascular status of this extremity must be determined prior to any treatment.

Roentgenograms. Anteroposterior and lateral roentgenograms must be obtained in order to evaluate the fracture(s) (Fig. 14–6). The joint above and the joint below must be visualized in two planes in order to fully assess the injury. Most fractures in the femoral shaft are evident on one of the two views.

Treatment. The ideal treatment of the femoral fracture in the child is use of traction until bony stability is achieved. Traction is followed by application of a

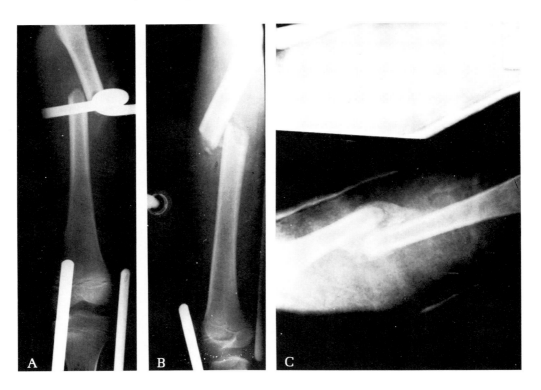

Fig. 14–6. Roentgenograms of fracture of femoral shaft in twelve-year-old child. A, Anteroposter view of fracture being treated by Russell's traction. B, Note fragment ends are deliberately overlapped (bayonet apposition) to accommodate for bone growth stimulation that usually occurs with this injury. C, After application of plaster of Paris spica cast once fracture becomes "sticky."

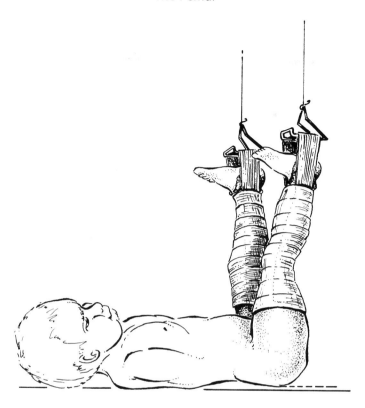

Fig. 14–7. Bryant's traction applied to treat fracture of right femoral shaft. When proper weight has been applied, the buttocks should clear the bed by one finger breadth. Potential of ischemic contracture during use of this method is sufficiently real to warrant constant attention to prevent this serious complication. Method is particularly effective when child weighs less than 40 pounds (usually five years of age or under).

spica cast. In the child up to about five years of age (or 40 pounds) the Bryant's type of double leg traction is effective (Fig. 14–7). In the use of this traction method, great attention must be given to the wrapping of the traction straps so as not to cause any unusual compression force. Sufficient weight on each traction system should be placed so that one finger breadth distance lies between the buttock and the bed. The potential of an ischemic contracture during use of this method is sufficiently real to warrant constant attention to prevent this serious complication.

In the child over five or six years of age up to approximately 14 years of age, Russell's traction works quite well for the femoral shaft fracture (Fig. 14–8). In the age group above fourteen years, the balanced skeletal traction must be utilized because of the weight of the extremity. The overlapping or bayonet apposition is to be preferred in the reduction of the femoral shaft fracture in any child up to the age of twelve. This allows compensation for bony overgrowth following increased vascularity from the fracture.

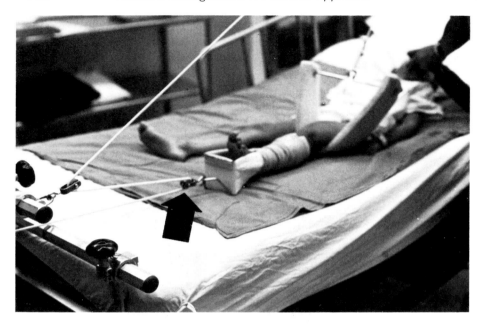

Fig. 14–8. Russell's traction. This method of treatment is effective for femoral shaft fractures in children from about five years of age (over 40 pounds) until about fourteen years of age. When fracture shows early union (approximately three to four weeks), a spica cast is applied until roentgenographic evidence of union is seen.

Traction is required from ten days to three weeks until the fracture shows signs of early union. The spica cast is then utilized for a total immobilization period of about ten weeks. The final decision to discontinue immobilization can be made only after roentgenographic evidence of union is seen. The cast brace may be used instead of the spica cast for the latter period of fracture immobilization (Fig. 14–9). It has the advantage of allowing general mobility for the child.

Supracondylar Femur Fractures

The supracondylar fracture of the femur in the child occurs most commonly with a dorsal angulation of the distal fragment.

Examination. The examination reveals a hyperextension deformity at the knee with a hyperextension appearance. Seldom is there a distal neurologic or vascular alteration.

Roentgenograms. Anteroposterior and lateral roentgenograms show interruption of the femoral cortex. The distal fragment is commonly displaced dorsally. The true supracondylar fracture occurs proximal to the distal femoral epiphyseal plate by approximately one to one and one-half inches.

Treatment. The supracondylar fracture of the femur occurs more commonly in the six- to fourteen-year-old age group and is well treated in Russell's type of traction. However, significant flexion of the knee must be maintained in order to keep the distal fragment reduced into a proper relationship with the

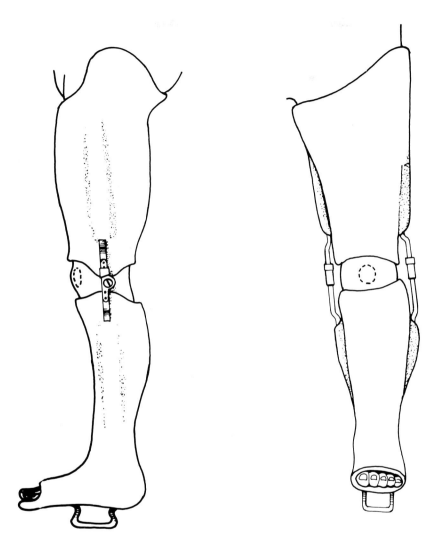

Fig. 14–9. Frontal and side views of cast brace used in treatment of shaft and supracondylar fractures of femur. This method may be used for proximal tibia as well as for tibial shaft. (Courtesy Raymond Bagg, M.D.)

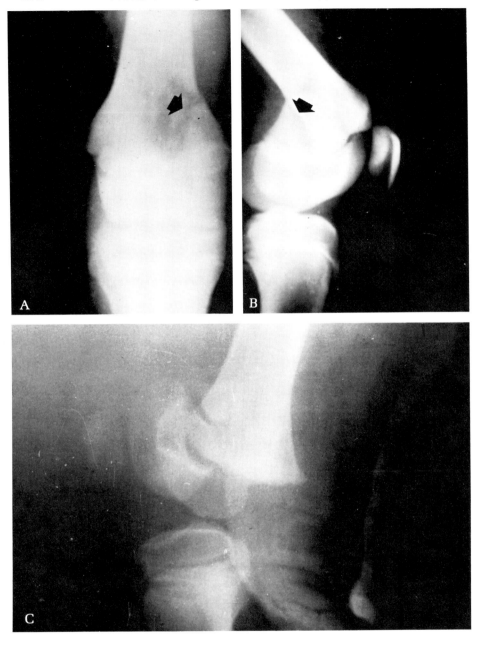

Fig. 14–10. Roentgeonograms of Type II epiphyseal slip of distal femur. A, Anteroposterior view. Segment of lateral metaphysis of femur (arrow) is attached to epiphysis. B, Lateral view showing epiphyseal slip was caused by flexion force. Also seen is spike of lateral femoral metaphysis attached to posterolateral epiphysis. An extension and adduction directed force should reduce and maintain this displacement in a long leg cast. Occasionally initial traction is necessary to reduce displacement. C, Lateral view of epiphyseal slip caused by extension force. It should be reduced and maintained by flexion force in a long leg cast. Occasionally initial traction may be necessary to reduce displacement.

proximal fragment; the gastrocnemius muscle will tend to hyperextend the distal fragment. Following two to three weeks of traction, stability has often been achieved, and a long leg plaster of Paris cast or a cast brace can then be applied. This will need to be maintained for at least two months until good evidence of early bony union is seen on a roentgenogram.

Separation of Distal Femoral Epiphysis

Examination. The separation of the distal femoral epiphysis has much the same appearance as the supracondylar fracture on examination and occurs in much the same way so far as the mechanism of injury.

Roentgenograms. The separation of the distal femoral epiphysis can be differentiated from the supracondylar fracture in the roentgenographic examination. Displacement of the distal femoral epiphysis from the metaphysis will be noted, the epiphysis having been separated from the shaft through the epiphyseal plate (Fig. 14–10). Often a small fragment of metaphyseal bone can be seen attached to the distal fragment. This occurs in the adolescent age group and attention must be given to determine that this fracture of the epiphysis is not in the so-called danger group of the Salter classification (see Chapter 2).

Treatment. In epiphyseal injuries, particularly types III and IV, absolutely perfect reduction must be accomplished and maintained. Usually a gentle manipulation under general anesthetic reduces this fracture, and it can be maintained in position either by use of a snug long leg cast (my preference) or by use of Russell's type traction.

A type II epiphyseal slip caused by flexion force (Fig. 14–9B) should be reduced and maintained by extension and adduction. One caused by extension force (Fig. 14–9C) should be reduced by a flexion force. Both types should be immobilized in long leg casts. Occasionally initial traction may be necessary to reduce the displacement.

REFERENCES

1. Adams, J. C.: Outline of Fractures, Including Joint Injuries, 6th ed. Baltimore, Williams & Wilkins Co., 1972.
2. Blount, W. P.: Fractures in Children. Baltimore, Williams & Wilkins Co., 1954.
3. Charnley, J.: Closed Treatment of Common Fractures, 3rd ed., 1961, (Fourth Reprint). Edinburgh & London, Churchill Livingstone, 1972.
4. Crock, H. V.: Blood Supply to the Lower Limb Bones in Man. Edinburgh & London, Churchill-Livingstone, 1967.
5. Ralston, E. L.: Handbook of Fractures. St. Louis, C. V. Mosby Co., 1967.
6. Rang, M. C.: Children's Fractures. Philadelphia, J. B. Lippincott Co., 1974.
7. Rockwood, C. A., and Green, D. P.: Fractures. Philadelphia, J. B. Lippincott Co., 1975.
8. Salter, R. B., and Harris, R. W.: Injuries involving the epiphyseal plate. J. Bone Joint Surg. 45-A:587, 1963.
9. Scully, T. J.: Ambulant, nonoperative management of femoral shaft fractures, Part I. Clin. Orthop. 100:195, 1974.
10. Scully, T. J.: Ambulant, nonoperative management of femoral shaft fractures, Part II. Clin. Orthop. 100:204, 1974.
11. Watson-Jones, R.: Fractures and Joint Injuries, 4th ed., 2V. Baltimore, Williams & Wilkins Co., 1952-1955.

15

THE KNEE

The condyles of the distal femur are so matched to the plateaus of the proximal tibia that with the collateral ligaments and the cruciate ligaments, the knee joint maintains a good stability. The motor control for flexion of the knee joint is accomplished predominantly by the hamstring tendons that arise from muscles in the posterior thigh. These insert just distal to the knee joint on the medial and lateral sides. Extension of the knee (and the factor that allows weight bearing of the body across the knee) is controlled by the quadriceps muscle inserting into the patella; the patellar tendon then extends from the patella down to and inserts into the tibial tubercle. The movement of the knee is like that of a complex ginglymus joint with a constantly changing axis of motion as the knee flexes and extends. As the knee moves into full extension, the femur internally rotates in relationship to the tibia in order to tighten the cruciate ligaments and thus increase the stability of the knee joint. As the knee begins to flex, the popliteus muscle unlocks this "screw home" mechanism and allows normal flexion to ensue.

Fracture of Patella

The patella may fracture from direct trauma to the patella itself. It may also fracture by an avulsion mechanism following an unusually forceful contraction of the quadriceps when the knee is simultaneously forcibly flexed.

Examination. On observation of the knee with a patellar fracture there may be no definite abnormality visible. There may be ecchymosis and swelling of the joint. To palpation there may be separation of the two fragments.

Roentgenograms. The anteroposterior and lateral roentgenograms are a distinct aid in determining the course of treatment (Fig. 15–1). On them there may be no evidence of separation of the bony fragments, although the bony fragments may be clearly separated.

Treatment. If no displacement of the fracture fragments has occurred, then a cylinder cast for four to six weeks should be sufficient treatment. However, should separation of the fragments occur, this indicates also a separation of the patellar tendon and hence loss of extension control across the joint. In this event operative intervention is necessary. The fragments may be replaced and a circumferential wire (circlage) placed about them to maintain reduction. If one of the fragments is unusually small, it can be simply excised and the patellar

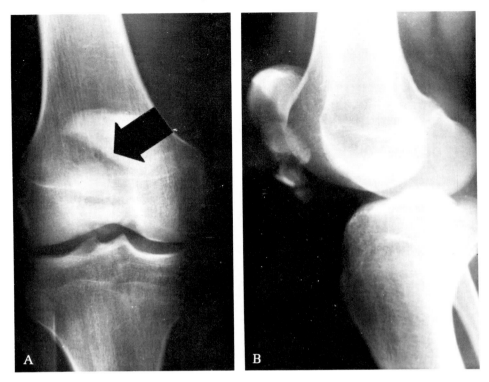

Fig. 15–1. Roentgenograms of fracture of patella. A, Arrow points to fracture line in comminuted patella. There appears to be only one sizable fragment to which the patellar tendon might be attached after excising the multiple small fragments. B, Lateral view delineates more clearly the comminution of this patella fracture. Operative treatment is the only satisfactory method of handling this fracture. Before retaining the large fragment, however, the surgeon must be certain the articular surface of the patella has not been irreparably damaged.

tendon attached to the raw fracture surface. In this event, care must be taken to bring the patellar tendon to the cartilaginous surface so as not to cause the patella to scoop into the patellar groove of the femur and scrape the cartilaginous surface. Most surgeons consider partial excision of the patella to be the better treatment when separation of fragments occurs and when the fragment to be retained provides 60% or more of the cartilage surface. If there are multiple fragments, they may all be excised and the patellar tendon may be repaired. Immobilization in a plaster of Paris cast after any of these procedures is recommended for about 6 weeks. Attention must be directed then to regaining as full a range of motion and as much quadriceps strength as possible.

Dislocation of Patella

The patella may dislocate in traumatic circumstances, particularly when the patellar tendon inserts laterally. Usually associated with the laterally inserting patellar tendon is a high-riding patella. This patella often does not require significant trauma to dislocate it. The dislocation may occur and spontaneous

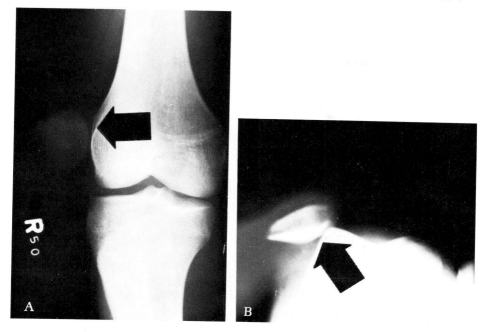

Fig. 15–2. A, Anteroposterior roentgenogram showing laterally dislocated patella (arrow). If dislocation occurs because of ligamentous and tendinous laxity, it will tend to recur. The dislocated patella secondary to trauma tends to maintain reduction once reduced and immobilized for four to six weeks. B, Skyline view of knee in which patella is dislocated laterally (arrow).

reduction may ensue. This possibility must be considered at the time of examination of any injured knee in which the cause of injury has not been recognized. Sometimes laxity of the tendons or ligaments may cause the patella to dislocate. Dislocations from laxity tend to recur.

Examination. If the knee is examined at the time that the patella is dislocated, the patella most commonly lies *lateral* to the lateral femoral condyle.

Roentgenograms. The roentgenograms clearly show the position of the patella lateral (or medial) to the femoral condyle (Fig. 15–2). The lateral roentgenogram shows a superimposition of the patella on the femoral condyles.

Treatment. A combination of meperidine and diazepam usually provides sufficient analgesia and relaxation for treatment of the patellar dislocation. Reduction of the patella is accomplished with hyperextension of the knee and a gentle but firm force to ride the patella up and medial to the lateral condyle of the femur. Once reduced, an elastic bandage is usually sufficient to maintain the reduction. However, a cylinder cast for four to six weeks is considered necessary by some.

Dislocation of Knee

Posterior dislocation of the knee occurs seldom. It is the product of severe trauma. The tibia is forcibly driven posteriorly from its position at 90 degrees of flexion on the femur. In order for this injury to have occurred, the cruciate ligaments must be traumatically severed or avulsed; the fibers of the medial collateral and lateral collateral ligaments separate in the body of the ligament or avulse from their respective insertions.

Examination. If the knee is dislocated, the examination shows the tibia to be in the popliteal space. There is likely obliteration of the pulses peripheral to this injury. There may well be injury of the posterior tibial and peroneal nerves.

Roentgenograms. The anteroposterior roentgenogram shows superimposition of the distal femoral condyles over the proximal tibia plateaus (Fig. 15–3). The lateral roentgenogram shows the position of the tibial plateaus posterior to the femoral condyles.

Treatment. Because of the potential for profound neurovascular damage of the knee, this dislocation must be reduced as quickly as possible. It is possible that reduction can be accomplished in the emergency room following ad-

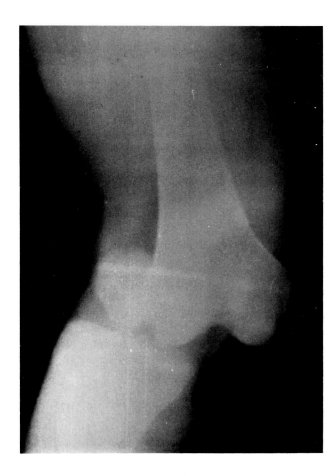

Fig. 15–3. Anteroposterior roentgenogram showing lateral dislocation of tibia on femur causing major ligamentous tearing. Any dislocation of the knee is fraught with potential concomitant vascular and nerve injury.

ministration of a combination of meperidine and diazepam to provide analgesia and relaxation. The reduction is accomplished with the knee partially flexed while a slow but steady anterior force is exerted by the surgeon's arm placed against the tibia from the popliteal space.

Should reduction not ensue, then a general anesthetic must be given and reduction must be accomplished as soon as feasible. It has been stated that reduction should be open if closed reduction is not possible. Closed reduction has been effected in each instance of my experience, and operation has not been necessary. The principle, however, is sound.

Following reduction of the dislocation, a long leg plaster of Paris cast should be applied with approximately 30 degrees of flexion and an anterior force supplied by posterior molding of the cast just distal to the popliteal space. The injured lower limb should be watched carefully over the first twenty-four to forty-eight hours to be certain that adequate circulation has been maintained. The plaster of Paris cast must be maintained in position for some six weeks. An active range in motion exercise program should be initiated at the time the cast is removed. The potential of collateral ligament instability of the knee joint following such an injury exists. However, experience at the Cook County Hospital has not shown the operative management to be superior to the closed management in preventing such laxity.

Fractures of Tibial Plateau

Fractures of the lateral tibial plateau are generally caused by an abduction injury of the lower leg on the knee; such an injury to the medial tibial plateau is caused by an adduction injury. These often occur with the knee partially flexed.

Examination. If the tibial plateau is fractured, on examination the leg will show an abduction or adduction position from the knee distally. Associated with this injury is a bloody effusion within the knee joint.

Roentgenograms. The anteroposterior roentgenograms should show fracture line(s) with depression of the involved plateau (Fig. 15–4). Should a significant plateau fracture be suspected but not confirmed on roentgenogram, tomographic views will aid in visualizing a break of the cortex or lowering of the plateau (Fig. 15–5).

Treatment. If the tibial plateau injury is such size as to be reducible and stable, then a long leg plaster cast to maintain reduction is the treatment of choice. If the fragment or fragments will not remain reduced and will leave an unstable joint ultimately, it is advisable to consider operative elevation of the tibial plateau and internal fixation where possible. This may require backpacking of bone secured from another site. Transverse bolts may aid in holding the plateau elevated. Following operation, the leg must be immobilized in a long leg cast for six weeks. Occasionally such comminution exists that the only treatment feasible is placing the limb in balanced skeletal traction. In this event, a distal tibial pin is used so that early flexion and extension of the knee can be begun in the splint. Weight bearing is inadvisable until evidence of union and stability is seen on a roentgenogram. An ischial weight bearing caliper allows bypass of weight from the pelvis to the heel of the shoe and is an excellent means of treatment after the initial immobilization.

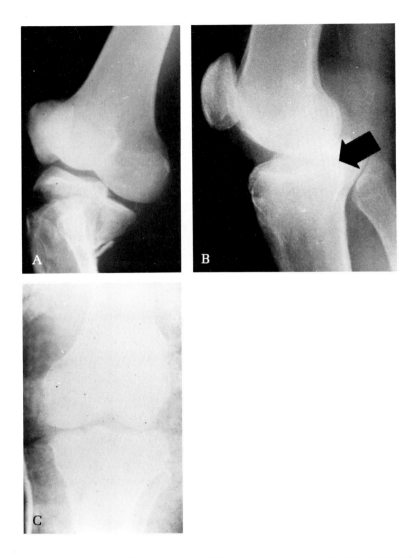

Fig. 15–4. Roentgenograms of comminuted tibial plateau fracture. A, Anteroposterior view. With varus angulation, some stabilizing soft tissue may be present along medial tibial cortex. B, Lateral view suggesting depression of tibial plateau (white line at tip of arrow). The other fracture lines are not clearly seen. C, Anteroposterior view after reduction and immobilization in a cast. A good reduction was obtained and three-point fixation was maintained by the cast. Some depressed plateau fractures require surgical elevation and bolt fixation and/or bone graft to secure reasonably congruous joint surfaces. Other plateau fractures may be treated in balanced skeletal tract accompanied by early mobilization, usually without weight bearing until roentgenographic evidence of union is present.

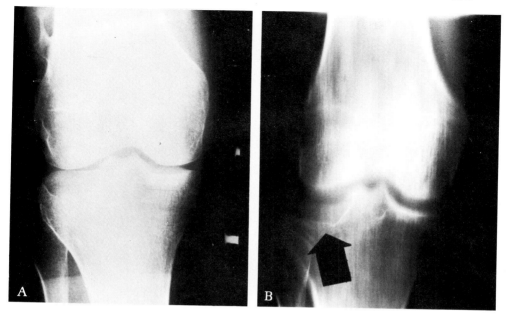

Fig. 15–5. Lateral fracture of tibial plateau. A, Anteroposterior roentgenogram showing treatment by long double upright orthosis. The fracture appears well managed at three weeks following injury. B, Anteroposterior tomogram. Arrow points to significant depression of lateral tibial plateau. This particular fracture would best be treated by operative elevation of depressed fragment.

One of the complications of the tibial plateau fracture is silent venous thrombosis. This is presumably due to the massive bleeding in the popliteal space and an inability of the veins to maintain patency in the face of this pressure.

KNEE INJURIES IN CHILDREN

Although ligamentous injuries and cartilage tears do occur in the child, they are much less common than they are in the adult. Generally, immobilization is a good initial treatment for any knee that has sustained significant injury. Ligaments will usually heal and any significant residual meniscal injury can be dealt with on an elective basis.

Fracture of Patella

The fracture of the patella in a child is not common because of the resilience of the tissues. However, it can occur, and if the fragments are displaced, they must be brought together and held with internal fixation such as the circlage wire. The roentgenograms of the opposite patella should be secured for comparison purposes. A bipartite patella may be confused with a fractured patella but is most commonly present bilaterally (Fig. 15–6). On examination there is no significant tenderness at the bipartite patella.

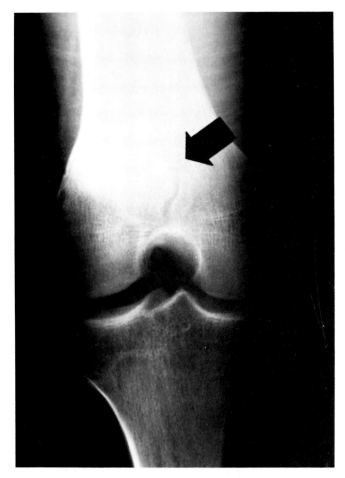

Fig. 15–6. Bipartite patella in a child. The arrow on anteroposterior roentgenogram points to radiolucent cartilage line.

Dislocation of Patella

Traumatic dislocation of the patella rarely occurs in the child. The subluxation of the patella, however, may occur, particularly in the high-riding patella or in the patella whose tendon inserts into a laterally positioned tibial tubercle. This must be considered in a knee injury with effusion but no evidence by history and examination for the cause of the effusion. A simple wrap with an elastic bandage is sufficient to support the subluxing patella until the effusion subsides.

Fractures of Tibial Spines

Occasionally an avulsion of tibial spine occurs in the child following known injury. The mechanism is probably one of an anteriorly or posteriorly directed force against the flexed proximal tibia which pulls the cruciate ligaments sufficiently tight to avulse a portion of the proximal epiphysis of the tibia.

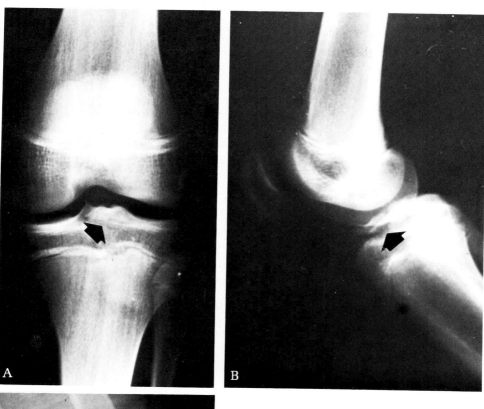

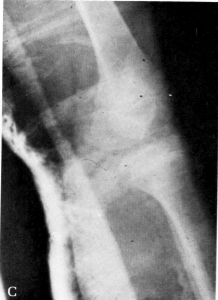

Fig. 15–7. Roentgenograms of tibial spine fracture in child. A, Arrow in anteroposterior view is pointing to fracture line scooped down into plateau below spinous process. B, In lateral view arrow points to fracture line beneath tibial spine. C, Lateral view after treatment of fracture by applying cast in full extension. Four to six weeks is usually sufficient immobilization. An occasional displaced fracture of tibial spine requires operative replacement to achieve joint congruity.

Examination. On examination, the knee with tibial spine fractures is irritable. There is a bloody effusion in the joint. There is no frank evidence of ligamentous laxity, although the knee cannot be freely examined. There is lack of full of extension capability of the knee.

Roentgenograms. The anteroposterior and lateral roentgenograms will show an avulsion of a portion of the proximal tibial epiphysis which may vary from a thin plate all the way to a major fragment (Fig. 15–7).

Treatment. Full extension of the knee with tibial spine fractures will often reduce the tibial spines back into position. The long leg plaster of Paris cast should be then applied with the leg in the hyperextended position. If the fragments will not reduce with the extended position, the treatment of choice is an arthrotomy with reduction of the fragments. The reduction is maintained by a suture placed through two small holes drilled in the anterior cortex and up across the epiphyseal plate into the knee at the tibial spines. The suture is passed over the avulsed segment of epiphysis and tied at the anterior tibia. Immobilization in a long leg plaster of Paris cast should be accomplished for four to six weeks. Once the roentgenogram shows evidence of union at the site of avulsion, a well-directed program of exercises for improving range of motion and strengthening the quadriceps is begun.

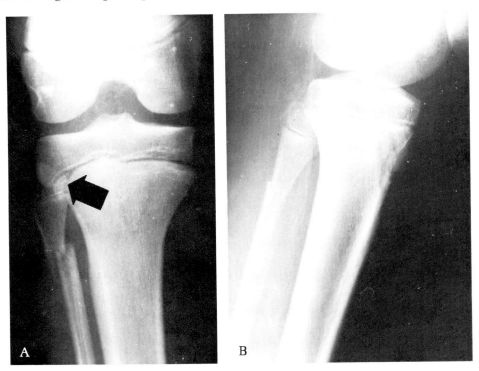

Fig. 15–8. Roentgenograms showing Type II epiphyseal separation of proximal tibial epiphysis. A, Anteroposterior view. The arrow points to fragment of metaphysis remaining attached to proximal epiphysis. Note that medial margin of epiphysis lies lateral to medial margin of tibial metaphysis, indicating some medial displacement of tibia distal to epiphyseal separation. B, Lateral view. Little, if any, anterior or posterior displacement of epiphysis is seen.

Epiphyseal Separation of Proximal Tibia

Separation of the proximal tibial epiphysis, particularly with a varus or valgus strain, is seen following significant trauma. This injury is most often seen in a child toward the end of his growth phase.

Examination. On examination, an obvious deformity with angulation present will be noted from the injury level distally toward the valgus or varus position. There is seldom an effusion within the knee joint. The patient cautiously offers the knee for examination.

Roentgenograms. The roentgenograms reveal separation of the proximal tibial epiphysis (Fig. 15–8). Careful review of the roentgenograms of the injured tibia with the comparison views of the uninjured tibia are essential to

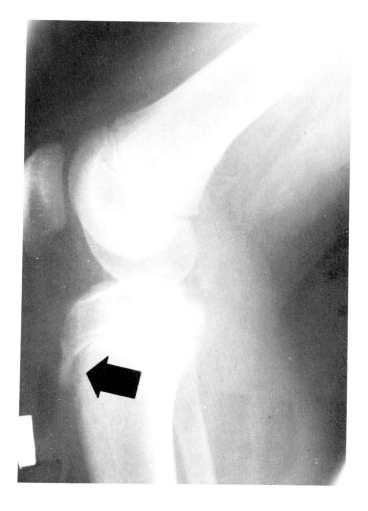

Fig. 15–9. Arrow points to slight anterior displacement of tibial tubercle following fracture at base. With the leg in full extension a cast was applied while molding the patella and the tibial tubercle. Significant displacement of the tibial tubercle requires reduction and fixation with small Kirschner wires.

be certain of the type of injury. These separations are often from the group II classification of Salter and Harris (see Chapter 2).

Treatment. Reduction of the epiphyseal separation of the proximal tibia is accomplished by slightly increasing the deformity and then exerting a gentle manual force against the apex of deformity. The distal leg is then brought back to the midline. Maintenance in a long leg walking cast for six weeks should be sufficient.

Avulsion of Tibial Tubercle

In the growing child, occasionally a forced hyperflexion with a simultaneous contraction of the quadriceps mechanism will avulse the apophysis of the tibial tongue. Although no longitudinal growth occurs from the tibial tubercle at this point, a continuation of growth should occur in order to allow appropriate contour to the anterior proximal tibia.

Examination. On examination, there is unusual prominence of the tibial tubercle on palpation.

Roentgenograms. The lateral roentgenogram reveals an elevation of the distal tongue of the tibial tubercle with a fracture across its waist (Fig. 15–9).

Treatment. A trial at closed reduction is indicated for the avulsion of the tibial tubercle. Maintenance of reduction is seldom possible, even when reduction is achieved. If reduction cannot be maintained, operative fixation is indicated. Percutaneous crossed Kirschner wires may be sufficient for maintaining reduction. If reduction is not possible, short of opening to the fracture site, then a suture or two may maintain the reduced position of this tongue of the tibial apophysis. Following the reduction and fixation, a long leg plaster of Paris cast with the leg in extension is the best means for immobilization. This should be held for four to six weeks before gradual motion is begun.

REFERENCES

1. Adams, J. C.: Outline of Fractures, Including Joint Injuries, 6th ed. Baltimore, Williams & Wilkins Co., 1972.
2. Blount, W. P.: Fractures in Children. Baltimore, Williams & Wilkins Co., 1954.
3. Charnley, J.: Closed Treatment of Common Fractures, 3rd ed., 1961, (Fourth Reprint). Edinburgh & London, Churchill Livingstone, 1972.
4. Crock, H. V.: Blood Supply to the Lower Limb Bones in Man. Edinburgh, Churchill-Livingstone, 1967.
5. Dehne, E. and Torp, R. P.: Treatment of joint injuries by immediate mobilization. Clin. Orthop. 77:218, 1971.
6. Ralston, E. L.: Handbook of Fractures. St. Louis, C. V. Mosby Co., 1967.
7. Rang, M. C.: Children's Fractures. Philadelphia, J. B. Lippincott Co., 1974.
8. Rockwood, C. A., and Green, D. P.: Fractures. Philadelphia, J. B. Lippincott Co., 1975.
9. Salter, R. B., and Harris, R. W.: Injuries involving the epiphyseal plate. J. Bone Joint Surg. 45-A:587, 1963.
10. Watson-Jones, R.: Fractures and Joint Injuries, 4th ed., 2V. Baltimore, Williams & Wilkins Co., 1952-1955.

16

THE LOWER LEG

The major weight bearing of the lower leg is performed by the tibia. The tibia and fibula, however, do form a both bone system such as has been previously discussed (Chapter 1). In the both bone system, when one of the bones fractures and displacement occurs, either an obligatory fracture in the other bone of the system or a ligamentous injury between the attachments of the two bones must occur.

The proximal portion of the tibia is composed predominantly of a highly vascular cancellous bone which gives way to a more compact cortical type of bone distal to the knee joint. The nutrient artery to the tibia enters about the junction of the proximal and middle thirds and turns proximally to supply the upper portion of the tibia and distally to supply the lower two thirds of the tibia. It is thought that this may be one of the contributing factors to nonunion of the tibial fracture, nonunion being more common following fracture in the distal one third of the tibia. The muscles for external control of the dorsiflexion of the foot and the toes arise from the anterior compartment of the lower leg. From the lateral compartment arises the peroneal muscles which control the eversion of the hindfoot and the pronation of the forefoot. The posterior compartment gives rise to the muscles which control the plantar flexion of the ankle, as well as the flexion of the toes. Neurovascular bundles traverse each of these compartments on their way to the foot.

Shaft Fractures of Tibia and Fibula

The fractures of the shaft of the tibia and fibula are most often the product of a direct force. When an indirect force with rotation occurs, it creates the spiral fracture.

The fractured tibia is the most commonly seen open fracture because this bone is subjected to the greatest violence in accidents. The tibia lies subcutaneous throughout its entire length with little if any soft tissue protection from an exterior blow.

Examination. Since the tibia is subcutaneous throughout its entire course, a deformity, as well as probable swelling, will be observed at the fracture site. If the fracture is an open one, the break in the skin and soft tissues will be observed.

Roentgenograms. The anteroposterior and lateral roentgenograms are helpful in determining not only the level of fracture but the specifics of the fracture itself (e.g., transverse, spiral, comminuted, see Chapter 1) (Fig. 16–1). Sometimes, because of the length of the lower leg, a second roentgenogram is required to allow visualization of the joint above and the joint below the fracture.

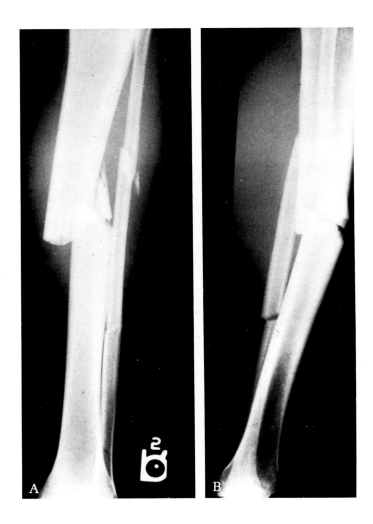

Fig. 16–1. Roentgenograms of transverse tibial shaft fracture. A, Anteroposterior view. There is minimal comminution. Periosteum is intact on concave side (lateral) of fracture. Thus reduction will be performed by increasing angulation and matching lateral cortices at fracture before straightening angulation. B, Lateral view. Concave side is posterior. In reducing this fracture, distal fragment will be moved in that direction to increase deformity and allow matching of posterior cortices before straightening angulation. Once angulation is corrected in anterior and lateral planes, correction can be maintained by three-point fixation in plaster of Paris cast.

Treatment. The specifics of the fracture of the lower leg will help determine the type of treatment program to be embarked upon. The open fracture must be treated immediately by operative means. The wound needs to be excised and copiously irrigated with saline solution, and if judged appropriate, some type of internal fixation should be used. A strictly transverse fracture can usually be reduced by increasing the angulation and matching the cortices before straightening them. The reduction can be maintained in a long leg cast. This immobilization will have to be maintained for approximately three months, the latter six weeks of which may well be in a walking cast. The early weight bearing patellar tendon bearing (PTB) cast is well adapted to treatment of this fracture.

The oblique fracture (Fig. 16–2), which will continually attempt to shorten, creates a different problem and often requires more than the long leg cast in

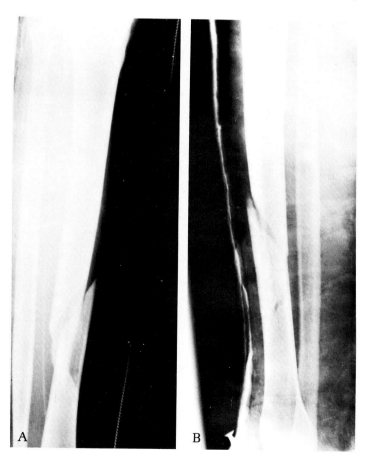

Fig. 16–2. Roentgenograms of foreleg in which oblique fracture is present. A, Anteroposterior view. Because of length of lower leg, a second roentgenogram was required to allow visualization of joint above and joint below fracture. Minimal tibiofibular diastasis at ankle could be explained by both bone principle. B, Lateral view. Note radiolucent line confirming partial fracture of distal fragment. This suggests injuring force of major magnitude.

order to maintain length. Early weight bearing in the patellar tendon bearing (PTB) cast can be utilized in this circumstance if the significant degree of shortening which almost invariably occurs will be acceptable. I have found open reduction and screw fixation of the long oblique fracture to be most effective as a means of maintaining reduction and length. Similar treatment for the spiral fracture can be accomplished to good effect. Reticence to operate at

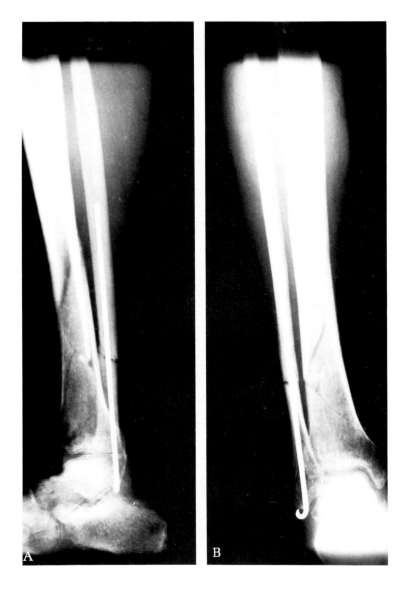

Fig. 16–3. Open moderately comminuted fracture of tibia and closed transverse fracture of fibula. A, Anteroposterior roentgenogram. B, Lateral roentgenogram. Treatment for this inherently unstable fracture included excision of wound, primary closure of tibial wound, and fixation of fibula with Rush pin to provide stability. Union of tibia ensued over six-month period.

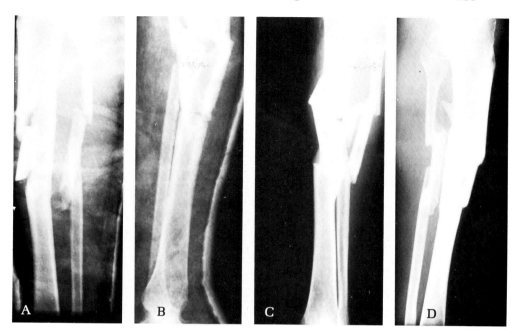

Fig. 16–4. Roentgenograms of comminuted tibial and fibular fractures in motorcycle rider who sustained multiple injuries. A, Anteroposterior view. Alignment of fracture as shown through plaster of Paris cast is relatively good. B, Lateral view. Note again relatively good alignment of this very comminuted fracture. C, Anteroposterior view ten months following injury. The fractures are well united without surgical intervention. D, Lateral view of healed fracture. A modest prominence of tibial spine at inferiormost fracture is only evidence for malunion.

the fracture site in the spiral fracture or the oblique fracture, which are unstable fractures, may lead to insertion of Kirschner wires through the tibia above and below the site of fracture with incorporation into the plaster cast. A Rush pin up the fibula may allow stability and maintain length (Fig. 16–3). Particularly is the use of the Rush pin up the fibula worth considering in the comminuted fracture of the tibia. This gives an effective means of maintaining length and stability. Most tibial fractures will require twelve to fourteen weeks of immobilization before evidence of union will be seen on the roentgenogram. An unusually comminuted fracture of the tibia is not necessarily a reason for operative treatment. In fact, it may create a contraindication to operative treatment (Fig. 16–4).

Fracture of Fibular Shaft

The isolated fracture of the fibular shaft occurs generally from a direct blow or from a rotary mechanism at the ankle which seems to be sufficiently resilient to sustain the injury at the ankle level, but not more proximally at the fibula. A special concern in the spiral fracture of the fibula is the potential of peroneal injury when the fracture extends sufficiently high in the fibula to enter the peroneal groove. Another matter of concern with a displaced fibular fracture can be a tibiofibular diastasis at the ankle.

Examination. Upon palpation, one finds point tenderness over the area of fibular shaft fracture. Occasionally the displaced fragment can be palpated.

Roentgenograms. The roentgenograms confirm the presence of the fracture of the fibula, often a spiral type (Fig. 16–5).

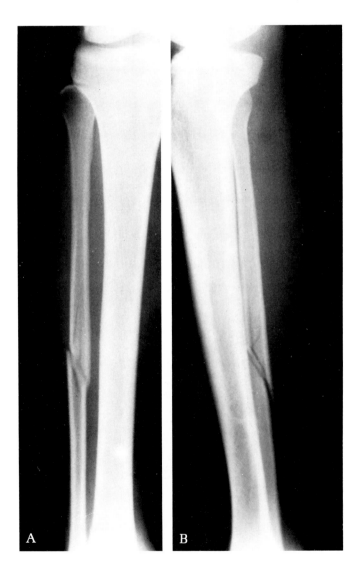

Fig. 16–5. A, Anteroposterior roentgenogram of isolated fracture of fibular shaft, often associated with fracture elsewhere in lower leg or with tibiofibular diastasis at ankle. B, Lateral roentgenogram of undisplaced fracture of fibular shaft. A simple elastic wrap may be sufficient treatment if no other bony or ligamentous injury accompanies it.

Treatment. The fibular shaft fracture is treated symptomatically. If sufficient comfort ensues, a simple elastic wrap is utilized. If the patient needs further support, a short leg plaster of Paris walking cast can be applied.

FRACTURES OF LOWER LEG IN CHILDREN

Commonly the injury to the foreleg in the infant and younger child produces a spiral fracture of the tibia. This type of fracture occurs by catching of the foot and often leaves an intact fibula. Between the ages of five and ten years transverse fractures of both bones from direct trauma are more common. The adolescent will more often have a comminuted fracture of the tibia and fibula and often with significant displacement.

Shaft Fractures of Tibia and Fibula

The mechanism of injury for shaft fractures of the tibia and fibula is variable and dependent upon the activity of the child at the time of the fracture, as well as upon the age of the child.

Examination. As previously noted in the discussion of fractures in the adult, the examination will reveal tenderness and deformity at the site of fracture.

Roentgenograms. The roentgenograms will confirm the fracture as to type (e.g., transverse, angulation, comminution, see Chapter 1). Intact periosteum on the concave side of the fracture will hold the key to maintenance of reduction (see Chapter 1).

Treatment. The deformity in the tibial shaft fracture can be increased toward the concave side, and the cortices of bone on the concave side of the distal and proximal fragments can be brought together. The distal segment is then moved away from the concave position to reduce the fracture. This maneuver tightens the periosteum and maintains reduction. The long leg plaster of Paris cast is utilized with three-point fixation to maintain the reduction (Fig. 16–6). The cast should be worn for six weeks and be replaced by a walking cast for an additional six weeks. The walking cast may be a long leg or a patellar tendon bearing cast depending upon the experience and preference of the treating physician.

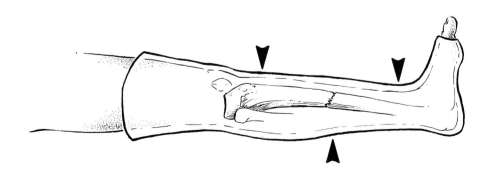

Fig. 16–6. Illustration of long leg cast applied to secure three-point fixation. This method utilizes intact soft tissue to maintain reduction while union of the fracture progresses.

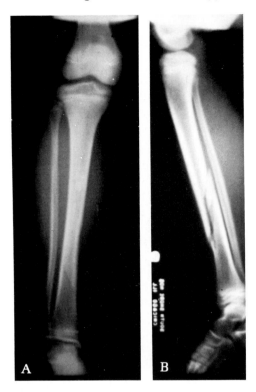

Fig. 16–7.   Roentgenograms of spiral fracture in tibia of child. A, Anteroposterior view. Note single oblique fracture line at junction of middle and distal one thirds. B, Lateral view, revealing full extent of spiral fracture. This fracture is not uncommon in children and can almost always be treated by closed means.

   The spiral fracture of the tibia, not uncommon in the younger child, is much like the aforementioned fracture of the tibia (Fig. 16–7). The fibula often is not fractured and thus maintains a certain amount of stability against which one may work. The leg should be immobilized in a long leg plaster of Paris cast for six weeks and then in a walking cast, either long leg or patellar tendon bearing depending upon the treating physician's choice, for an additional six weeks. Occasionally a fracture in the child needs internal fixation (Fig. 16–8).

The Greenstick Fracture

   The tibia in the growing child is subject to many forces of stress. The greenstick fracture may angulate a shaft of the tibia or fibula. As in the greenstick fracture of the forearm, too great an angulation in the shaft is generally not acceptable because it occurs at the center of the shaft. Little chance exists for correction through growth, but the tendency for the weight bearing bones to correct such angular deformity appears greater in the lower limbs than in the upper limbs (by Wolff's Law).

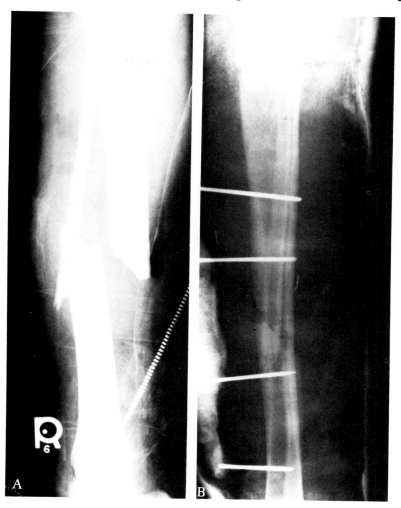

Fig. 16–8. Lateral roentgenograms showing fairly transverse fracture of tibia in a child. If fracture is stable after reduction, the leg can be immobilized in a long leg cast. A, Before reduction. B, After reduction. Because of instability following reduction, Kirschner wires were placed into the proximal and distal fragments and incorporated in the cast.

Examination. On examination, one notes pain and an angular deformity of the lower leg at the fracture site.

Roentgenograms. The anteroposterior and lateral roentgenograms confirm the angulation of the leg without complete separation of the cortices of the tibia and fibula.

Treatment. A long leg plaster of Paris cast can be applied to most types of greenstick fractures in the tibia without reduction of the angulation. An angulation greater than 20 degrees should be corrected by manipulation under anesthesia. After five or six weeks the long leg cast can be replaced by a walking cast for four more weeks. The torus greenstick fracture, which is purely a buckling of the cortex, can be treated by a weight bearing cast for eight weeks.

REFERENCES

1. Adams, J. C.: Outline of Fractures, Including Joint Injuries, 6th ed. Baltimore, Williams & Wilkins Co., 1972.
2. Blount, W. P.: Fractures in Children. Baltimore, Williams & Wilkins Co., 1954.
3. Charnley, J.: Closed Treatment of Common Fractures, 3rd ed., 1961., (Fourth Reprint). Edinburgh & London, Churchill Livingstone, 1972.
4. Crock, H. V.: Blood Supply to the Lower Limb Bones in Man. New York, Edinburgh, Churchill-Livingstone, 1967.
5. Dehne, E., and Torp, R. P.: Treatment of joint injuries by immediate mobilization. Clin. Orthop. 77:219, 1971.
6. Scully, T. J.: Ambulant, nonoperative management of femoral shaft fractures, Part I. Clin. Orthop. 100:195, 1974.
7. Scully, T. J.: Ambulant, nonoperative management of femoral shaft fractures, Part II. Clin. Orthop. 100:204, 1974.
8. Rang, M. C.: Children's Fractures. Philadelphia, J. B. Lippincott Co., 1974.
9. Rockwood, C. A., and Green, D. P.: Fractures. Philadelphia, J. B. Lippincott Co., 1975.
10. Watson-Jones, R.: Fractures and Joint Injuries, 4th ed., 2 V. Baltimore, Williams & Wilkins Co., 1952-1955.

17

THE ANKLE

The ankle joint is a remarkably stable joint allowing only dorsiflexion and plantar flexion. The inversion and eversion motions which are often considered to be ankle motions are in fact purely subtalar motions. The ankle stability is maintained by a mortise whose medial wall is the malleolus. The lateral wall of the mortise is the lateral malleolus. The superior weight bearing surface with which the dome of the astragalus articulates is the distal tibial articular surface, often called the tibial plafond. The malleoli are not of equal length, the medial malleolus being three-eighths to one-half inch shorter than the lateral mal-

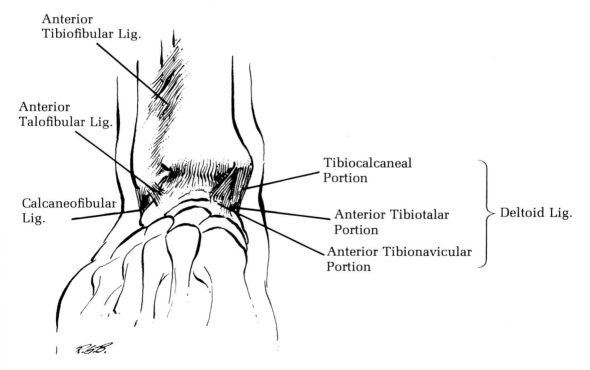

Fig. 17–1. Illustration of anterior ankle. A more extensive concept of ligaments and their relationship to ankle is shown. In addition to lateral and medial ligaments, note tibiofibular ligament immediately superior to ankle joint.

leolus. In addition, the lateral malleolus is positioned more posteriorly than the medial malleolus. The tibiofibular relationship at the ankle is maintained by strong anterior and posterior tibiofibular ligaments which lie one-fourth to one-half inch proximal to the joint surface of the tibial plafond (Fig. 17–1). The ankle capsule encloses the entire ankle joint about its periphery in such a fashion as to allow the full dorsiflexion and plantar flexion motions necessary for ambulation and other active ankle use (Fig. 17–2). From the tip of the medial malleolus, the medial collateral ligament passes anteriorly to the medial wall of the neck of the talus, inferiorly into the medial os calcis, and posteriorly into the wall of the os calcis. On the lateral side, the lateral collateral ligament fibers provide stability by attachment from the tip of its malleolus down into the lateral os calcis inferiorly as well as posteriorly. The tendons for dorsiflex-

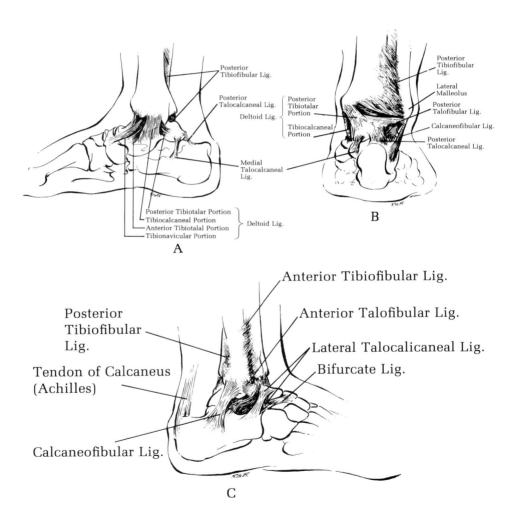

Fig. 17–2. Ligaments of ankle. A, Medial aspect of medial (deltoid) ligaments. B, Posterior aspect. C, Lateral view.

ion of the foot and of the toes pass from the anterior compartment of the lower leg across the anterior ankle and into the foot. Associated with these tendons at the central point of the ankle are the anterior tibial artery and veins, as well as the distal extension of the deep peroneal nerve. The lateral compartment tendons, namely, the peroneal tendons, pass posterior to the lateral malleolus in anatomic grooves. They are accompanied by a small peroneal artery. Posterior to the medial malleolus pass the tendons of the posterior tibial, the flexor digitorum communis, and the flexor hallucis longus muscles. The posterior tibial artery, veins, and nerve lie between the tendons of the flexor communis and the flexor hallucis longus.

Ligamentous Injury

The ankle sprain or strain is undoubtedly the most common injury at the ankle. An inversion force tends to be the most common cause of this injury. The

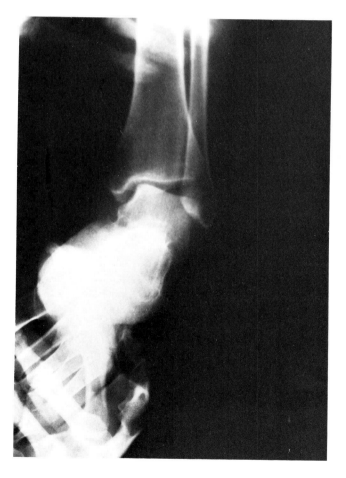

Fig. 17–3. Anteroposterior roentgenogram with inversion stress to display hidden lateral collateral ligament tear requiring active treatment. A plaster of Paris cast with eversion positioning is often sufficient treatment.

medial malleolus does not extend as far distally as the lateral malleolus and thus offers less buttress against the inversion injury. The inversion type injury is therefore more common than is the eversion injury at the ankle. The eversion sprain, as well as the plantar flexion sprain, however, does occur.

Examination. Examination gives the best clue as to the ligamentous injury present and its extent. In the inversion injury, palpation at the tip of the malleolus and at the points of insertion of the lateral collateral ligament allows one to ascertain the major area of ligamentous injury. Recreation of the force of injury will recreate this specific pain. Extensive swelling and ecchymosis will often be seen localized to the area of the ligamentous injury. Examination in the eversion injury reveals pain and tenderness localized to the tip of the medial malleolus or along its course to insertion on the medial talar neck and/or the medial os calcis. The strain or sprain in the plantar flexion injury produces pain at the anterior ankle joint.

Roentgenograms. Roentgenographic examination of the ankle with a soft tissue lesion is usually not revealing of bony abnormality. Any roentgenographic examination of the ankle must include the anteroposterior view, the lateral view, and the mortise view as baseline studies. The inversion stress roentgenograms of both ankles may be helpful to further assess a subluxation of the talus concomitant to a massive lateral collateral ligament tear (Fig. 17–3) (the normal ankle is used for comparison).

Treatment. In treatment of sprains, which are in essence partial collateral ligament tears, the ankle is immobilized in such a position as to approximate the torn ligamentous fibers. Thus the inversion injury would be immobilized with an eversion effect; the eversion injury would be immobilized with inversion; and the plantar flexion injury would be immobilized with the ankle dorsiflexed. In the less serious injury, an elastic bandage is usually sufficient for stabilizing the ankle. Occasionally, however, a more significant injury has occurred which can be well treated by use of the Gibney boot, a basketweave effect produced with adhesive plaster (Fig. 17–4). Either of these two methods should be used for about ten days and may require the use of crutches at the same time. If the injury is deemed more serious than this, a walking cast is most effective for approximately three weeks. A short leg walking cast is sufficient for the immobilization, but often a patient with an ankle injury is more comfortable if the potential rotary effect from the knee is negated by extending the cast to a point just above the knee.

Dislocation of Ankle

Dislocation of the ankle may occur into the space anterior to the ankle mortise or the space posterior to the ankle mortise without incurring a fracture. The mechanism of injury for either of these dislocations would be a direct force in the direction toward which the dislocation occurs, associated with dorsiflexion of the ankle in the posterior dislocation and plantar-flexion of the ankle in the anterior dislocation. The most common dislocation, however, occurs in association with a fracture. When associated with fracture of the malleolus, the dislocation may occur toward the medial or toward the lateral side (Fig. 17–5). The force in this instance is toward the direction of the dislocation and is a direct force.

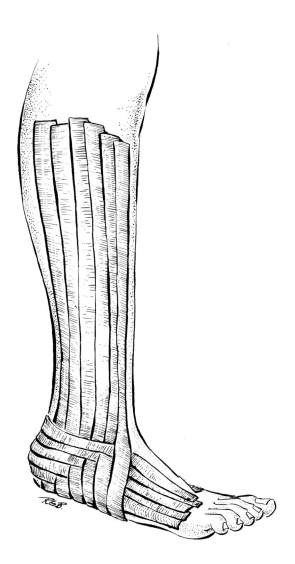

Fig. 17–4. Gibney boot for immobilizing lesser sprains and strains. The patient can hold a gauze strip under the metatarsal heads to position the ankle for reversing the stretch of the injury while adhesive strips are applied.

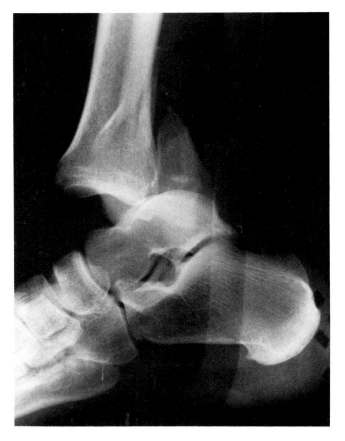

Fig. 17–5. Dislocation of ankle in association with fracture of distal fibula, as well as torn tibiofibular ligaments, ankle capsule, and medial collateral ligaments. Tibiotalar dislocation alone does occur but is not a common injury.

Examination and Roentgenograms. On examination of the dislocated ankle, the direction of dislocation can be determined by simple observation and palpation. The tibia is prominent in the direction away from the talus dislocation.

Treatment. Treatment of dislocation of the ankle without fracture often requires an anesthetic in order to achieve sufficient relaxation to relocate the talus into the mortise. Nothing is to be lost, however, from making the effort to reduce this dislocation, using analgesia and relaxation from meperidine and diazepam. The reduction is accomplished by longitudinal traction force plus a force directed in the direction of the ankle mortise from the dislocated talus. Thus the posterior dislocation would require an anterior force with some minimal dorsiflexion and plantar flexion movements as an assist to slide the talus under the margin of the posterior plafond and into the mortise. The anterior dislocation is reduced by a posterior force with longitudinal traction while simultaneously attempting to distract the talus in a plantar direction.

Once the dislocation has been reduced, a short leg walking plaster of Paris cast should be applied, and the patient should avoid weight bearing on the affected limb for several days. The time of immobilization for this particular injury is generally six weeks.

Fracture-Dislocation of Ankle

When a fracture occurs, the dislocation is more commonly medial or lateral and is more unstable because the fracture of the malleolus occurs in conjunction with a tear of the collateral ligament from the opposite malleolus. With vital structures coursing across the ankle joint and having specific bounds within which they must traverse, the potential of vascular and/or nerve injury in the dislocated ankle must be recognized. The examination must include neurologic and vascular assessment prior to any treatment.

Treatment. When fracture of one or both of the malleoli has occurred at the time of the dislocation, (Fig. 17–6) the relocation is easy, but there is danger of instability and redislocation. Because of this, it is felt that relocation of the ankle should be followed by operative repair of the ligaments or internal fixation of the reduced malleolus on the side away from the dislocation. The fractured malleolus away from the side of dislocation then assumes the position of stability for this ankle. A long leg plaster of Paris cast should be utilized in this circumstance for the first six weeks. If roentgenograms then show sufficient early union, the long leg cast may be replaced with a short leg walking cast for an additional four to six weeks.

Inversion Fractures of Malleolus

The force creating the inversion injury may avulse the lateral malleolus at some point distal to the tibial plafond (Fig. 17–7). Should the force continue

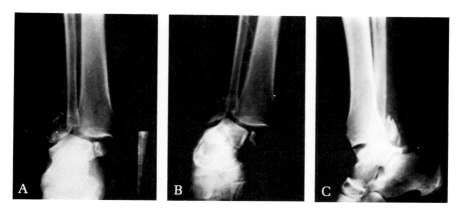

Fig. 17–6. Roentgenograms showing posterolateral fracture-dislocation at tibiotalar joint, probably from severe plantar flexion force to foot. A, Anteroposterior view. B, Mortise view. Little additional information is gained. Medial and lateral malleoli have been fractured at level slightly superior to tibial plafond—in fact suggesting little if any eversion or inversion forces in original injury. C, Lateral view showing talus to be partially dislocated posteriorly but without fracture of posterior tibial plafond. Posterior tibia is overlaid on talus because lateral dome of talus is lying lateral and superior to its usual relationship to tibia (see A and B).

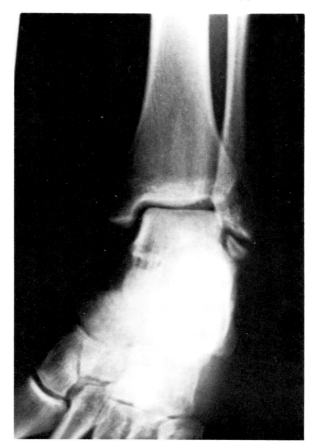

Fig. 17–7. Nonunion in pull-off fracture of lateral malleolus occurring at level below joint line and probably caused by inversion force. Since the medial malleolus does not extend as far inferiorly as does the lateral malleolus, it does not provide as firm support against injury. Hence isolated tears of lateral ligament are more common than are those of medial ligament.

unabated after the avulsion fracture of the lateral malleolus, the next injury to occur will be the push fracture of the medial malleolus. The push fracture starts at the level of the plafond and works obliquely and proximally toward the medial tibial cortex (Fig. 17–8). Thus, dependent upon the inversion stress, there may be a single fracture of the lateral malleolus or a bimalleolar fracture in which the lateral malleolar fracture occurs by traction and the medial malleolar fracture is caused by a push mechanism from the talus. When a medial malleolar fracture begins at the level of the tibial plafond and works more proximal and no lateral malleolar fracture is present, it can be assumed that a separation of at least a portion of the fibers of the lateral collateral ligament of the ankle must also have occurred.

Roentgenograms. Roentgenograms must include the anteroposterior, the lateral, and the mortise views in order to appropriately assess any ankle injury.

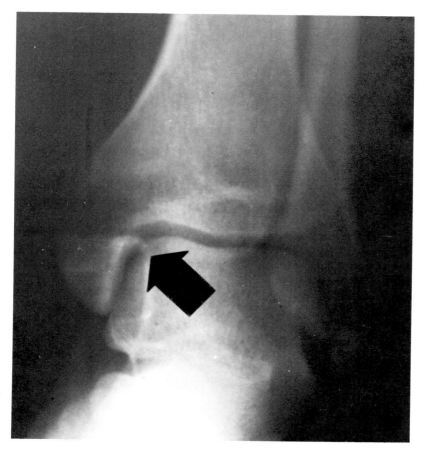

Fig. 17–8. Anteroposterior roentgenogram of fracture of ankle. The medial malleolar fracture line starts at plafond level and runs supermedially (arrow), typical of fracture caused by push-off mechanism.

Should a rotational force be added to the inversion force (more commonly one of internal rotation), a spiraling effect may be seen in the fracture lines of both malleoli. In this instance, the previously described traction injury occurring distal to the tibial plafond associated with the "knock off" injury occurring from the level of the tibial plafond proximal may not be seen.

Treatment. In the treatment of the inversion injury of the malleolus, the inversion deformity is increased slightly and reduction is completed by an eversion movement of the foot and ankle into the normal position. A long leg plaster of Paris cast is most comfortable for the patient following this maneuver. Sometimes the analgesia and relaxation following administration of meperidine and diazepam are sufficient for performing this maneuver. More commonly a general anesthetic will be necessary. Should the roentgenograms following reduction show full reduction with restoration of the mortise, this may be left as is in anticipation that the fragments will unite. A long leg cast will be needed for six weeks and a short leg walking cast for an additional four to six weeks. If reduction is not in evidence on the anteroposterior, mortise, and lateral views, then open reduction will be necessary, followed by appropriate internal fixation.

To reduce the inversion injury in which a rotational force has also been in effect, the causative rotational force is reversed at the same time as moving the foot and ankle into the eversion position. Again, the roentgenograms must confirm restoration of the mortise and contact of the malleolar fragments in order to anticipate union with good stability. If the roentgenograms following manipulation fail to show adequate reduction, then open reduction and appropriate fixation will be necessary. Immobilization is for the same period as for the simple fracture.

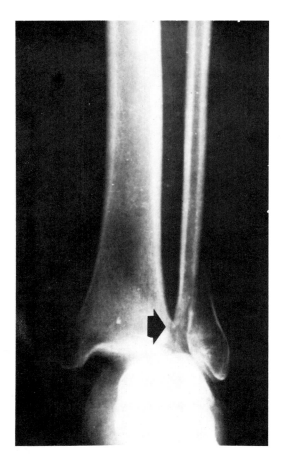

Fig. 17–9. Mortise view roentgenogram of ankle that has sustained an eversion injury caused by tearing of medial collateral ligament and "push off" of lateral malleolus. If the fracture of the lateral malleolus is accurately reduced, a stable ankle should ensue, since innermost part of tibiofibular ligament is intact as evidenced by lack of displacement (arrow).

Eversion Fractures of Malleolus

The eversion injury occurs when a force everts the foot and ankle, blocking the talus against the lateral malleolus. If the lateral malleolus is fractured by the "knock-off" mechanism, the fracture line may occur anywhere from the tibial plafond level proximally (Fig. 17–9). Should the fracture line occur proximal to the tibiofibular ligament insertion, the tibiofibular ligament is generally torn. This requires special consideration. Once the force has created the fracture of the lateral malleolus, it can cause a traction fracture of the medial malleolus at some point distal to the level of the tibial plafond (Fig. 17–10). Should the medial malleolus not fracture in this injury, then it is obligatory for at least a portion of the medial collateral ligament to tear.

The eversion injury may be associated with a rotational force, most commonly an external rotational force. The injuries created in this instance differ in that a spiral type of fracture may occur at either malleolus or in the distal fibula. If any significant plantar flexion is present at the time that this rotational force occurs, not only is the medial malleolus fractured, but the lateral malleolus and the posterior portion of the tibial plafond can also be fractured. This is the so-called trimalleolar fracture (Fig. 17–11).

Roentgenograms. For full evaluation of the eversion fracture, roentgenograms must include the anteroposterior, lateral, and mortise views. Careful study of these roentgenograms will help evaluate the mechanism of the injury and determine the method of treatment of the particular injury.

Treatment. The pure eversion injury can often be treated by reversing the force and inverting the ankle. Should adequate reduction occur with this

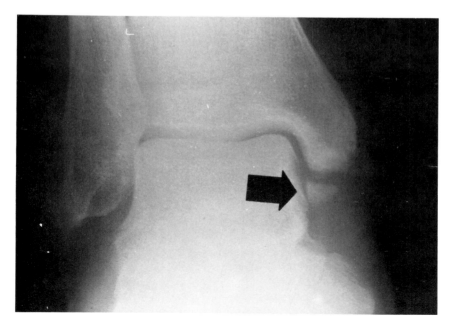

Fig. 17–10. Medial malleolus "pulled off" by eversion injury producing fracture of malleolus below tibial plafond (arrow).

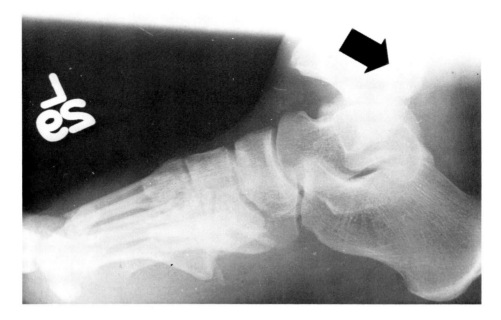

Fig. 17–11. Lateral roentgenogram revealing displaced fracture of posterior tibial plafond associated with posterior dislocation of astragalus on tibia (arrow). Since this appears to be an unstable fracture-dislocation, it was treated by open reduction and internal fixation with screw.

maneuver, reduction can be maintained in a long leg cast for six weeks and in a short leg walking cast for an additional six weeks. However, it is not necessarily likely that the medial malleolus will reassume a position of contact adequate for union. Because of this lack of contact after reduction, the eversion injury often requires operation with internal fixation of the medial malleolus. Immobilization is the same with or without operation.

When a rotational element is judged to have been present along with the eversion, closed reduction should be tried after administering an analgesic or anesthetic. Following attempted reduction, if roentgenograms do not show adequate contact at the fractured medial malleolus or if the mortise is not fully reestablished, then open reduction is indicated, followed by internal fixation of the medial malleolus. Occasionally, the lateral malleolus must also be internally fixed; fixation can be done with a longitudinal screw up the fibula.

When tibiofibular diastasis is present with separation of the distal fibula away from the tibia, then a transfixing screw must be placed across the fibula and into the tibia. This will secure the best possible ankle mortise. Before weight bearing is allowed at six weeks, the tibiofibular screw should be removed.

In the trimalleolar fracture (Fig. 17–12) when more than one third of the surface of the tibial plafond is fractured, it is important to reduce the posterior tibial joint surface perfectly. If reduction is not perfect, the posterior tibial plafond must be reduced openly and screw fixation must be used to maintain the reduction. Once the posterior tibial plafond is reduced and fixed, the lateral

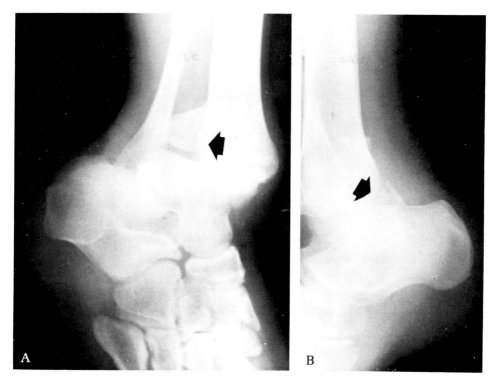

Fig. 17–12. Roentgenograms of fracture-dislocation of right ankle. A, Anteroposterior view. Arrow points to posterior tibial plafond fragment. Distal fibula is widely separated from its usual relationship to tibia, and astragalus is laterally displaced. The tibiofibular relationship must be reestablished and the fibula internally fixed to the tibia. B, Lateral view. Arrow points to "posterior" malleolar fragment. Note talus lies posterior to its usual relationship with tibial plafond. Because this tibial fragment is at least one third of the plafond joint space, it needs to be openly reduced and internally fixed to recreate stability of ankle joint.

malleolar fracture may be reduced spontaneously. In this situation, the medial malleolar fracture often still requires screw fixation.

In any of these injuries treated by closed or open means, the long leg plaster of Paris cast must be used for six weeks and then be replaced by a short leg walking cast for an additional period of four to six weeks.

Tibiofibular Diastasis

The tibiofibular diastasis may occur by an inversion force without fracture. This is not common but is seen. The injury can be determined upon examination by an attempt to slide the talus from medial to lateral without allowing inversion and eversion. In this instance the medial-lateral sliding of the talus can be palpated. The anteroposterior and lateral roentgenograms usually are not helpful (Fig. 17–13A,B). The mortise view will show separation of the fibula from the tibia (Fig. 17–13C). A transfixing screw must be inserted to reestablish the integrity of the mortise (Fig. 17–13D&E). Following insertion of

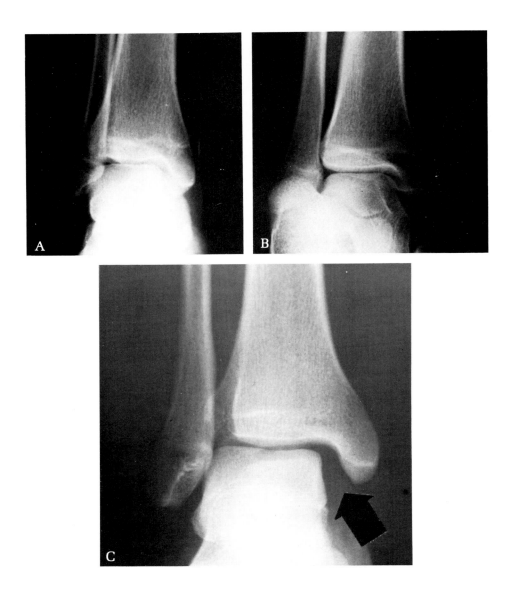

Fig. 17–13. Roentgenograms of ankle following eversion injury. A, Anteroposterior view. B, Mortise view. There is perhaps a suggestion of widening of mortise. C, Mortise view ten days later revealing tibiofibular diastasis and widening of joint space between medial malleolus and medial talus (arrow). A fracture of fibula at mid and distal thirds was also present.

the transfixing screw, a long leg plaster of Paris cast is used. The screw is removed at six weeks, just prior to initiation of weight bearing. Once removal of the screw is accomplished in six weeks, the patient should be in a walking cast for about four weeks.

Chip Fractures of Dome of Talus

With either the inversion or the eversion injury a small chip of cartilage and bone may be knocked off the superior margin of the talus. In the inversion injury the chip is usually knocked off the posterolateral side, and in the eversion injury the chip is from the posteromedial side. This injury cannot occur without some ligamentous tearing, since an unusual mobility of the talus must be present for this chip fracture to occur.

Examination. Upon examination, the ankle is extremely tender and swollen. Aspiration of the joint will return bloody fluid that often has fat droplets on its surface.

Roentgenograms. Careful study of the anteroposterior, lateral, and mortise roentgenograms may reveal a small flake on the dome of the talus (Fig. 17–14). When the fracture is not seen on the films, but is suspected, additional mortise views with the foot in varying degrees of plantar and dorsiflexion may bring the chip fracture into relief.

Treatment. The treatment of choice for the chip fracture is arthrotomy with removal of the fractured chip. The postoperative course is usually benign. The patient is placed in a walking cast for six weeks, and mobilization is gradually begun.

Dislocation of Talus

Although not a common injury, an isolated dislocation of the talus can occur. Particularly can this occur at the time of forced dorsiflexion of the ankle. In this injury the talus is forced into a position posterior to the ankle.

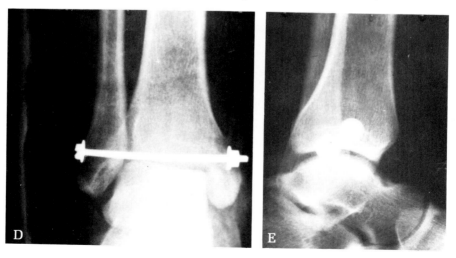

Fig. 17–13. (Cont'd)   D, Anteroposterior and E, Lateral views following reduction of diastasis and bolt fixation.

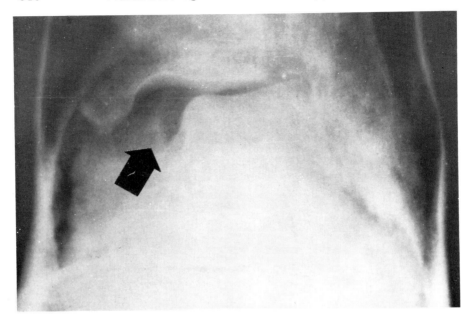

Fig. 17–14. Chip fracture off dome of talus (arrow) caused by an eversion injury which "pushes" the lateral malleolus off and tips the talus within the mortise.

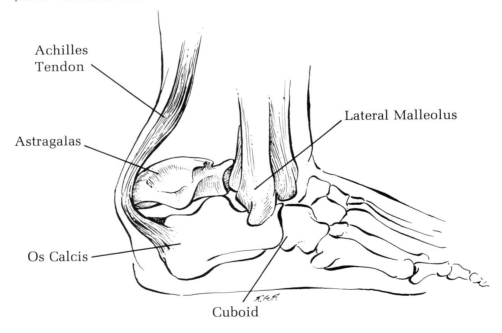

Fig. 17–15. Illustration showing astragalus dislocated posteriorly from between tibia and os calcis. This is caused by a very strong dorsiflexion force which effectively "squeezes" the talus posteriorly. The talus is an entirely intra-articular bone, and thus its blood supply is precarious (see Fig. 18–2).

Examination. Examination reveals the fullness of the posterior ankle and a painful foot with any attempted movement.

Roentgenograms. The anteroposterior roentgenograms will confirm the absence of the talus from the mortise. On the lateral view the talus is seen posterior to the ankle joint (Fig. 17–15). It not only separates from the articulation with the tibia, but also from the navicular and the os calcis.

Treatment. Reduction of a dislocation of the talus usually requires a general anesthetic. Efforts at closed reduction must be made first. This is done by longitudinal traction on the foot and the heel with the foot dorsiflexed and with an assistant providing gentle force from posterior toward anterior on the body of the talus. Occasionally, the talus will slip back into joint with this maneuver, particularly with some gentle dorsiflexion plantar flexion "jiggles." However, should closed reduction not ensue, then open reduction must be accomplished. Dislocation of the talus can only occur by significant ligamentous tearing. Included in this separation may be the loss of the major blood supply to the talus, which is an entirely intra-articular bone.

Following reduction, either closed or open, a short leg plaster of Paris cast may be used for six weeks. Three of these weeks may be with a walking heel.

Long-term observation of the patient after a dislocation of the talus is indicated. Avascular necrosis is not an uncommon complication from this injury.

ANKLE INJURIES IN CHILDREN

The ankle fractures that are typically seen in adults do not occur in children. Epiphysial fractures more commonly occur from similar injuring forces in the child (see Chapter 2). The transversely directed force will less often cause a growth disturbance than will the longitudinal thrust.

Sprains

Sprains of the ankle in the child are fairly uncommon, although the adolescent athlete begins to show the ankle sprain as typically seen in the adult. When a sprain is present, examination reveals point tenderness over the area of ligamentous injury. Roentgenograms may not be particularly helpful in diagnosis, except to rule out fracture.

An elastic wrap is usually sufficient treatment for the ankle sprain of the child or the adolescent. However, when a more severe sprain is diagnosed, the adolescent must be given the same consideration of aggressive treatment as the adult.

Epiphyseal Separation at Ankle

The more common injury at the ankle of the child, particularly from the ages of three to twelve years, is an injury of the tibial epiphysis. The mechanism of injury can be inversion, eversion, rotational, forced dorsiflexion, or forced plantar flexion.

Examination. On examination, a deformity consistent with the specific injury is noted in the ankle. There is often swelling within the ankle joint. All movement of the ankle is guarded.

Roentgenograms. Roentgenograms must include the anteroposterior, lateral,

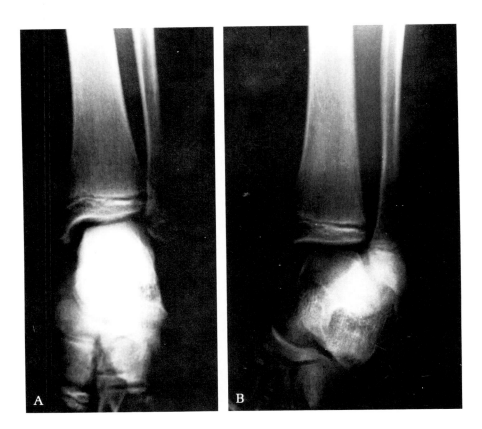

Fig. 17–16.   A, Anteroposterior and B, Mortise views necessary in securing roentgenograms of child's ankle. The uninjured ankle should always be seen in as similar a view as possible for comparison. A lateral view is also needed.

and mortise views (Fig. 17–16), as well as comparison views of the opposite ankle. When an epiphyseal injury is present, it must be evaluated as to its grouping within the classification as outlined by Salter and Harris (see Chapter 2). A type II separation through the epiphyseal plate with a portion of the metaphysis remaining attached to the concave side will be most common (Fig. 17–17). However, attention must be paid to the possibility of occurrence of the type III (Fig. 17–18) or type IV injury (Fig. 17–19A).

Treatment.   In most instances treatment for the epiphyseal separation at the ankle is closed reduction under general anesthetic. The long leg plaster of Paris cast is applied, and the roentgenograms are reviewed to determine adequacy of reduction. If the injury is determined to be of the type III or type IV epiphyseal injury, then nothing less than perfect reduction is acceptable. In the event of lack of perfect reduction, then gentle open reduction and pin fixation must be accomplished for maintenance of reduction. This is followed by a long leg cast for four weeks and a short leg walking cast for four weeks. All metal fixation across the epiphyseal plate, used to maintain reduction, should be removed at four to six weeks.

The lack of sufficient evaluation of the injury may well be shown by the mute evidence of ankle deformity in later years (Fig. 17–19B,C).

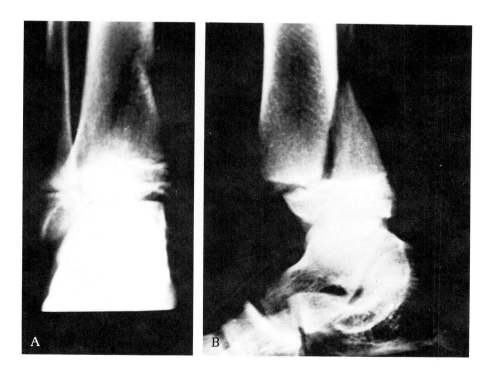

Fig. 17–17.   A, Anteroposterior and B, Lateral roentgenograms of Type II epiphyseal injury in a thirteen-year-old. This will likely result in no growth disturbance if gently reduced and immobilized in a cast for about six weeks.

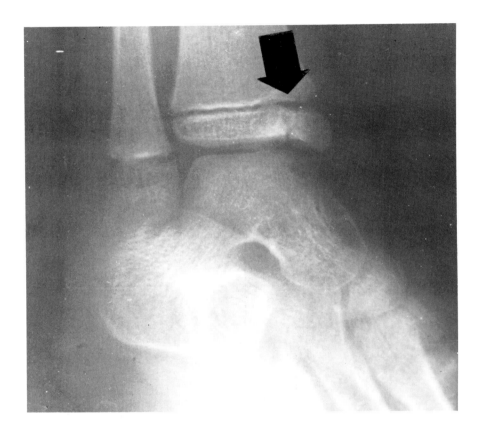

Fig. 17–18.   Mortise view roentgenogram showing Type I epiphyseal injury to distal fibula (note lateral margin of fibular epiphysis lies slightly medial to metaphyseal margin). Type III fracture through tibial epiphysis with some moderate displacement of medial malleolar segment is pointed out by arrow.

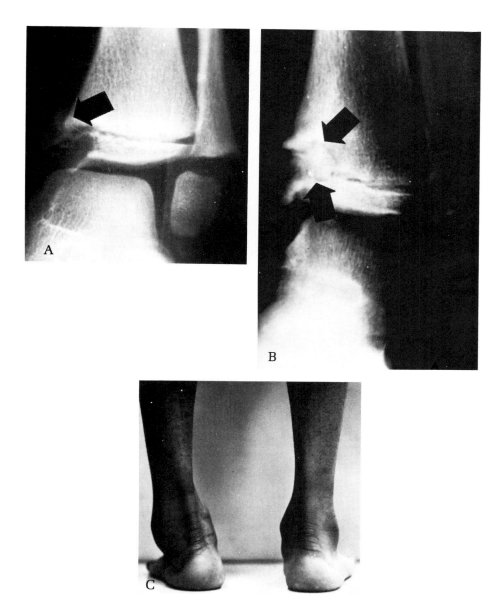

Fig. 17–19. Type IV epiphyseal injury. A, Anteroposterior roentgenogram of injured ankle of a twelve-year-old. Note medial malleolar fracture crossing epiphyseal plate into metaphysis of distal tibia (arrow). B, Consequences of inadequately recognized and thus poorly treated injury. Anteroposterior roentgenogram two years following injury shows two separate levels of epiphyseal plate on medial tibia distally. Note obliquity of joint line. C, Posterior view of both ankles three years after injury, showing that growth activity of medial tibial epiphysis was diminished.

Chip Fracture of Talus

The chip fracture of the talus occurs in the child as often as it does in the young adult. The examination reveals fullness of the ankle joint with point tenderness toward the side of the injury.

The roentgenograms must include anteroposterior, lateral, and mortise views. The chip will most likely be seen in one of these views. However, if this is the suspected diagnosis and the chip is not seen, then mortise views with the foot in various degrees of plantar-flexion and dorsiflexion are indicated.

The treatment of choice is arthrotomy with excision of fragment. Following arthrotomy, the patient is kept in a short leg walking plaster of Paris cast for four weeks.

REFERENCES

1. Adams, J. C.: Outline of Fractures, Including Joint Injuries, 6th ed. Baltimore, Williams & Wilkins Co., 1972.
2. Blount, W. P.: Fractures in Children. Baltimore, Williams & Wilkins Co., 1954.
3. Charnley, J.: Closed Treatment of Common Fractures, 3rd ed., 1961, (Fourth Reprint). Edinburgh & London, Churchill Livingstone, 1972.
4. Ralston, E. L.: Handbook of Fractures. St. Louis, C. V. Mosby Co., 1967.
5. Rang, M. C.: Children's Fractures. Philadelphia, J. B. Lippincott Co., 1974.
6. Rockwood, C. A., and Green, D. P.: Fractures. Philadelphia, J. B. Lippincott Co., 1975.
7. Salter, R. B., and Harris, R. W.: Injuries involving the epiphyseal plate. J. Bone Joint Surg. 45-A:587, 1963.
8. Watson-Jones, R.: Fractures and Joint Injuries, 4th ed., 2V. Baltimore, Williams & Wilkins Co., 1952-1955.

18

THE FOOT

For functional purposes, the foot is composed of the hindfoot and the forefoot. The bones of the hindfoot are the astragalus (or talus), the navicular, the cuneiforms, the os calcis, and the cuboid. The significant motions that occur in the hindfoot are inversion and eversion at the subtalar joint supported by the relationship of the anterior talus to the navicular and by the anterior os calcis to the cuboid.

The forefoot bones are the metatarsals and the phalanges. Supination and pronation of the forefoot occur across the midtarsal joints—that is, the junction between the tarsal bones and the bases of the opposing metatarsals. The ligamentous structures of the foot are remarkably complex and strong. They provide support to the longitudinal arch which will allow total weight bearing to be accomplished between the prominence of the os calcis posteriorly, the lateral aspect of the midfoot, and the metatarsal heads anteriorly.

Fracture of Talus

Fracture of the neck of the talus occurs particularly with a sharp dorsiflexion move which traps the neck of the talus between the os calcis below and the anterior surface of the tibial plafond above.

Examination. The examination of the foot in which the talus has been fractured reveals a generally swollen hindfoot with severe pain in the anterior region of the ankle. No specific finding on examination will identify the exact nature of the injury.

Roentgenograms. The roentgenograms must include the anteroposterior and lateral views of the *foot* (Fig. 18–1). The fracture may be in such a position as to remove the blood supply from the head or from the dome of the talus. The blood supply to the talus enters predominantly from the neck dorsally, from the tarsal sinus on its inferolateral side, and at its posterior-most margin (Fig. 18–2).

Treatment. Treatment of the simple undisplaced fracture of the talus should be by immobilization in a short leg cast for eight weeks. In the event of significant displacement, manipulation must be accomplished to provide adequate contact between the fracture fragments. A good reduction of the fracture of the talus is essential to provide proper mechanics for future weight bearing and to prevent nonunion.

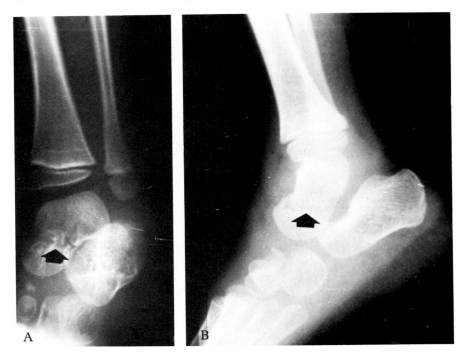

Fig. 18–1. A, Anteroposterior oblique roentgenogram demonstrating neck fracture of astragalus (arrow) in a seven-year-old. Without displacement there may well be intact blood supply to both fragments. B, Lateral roentgenogram showing relatively undisplaced fracture of talus (arrow).

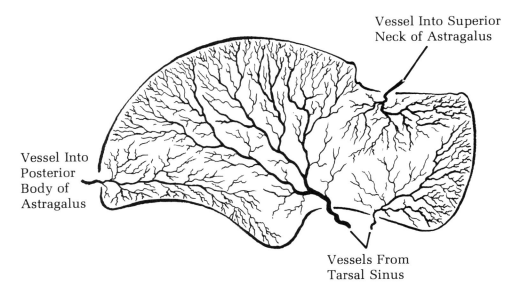

Fig. 18–2. Lateral view of astragalus showing its major sources of blood supply—dorsal neck of talus, inferior tarsal sinus, and posterior tongue of talus.

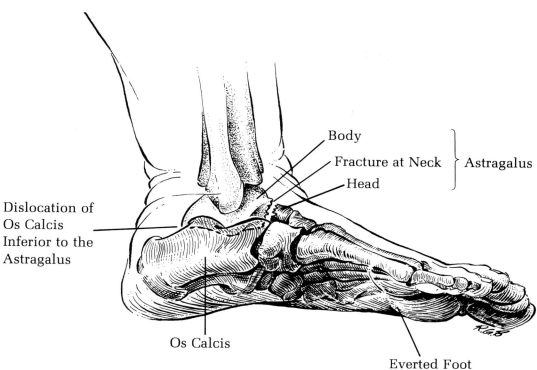

Fig. 18–3. Illustration of fracture-dislocation of foot on talus. Note fracture through neck of talus. The anterior talus has retained its relationship to the os calcis, the navicular, and the cuboid. This entire group moves as a unit in effect dislocating the foot away from the body of the talus, which remains in the ankle mortise.

    When any significant displacement of the distal fragment occurs, its surrounding hindfoot (os calcis, cuboid, and navicular) moves with it (Fig. 18–3). The ligaments between the posterior talus and the os calcis have been torn. The body of the talus remains in the ankle mortise. Reduction must be accurate. If this cannot be achieved by closed methods, then operative reduction and fixation are indicated.

Fracture-Dislocation of Astragalus

    On occasion, a strong dorsiflexion force fractures the neck of the talus and forces the body of the talus out of the ankle joint and into the space posteriorly.

    Examination. A fracture-dislocation of the astragalus is not easily determined from the physical examination. The usual concavity at each side of the Achilles tendon at the ankle may be absent; instead, the depressions may appear full to visualization and palpation.

    Roentgenograms. The diagnosis of a fracture-dislocation of the astragalus is confirmed particularly on the lateral roentgenogram of the foot (Fig. 18–1). The body of the talus will be posterior to the ankle joint while the anterior talus lies in its usual relationship to the navicular.

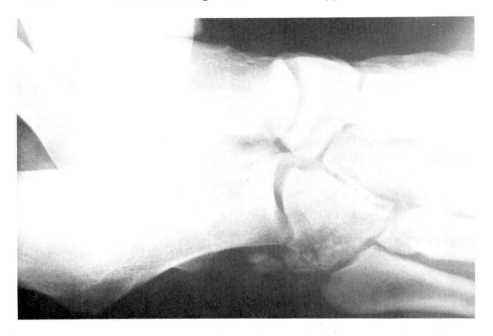

Fig. 18–4. Oblique lateral roentgenogram demonstrating comminuted yet relatively undisplaced fracture of cuboid. A short leg cast for eight to ten weeks will be sufficient treatment—the later four to six weeks should be weight bearing.

Treatment. A general anesthetic is necessary for treatment of the fracture-dislocation of the astragalus. Closed manipulation is attempted while traction is placed longitudinally to open the joint space from which the body of the talus comes. Concomitantly an assistant places a firm posterior-to-anterior force against the body of the talus to maneuver it back into the ankle joint. If reduction is accomplished, the foot and ankle should be placed in a plaster cast in the position of stability, in slight plantar flexion. If closed reduction is not possible, open reduction is indicated. Internal fixation by Kirschner wires will be necessary to maintain the reduction. Fractures of the astragalus generally require three months of immobilization for union, the first six weeks in a short leg nonweight bearing cast and the last six weeks in a short leg walking cast. Nonunion of this fracture is not uncommon. Roentgenographic evidence of fracture union must be present before stopping the immobilization. Treatment for this nonunion is by either bone graft or a triple arthrodesis. Because of the precarious nature of the blood supply into the talus, the future possibility of avascular necrosis must be considered. Continued examination and serial radiographic studies should be made periodically for two years.

Fractures of Tarsal Bones

Any of the tarsal bones may be fractured. These injuries are usually chip fractures, and the mechanism of injury is variable.

Examination. The examination will often identify the level of the injury because of point tenderness but will not identify the specific injury.

Roentgenograms. The roentgenogram must include anteroposterior, lateral, and oblique views of the foot in order to show any fracture line within the tarsal bones (Fig. 18–4).

Treatment. Simple immobilization for about four weeks is sufficient for most of the avulsion chip fractures in the tarsal bones. More consequential fractures may need longer immobilization.

Fracture of Os Calcis

The mechanism of injury for most fractures of the os calcis is a crushing injury from a fall onto the heel with the patient in an upright position. Ralston offers as practical a classification as any: (1) isolated fracture with no joint injury, (2) comminuted fracture with minimal joint involvement, and (3) comminuted fracture with severe crushing and joint involvement.

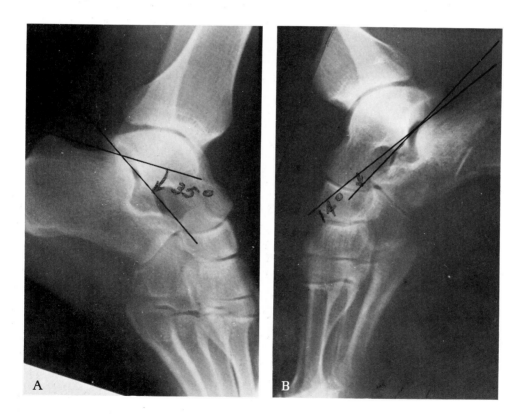

Fig. 18–5. A, Lateral roentgenogram of normal hindfoot marked to illustrate Böhler's angle, the angle at which a line from the anterior-superior articular point of the os calcis to the posterior-superior articular point intersects a line from the posterior-superior articular point to the posterior-superior prominence of the os calcis. This should be 30 to 40 degrees in the normal foot. B, Lateral roentgenogram of hindfoot in which Böhler's angle has been decreased significantly, indicating crush fracture of os calcis.

The os calcis may fracture by two or three major mechanisms. One forces an explosion type of fracture when the os calcis is caught between the talus above and the ground or weight bearing surface below. The fractures of the os calcis involving the joint surface almost invariably produce continuing pain while those not involving the joint are less likely to cause prolonged difficulty.

Examination. Examination of the foot with the os calcis fracture reveals a broadened hindfoot (medial to lateral). Ecchymosis is often evident. There is marked tenderness in response to any attempt at examination. Dorsiflexion and plantar flexion of the ankle are seldom painful, as this motion does not involve the os calcis.

Roentgenograms. The roentgenographic studies must include the anteroposterior view of the foot, the lateral view of the foot, and an os calcis view. On the normal lateral view, Böhler's angle is 30 to 40 degrees (Fig. 18–5A). This is the angle formed by intersection of the line from the posterior-superior prominence of the os calcis to its posterior-superior articular surface with the line from the superior surface of the anterior articulation to this posterior-superior articular surface. In the crushing fracture involving the joint, Böhler's angle will be reduced significantly (Fig. 18–5B).

Treatment. Occasionally, two or three *major* bony fragments may be identified in the os calcis that has been fractured. In this instance, there may be an indication for reduction. This reduction may be performed by closed means, primarily by side-to-side compression, with the patient under a general anesthetic.

A second method is one in which Böhler's angle may be restored, at least partially, by a Steinmann pin into the posterior os calcis. The posterior fragment is manipulated into a more plantar position while the anterior os calcis is also brought into a plantar position (Fig. 18–6A). The pin is then drilled forward to the anterior tip of the os calcis to maintain the reduction. This may restore Böhler's angle and allow for less long-term joint difficulty.

Another method for improving the tuber angle of Böhler is to pass a Steinmann pin transversely through the posterior os calcis and place a plantar force against this pin. At the same time as the plantar force is applied to the pin, the forefoot is manipulated into a plantar flexed position in order to bring the anterior os calcis into a more anatomic position. A short leg cast incorporating the os calcis pin can then be applied.

Burdeaux and McReynolds make a surgical approach to the fractured os calcis from the medial side. The large cortical fragment is held in place while any laterally displaced fragment is levered back into its relationship with this medial fragment. A two- or three-point staple is used to stabilize the fragments (Fig. 18–6B).

The os calcis must be protected from weight bearing for at least eight weeks and oftentimes as long as twelve weeks before sufficient bony union of the fragments has occurred to prevent settling. The long-term results in many of the os calcis fractures are poor. Pain is a not uncommon accompaniment to the os calcis fracture that has left the talocalcaneal joint incongruous. Operative procedures such as the triple arthrodesis often are necessary before comfort ensues. In fact, because of many poor results from the os calcis fractures, some orthopaedic surgeons recommend that triple arthrodesis be performed primarily or at six weeks following the injury.

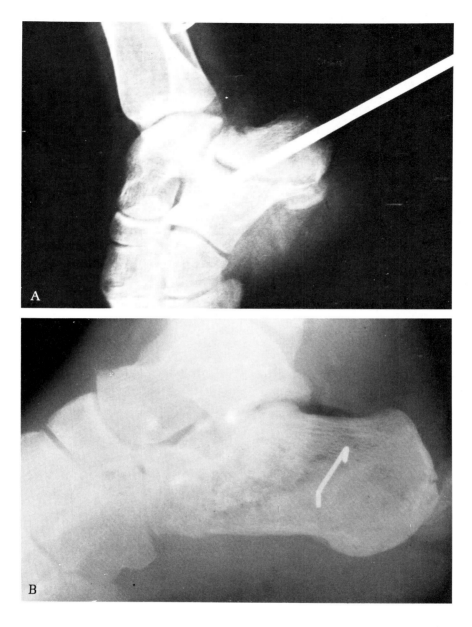

Fig. 18-6. Management of fracture of os calcis. A, Heavy Steinmann pin is drilled into the posterior fragment. The posteriorly protruding pin is pushed inferiorly while the forefoot is plantar flexed. The Steinmann pin is then drilled on into the reduced anterior fragment. Cast fixation should be added. The pin can be removed at six weeks but immobilization in cast is indicated for three months. B, Burdeaux and McReynolds use medial approach to os calcis. The major cortical fragment can be fixed by two- or three-point staple to achieve relatively congruous superior calcaneal joint surface. This method also requires cast immobilization for eight to twelve weeks.

Dislocations at Tarsometatarsal Joint

Dislocation at the tarsometatarsal joint is a particularly difficult injury because of the problems in diagnosing as well as in adequate treatment. The mechanism of injury is usually a rotational one with sharp dorsiflexion of the foot.

Examination. On examination of the foot with a dislocation at the tarsometatarsal joint, there is deformity to observation and to palpation. There is usually sharp pain at the tarsometatarsal level.

Roentgenograms. Anteroposterior, lateral, and oblique roentgenograms of the foot must be taken (Fig. 18–7). In order to properly assess these, comparison views of the opposite foot may be necessary. The notches and grooves in the tarsometatarsal articulation are such that they demand that each metatarsal base fit properly to its opposing tarsal space.

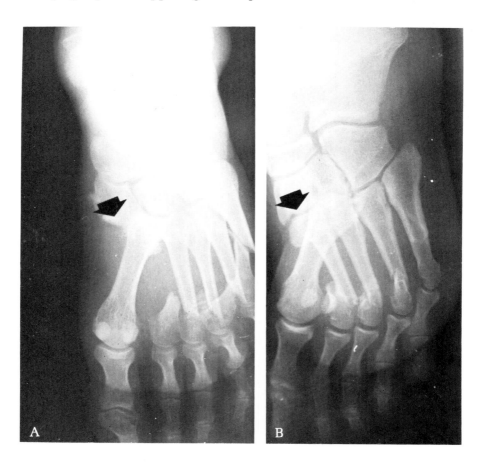

Fig. 18–7. A, Anteroposterior roentgenogram showing dislocation of first tarsometatarsal joint (arrow) accompanying fractures of necks of second through fifth metatarsals. B, Oblique view showing dislocation of first tarsometarsal joint (arrow). This is an unstable injury; the key to maintaining reduction, once obtained, is Kirschner wire(s) from distal to proximal across tarsometatarsal joint.

Treatment. Dislocations at the tarsometatarsal joint are often difficult to reduce but must be accurately reduced and early in order to get satisfactory results. In many instances following reduction, stability is not present, and crossed Kirschner wires may be necessary to maintain the reduction. Immobilization in a plaster of Paris cast for eight weeks should also be utilized.

It is to be emphasized that the late treatment of the tarsometatarsal dislocation is unsatisfactory. Satisfactory treatment requires proper primary diagnosis accompanied by effective early treatment.

Fracture of Fifth Metatarsal Base

Fracture of the base of the fifth metatarsal occurs particularly after an inversion force to the foot, since the tendon of the peroneus brevis attaches to it.

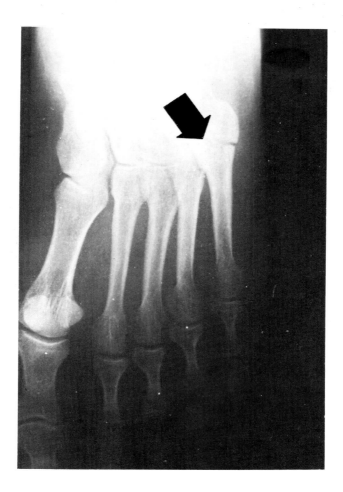

Fig. 18–8. Anteroposterior roentgenogram showing fracture of base of fifth metatarsal bone (arrow). The peroneus brevis tendon attaches here and can be a factor creating mobility of the fragment along with distress. Immobilization with a walking cast until union is adequate is excellent treatment.

Examination. Usually the diagnosis can be made on examination. There will be point tenderness at the bony prominence of the fifth metatarsal base accompanied by overlying ecchymosis.

Roentgenograms. The roentgenograms (Fig. 18–8) can confirm the diagnosis, but an anteroposterior roentgenogram of the opposite foot may be required to rule out an accessory ossicle.

Treatment. The fracture of the base of the fifth metatarsal is uncomfortable and may best be treated in a symptomatic fashion. An elastic wrap may be sufficient treatment when combined with the use of crutches. However, the patient may prefer a short leg plaster of Paris walking cast. The fracture will unite without event but usually takes about six weeks to show evidence of adequate union.

Fracture of Metatarsal Shaft and Neck

The metatarsal shaft and neck are fractured most commonly by direct injury. If the injury and displacement are sufficient, future difficulty may follow, particularly when accurate reduction is not accomplished.

Examination. Upon examination, a deformity may be seen in the forefoot. Often swelling is present and hides any specific bony deformity.

Roentgenograms. The anteroposterior and oblique roentgenograms (Fig. 18–7) will show the extent of displacement of the metatarsal shaft and neck.

Treatment. Manipulation of the displaced metatarsals into position can usually be accomplished following administration of meperidine and diazepam as an analgesic-relaxant combination. The major effort is to position fragments to relieve any plantar or superficial bony prominence. A short leg plaster of Paris cast is applied for four to six weeks with specific padding to retain the reduction. Of importance is the tipping of the metatarsal heads sufficiently to allow adequate weight bearing; however, they must not be forced to carry more than their share. Occasionally, traction to the distal phalanges from an outrigger device applied to the cast is necessary to maintain adequate reduction.

Fatigue Fracture of Metatarsal

The fatigue fracture of the metatarsal bone usually occurs along the distal shaft or neck of the second, third, or fourth metatarsal bone. It is occasioned by unaccustomed physical activity such as lengthy marches and for this reason has also been called the *march* fracture. The patient knows of no specific mechanism of injury.

Examination. Examination of the foot with a fatigue fracture will reveal joint tenderness with compression at the site of the fracture.

Roentgenograms. The roentgenograms (Fig. 18–9) may not reveal the fatigue fracture until some periosteal new bone is formed. In this event a high suspicion must be present.

Treatment. In any event treatment of the fatigue fracture is protection of the foot from weight bearing. This may be accomplished by a short leg plaster of Paris walking cast for from four to six weeks or by the use of crutches and restricted weight bearing.

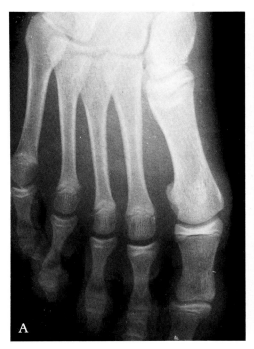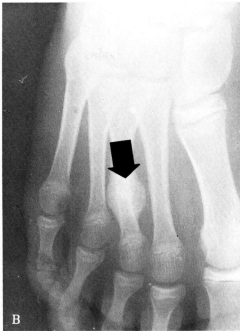

Fig. 18–9. Roentgenograms showing midfoot of sixteen-year-old male who complained of pain in this area for ten days. A, Anteroposterior view. Even a retrospective study fails to reveal evidence of bony injury. B, Anteroposterior view taken six weeks later and revealing large callus along third metatarsal shaft (arrow). In the interim this had been treated as a march fracture by applying a walking cast.

Phalangeal Fractures

Fractures of the phalanges occur generally from direct injury.

Examination. On the examination of the foot with phalangeal fractures longitudinal compression of the digit involved will cause pain at the point of fracture. Deformity may be present but is not necessarily evident on examination.

Roentgenograms. The roentgenograms will confirm the phalangeal fracture on anteroposterior and lateral views. There is often displacement of fragment(s), but of no major concern.

Treatment. Treatment of the phalangeal fracture is most easily provided by taping the fractured toe to an adjacent toe, having placed a piece of lamb's wool between the toes so taped.

Phalangeal Dislocation

Dislocations may occur at any of the interphalangeal joints. The creating force usually causes an angular or rotary force at the involved joint.

Examination. The diagnosis of a dislocated interphalangeal joint is usually evident on visualization or palpation.

Roentgenogram. The roentgenogram will show loss of the usual joint relationships at one of the interphalangeal joints (Fig. 18–10).

Treatment. Following digital block, reduction can generally be accomplished by traction. Once reduced, immobilization can be best accomplished by taping the involved digit to the largest adjacent digit.

INJURIES OF THE FOOT IN CHILDREN

Because the child's foot is more flexible and resilient than the adult's, any injury that is sustained is often transmitted to the foreleg above. However, fractures can occur to any bone of the foot. The blood supply to the astragalus can be a critical factor in complications following fracture of that bone. Most fractures of the foot in the child heal without event following closed reduction and immobilization.

Fracture of Astragalus

Fractures of the astragalus occur in children usually with a sharp forced dorsiflexion of the foot. The talar fracture in the child is not typically displaced.

Examination. Examination of the foot reveals tenderness to palpation over the instep and swelling, but seldom is there evidence of deformity.

Roentgenograms. The roentgenograms include the anteroposterior and lateral roentgenograms of the foot (Fig. 18–1). They should show evidence of a break in bony continuity of the talus. Most commonly there is no displacement.

Treatment. Immobilization in a plaster of Paris walking cast for six to eight weeks is usually sufficient in the child. Occasionally in the older child the displacement of the talus occurs and must be treated the same as the fracture in the adult.

Fracture of the Os Calcis

The os calcis fracture in the child is extremely rare and may be treated by a short leg plaster of Paris cast for eight weeks, the last three of which may be with a walking heel.

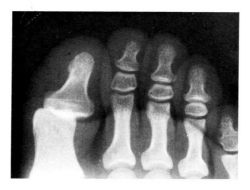

Fig. 18–10. Anteroposterior roentgenogram of interphalangeal dislocation. Reduction can often be accomplished by traction to a toe in which a digital block has been performed. Immobilization is accomplished by taping the involved toe to the largest adjacent toe.

Metatarsal and Phalangeal Fractures

Metatarsal and phalangeal fractures in the child are rare because of the resilience of the immature bone of the child. These may be treated by taping the toes together; usually several days of treatment are sufficient for the symptoms to disappear.

REFERENCES

1. Adams, J. C.: Outline of Fractures, Including Joint Injuries, 6th ed. Baltimore, Williams & Wilkins Co., 1972.
2. Blount, W. P.: Fractures in Children. Baltimore, Williams & Wilkins Co., 1954.
3. Burdeaux, B. D. Jr., and McReynolds, I. S.: Open reduction and internal fixation with metallic staples, for severe fractures of the os calcis., J. Bone Joint Surg. 49-A:1475, 1967.
4. Charnley, J.: Closed Treatment of Common Fractures, 3rd ed., 1961. (Fourth Reprint). Edinburgh & London, Churchill Livingstone, 1972.
5. Essex-Lopresti, P.: Results of reduction in fractures of the calcaneum. J. Bone Joint Surg. 33-B:284, 1951.
6. Essex-Lopresti, P.: The mechanism, reduction technique, and results in fractures of the os calcis. J. Bone Joint Surg. 34-B:395, 1952.
7. Giannestras, N. J.: Foot Disorders. Philadelphia, Lea & Febiger, 1973.
8. Ralston, E. L.: Handbook of Fractures. St. Louis, C. V. Mosby Co., 1967.
9. Rang, M. C.: Children's Fractures. Philadelphia, J. B. Lippincott Co., 1974.
10. Rockwood, C. A., and Green, D. P.: Fractures. Philadelphia, J. B. Lippincott Co., 1975.
11. Watson-Jones, R.: Fractures and Joint Injuries, 4th ed., 2V. Baltimore, Williams & Wilkins Co., 1952-1955.

INDEX